BODYWEIGHT WORKOUTS FOR BEGINNERS

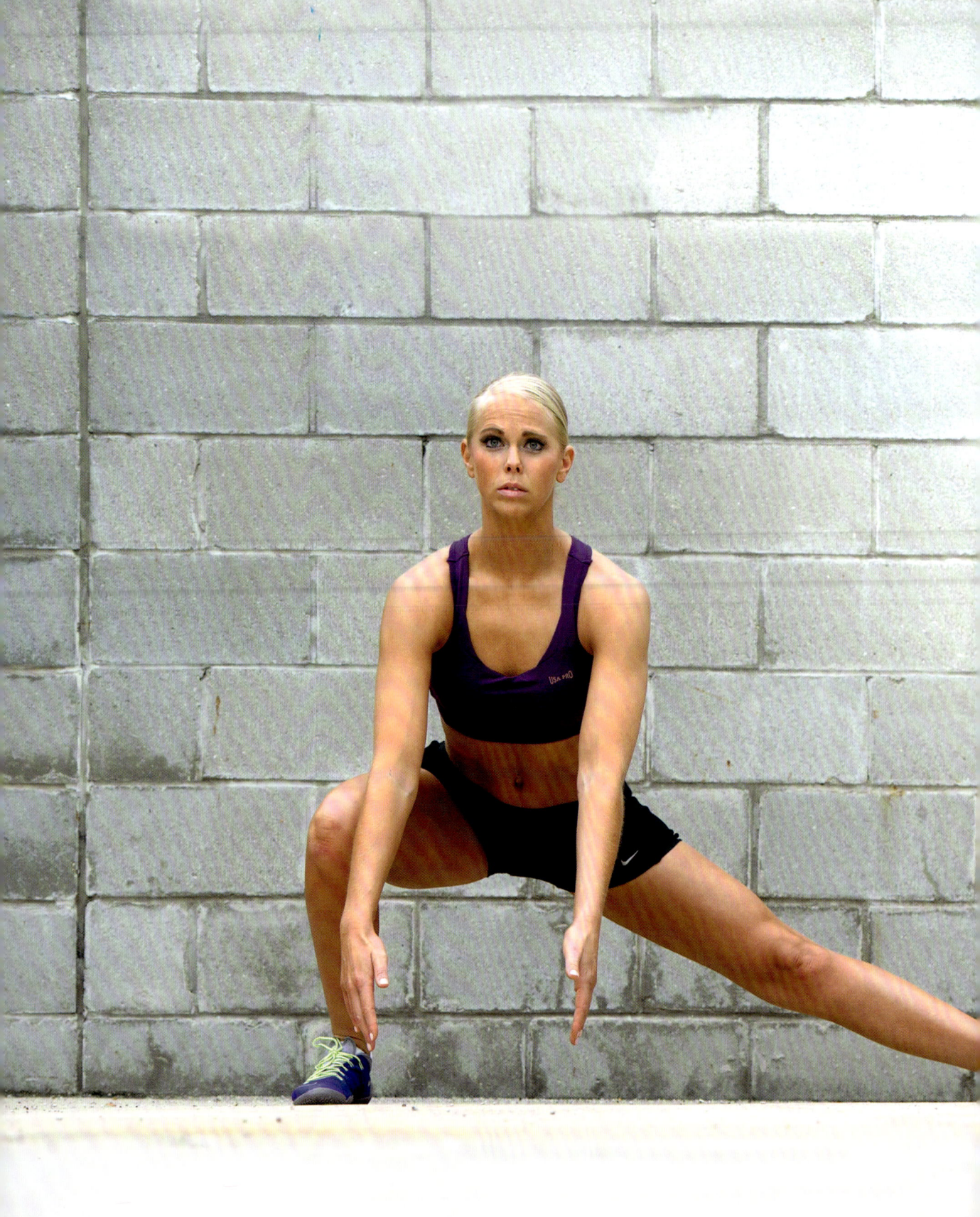

BODYWEIGHT WORKOUTS

WORKOUTS FOR BEGINNERS

SEAN BARTRAM

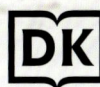

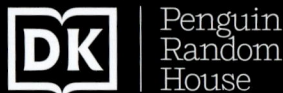

Publisher Mike Sanders
Art & Design Director William Thomas
Editorial Director Ann Barton
Photographer Matt Bowen
Proofreader Rick Ball
Indexer Celia McCoy

First American Edition, 2024
Published in the United States by DK Publishing
1745 Broadway, 20th Floor, New York, NY 10019

Updated and reprinted from *High Intensity Interval Workouts
for Women* and *Bodyweight Workouts for Men*

The authorized representative in the EEA is Dorling Kindersley
Verlag GmbH. Arnulfstr. 124, 80636 Munich, Germany

A catalog record for this book
is available from the Library of Congress.
ISBN 978-0-7440-9249-3

DK books are available at special discounts when purchased
in bulk for sales promotions, premiums, fund-raising, or
educational use. For details, contact SpecialSales@dk.com

Printed and bound in China

www.dk.com

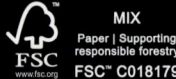

MIX
Paper | Supporting
responsible forestry
FSC™ C018179

This book was made with Forest
Stewardship Council™ certified
paper – one small step in DK's
commitment to a sustainable future.
Learn more at
www.dk.com/uk/information/sustainability

For Mum
(1956–2020)

Love you more.

CONTENTS

UPPER-BODY EXERCISES

CORE EXERCISES

ROUTINES

PROGRAMS

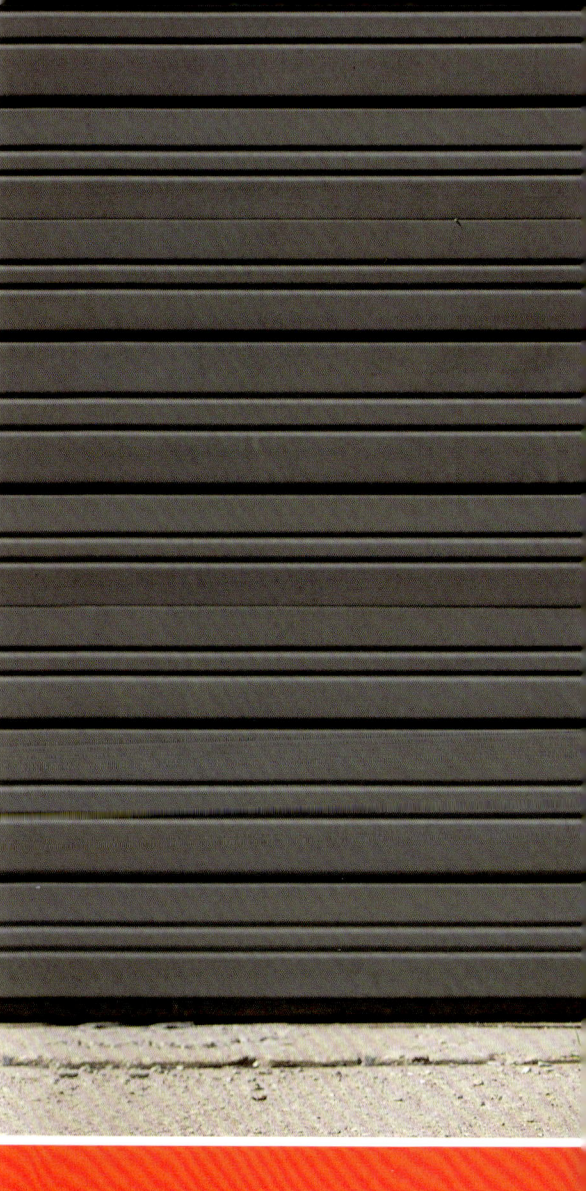

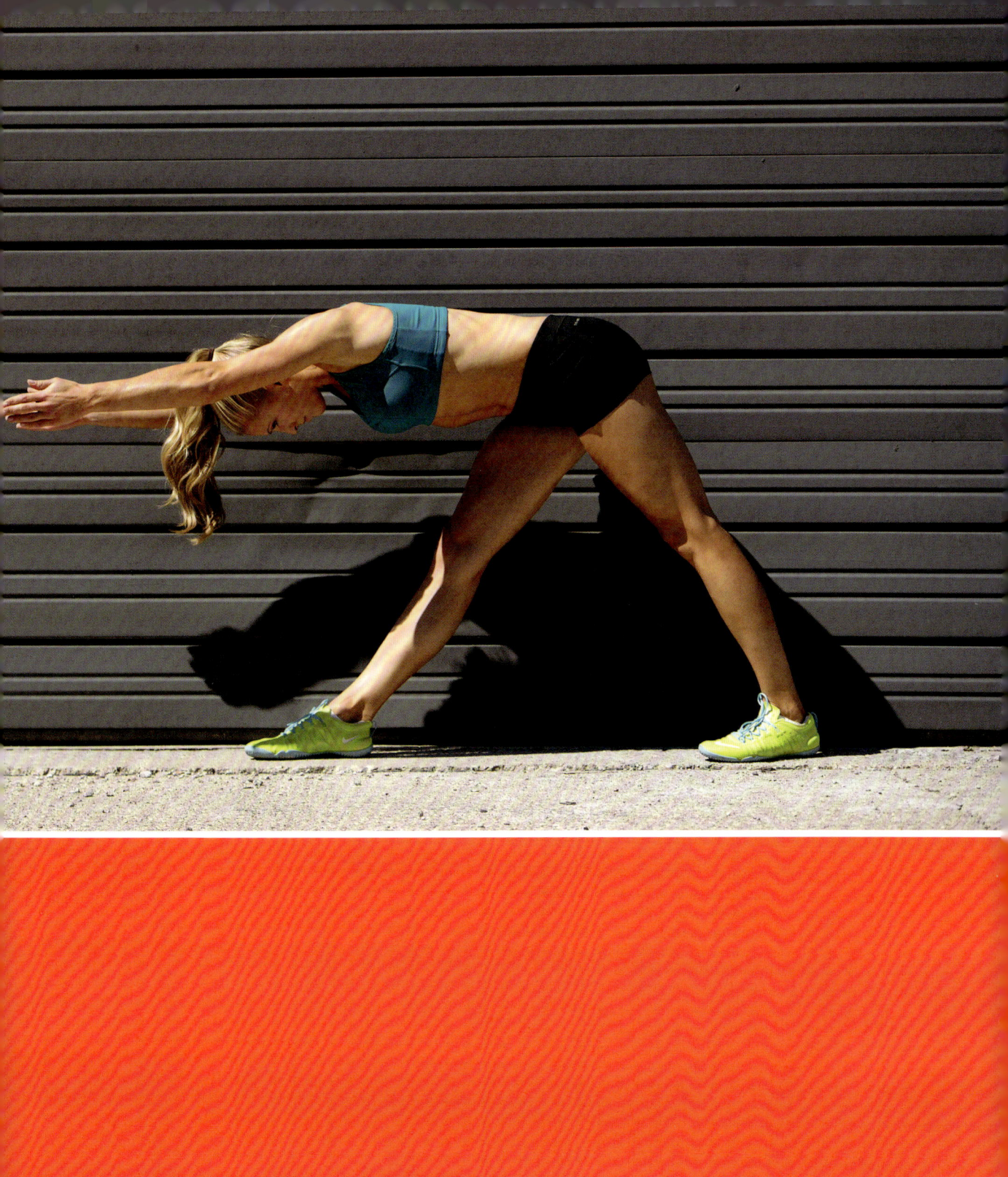

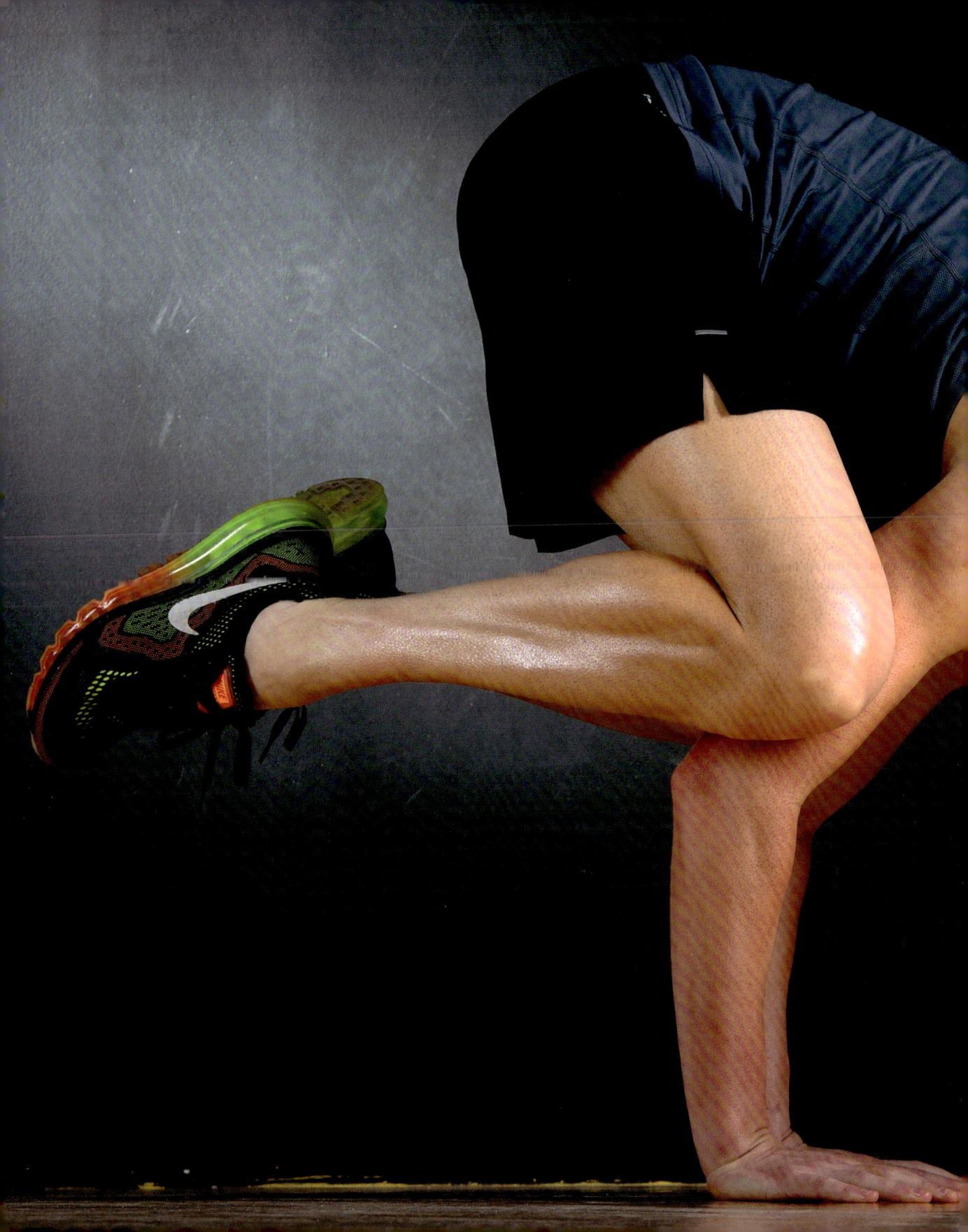

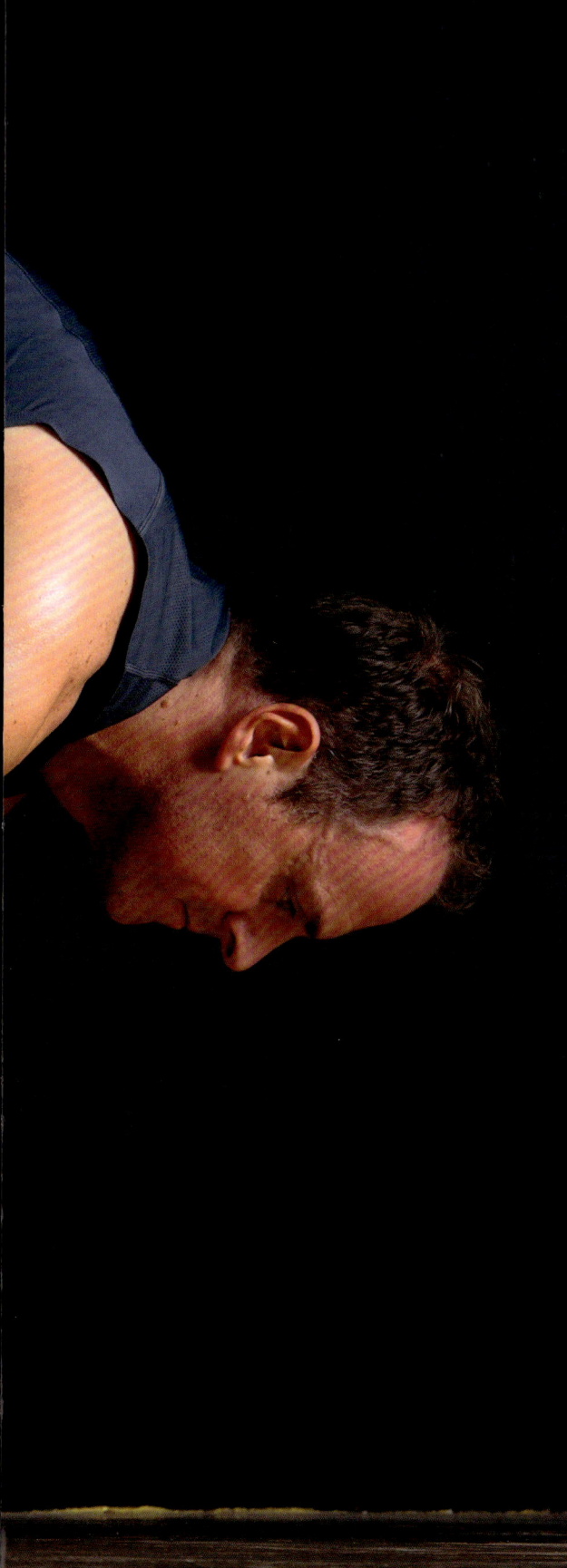

INTRODUCTION

As a resident of Indianapolis, Indiana, home of the Indy 500, I've learned to love racing. In the world of auto racing, a "homologation special" refers to a car pieced together from special parts to create a unique, limited-production, high-performance vehicle. *Bodyweight Workouts for Beginners* is a homologation special in book form: It fuses the best of two of my previous titles—*Bodyweight Workouts for Men* and *High Intensity Interval Training for Women*—with some great new content to create a one-of-a-kind vehicle for change. This new book will empower you with the knowledge and ability to get a great workout anywhere, anytime, using your body as the machine.

What's the difference between bodyweight resistance training and HIIT? Candidly, not much. HIIT can be bodyweight resistance training—and bodyweight resistance training can be HIIT. So why not fuse the concepts to build lean muscle, decrease body fat, and increase performance? In the following pages, you'll learn to first build strength and confidence with slow, controlled movements before adding explosive intensity to burn fat.

In my fitness career, I've been incredibly fortunate to train people from all walks of life. Those clients have included everyday people like you and me, as well as professional athletes from football, racing, dancing, cheerleading, gymnastics; men and women of the armed forces; and first responders. No matter the client, the goals are always the same: efficiency, increased strength and endurance, decreased body fat percentage, and a workout that can be performed anywhere.

Bodyweight Workouts for Beginners will teach you how to perform the 60 exercises with correct form and includes modifications to make movements easier and more challenging. It will take you on a journey to a leaner, stronger body with 30 routines and three 4-week workout programs designed to level up your fitness.

I expect you to work hard and curse my name occasionally, but also begin to move more athletically, improve performance, and gain strength, tone, and definition.

Above all else, I want you to have fun!

BODYWEIGHT BASICS

WHAT IS BODYWEIGHT RESISTANCE TRAINING?

Bodyweight exercises are strength-training exercises that don't require the addition of free weights such as dumbbells or barbells. Your own weight provides the resistance for the movements.

Examples of traditional bodyweight resistance exercises include push-ups and pull-ups. The beauty of this training is that for every exercise, there's a simple yet effective way to increase or decrease the exercise's challenge. Take the push-up, for example. To make the exercise less difficult, you can perform a kneeling push-up. To make it more difficult, you have a multitude of options, such as changing your hand positions, establishing stops throughout the motion, and elevating your feet. These variations not only increase the exercise's difficulty, but also extend the range of motion and recruit more muscle fibers.

In general, increasing the number of repetitions will improve endurance, while strength gains are made by increasing the intensity of the exercise by decreasing leverage, by working at the ends of range of motion, or by adding dynamic tension.

Organizations such as the World Calisthenics Organization and competitions such as Battle of the Bars showcase the elite performance that can be garnered from bodyweight resistance training. Practitioners such as Frank Medrano, Denis Minin, Lain Malle, and Jess St. John defy gravity on YouTube and other social media sites with physics-bending feats of strength created by utilizing the same techniques presented in this book.

Despite what an entire industry tries to promote, you do not need to pick up a weight to gain strength, increase lean muscle mass, and improve athletic performance.

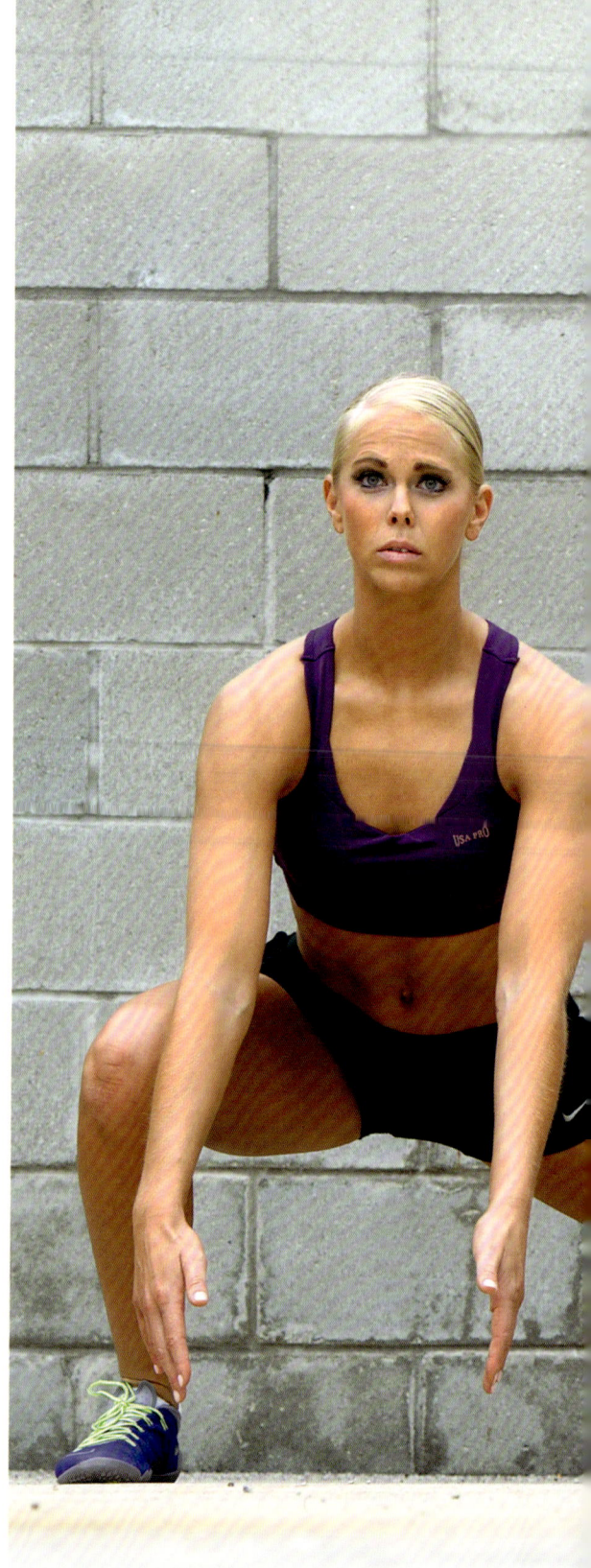

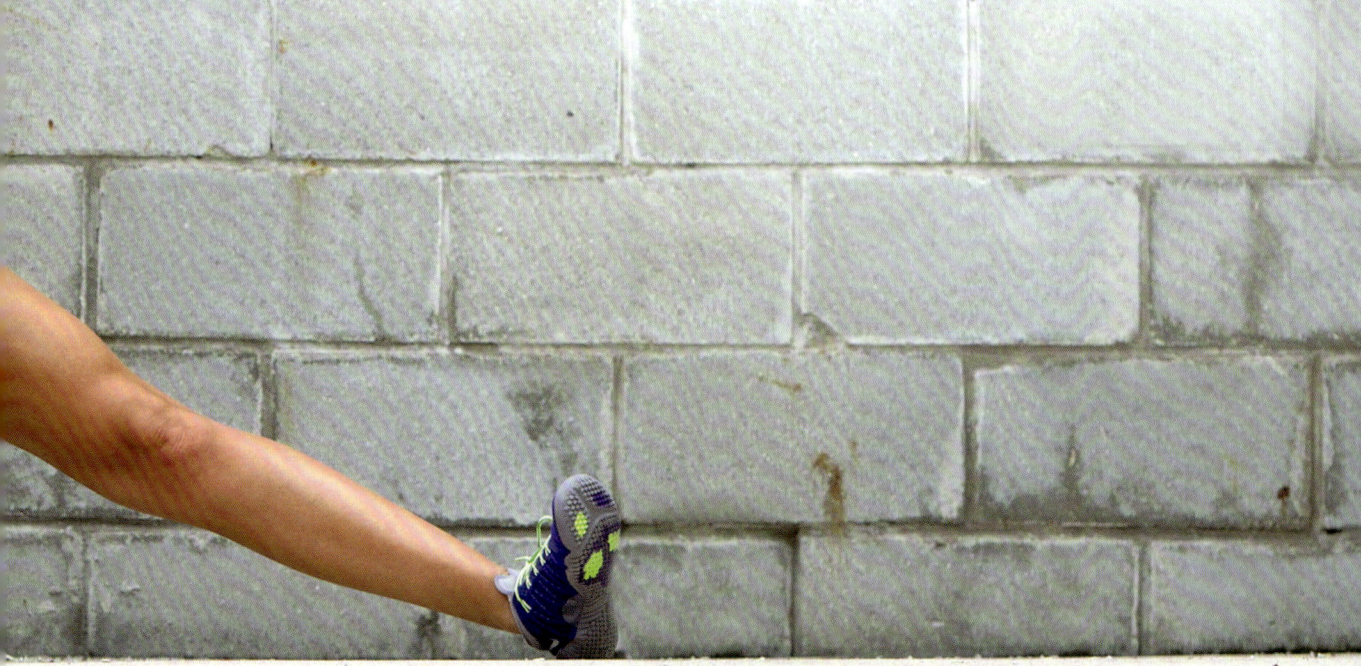

BENEFITS OF BODYWEIGHT RESISTANCE TRAINING

VERSATILITY	CONVENIENCE	COST	EFFICIENCY
While every exercise can be adapted to provide a greater challenge to the practitioner, the basic exercises are also perfect for beginners.	Because your body supplies the resistance for the exercises, bodyweight training can be undertaken anytime, anywhere— your home, a hotel room, a gym, or in the great outdoors.	Bodyweight resistance training will cost you nothing. You can keep those monthly gym fees, so it might even save you money.	We all live busy lives; time is our most precious commodity. Combining strength and cardio workouts saves time and reduces the transition time between exercises. Most workouts take only 10 to 45 minutes.

ADVANTAGES OF BODYWEIGHT RESISTANCE TRAINING

Let's be honest. While we work out for the health benefits, a big plus is looking great and feeling good. Being fit, lean, and healthy boosts self-confidence and makes you want to spend more time training.

I suspect you're interested in decreasing body fat, gaining strength, adding lean muscle, and improving your athletic performance. The exercises and programs in this book will help you meet those goals.

ADAPTABILITY

For years the fitness industry portrayed bodyweight exercise as little more than a warm-up, endurance, or cardio workout. The theory was that gaining strength required lifting heavy, progressively, and with attention to load, not reps. But why can't bodyweight exercises be progressive? Take standard push-ups. Perform as many repetitions as possible in a given time, and it's only about endurance. Increase the time it takes to perform each rep, however, and/or the dynamic tension (the muscular force required to execute that rep), and it makes the exercise more challenging and builds both strength and lean muscle mass, just like adding weight to a barbell. Applying these basic principles to every bodyweight exercise allows you to adapt the resistance and force required.

BUILD LEAN MUSCLE AND BURN FAT

You'll work multiple muscle groups at once via compound exercises. The minimal equipment and space required make it easy to transition between exercises, reducing rest time and allowing for a high intensity interval training type of workout. Alternating sets with minimal or no rest forces the body to produce muscle-building and fat-burning hormones like HGH and testosterone. This also stimulates excess post-exercise oxygen consumption (EPOC, also known as the "afterburn"), the measurable increased rate of oxygen intake following strenuous activity intended to erase the body's oxygen debt. Fatty acids are released as fuel for recovery. EPOC can boost fat burning by up to 48 hours.

INCREASE ATHLETIC PERFORMANCE

Alternating between exercises, working multiple muscle groups per exercise, and the lack of equipment all allow you to keep your body in a state of confusion, preventing it from adapting to a steady workload. Build in easy and simple ways to add or remove challenge and variety through exercise adaptations, and there really are an endless number of ways you can apply the techniques, exercises, and workouts found in this book.

CORE STRENGTH

Consisting of at least 29 muscles, your core is more than just six-pack abs. Every bodyweight exercise featured in this book engages the core either as a primary muscle or for stabilization. This will not only carve the kind of killer core usually featured on models on the front covers of fitness publications, but will also improve your posture and athletic performance.

SYMMETRY

There's no better way to develop a natural, symmetrical, and functional physique. You'll build the lean, athletic, and perfectly proportioned body of a Spartan warrior, gymnast, or martial artist. Research suggests that body symmetry can indicate biological fitness and longer life expectancy—not to mention that studies have shown that humans find symmetrical people more attractive!

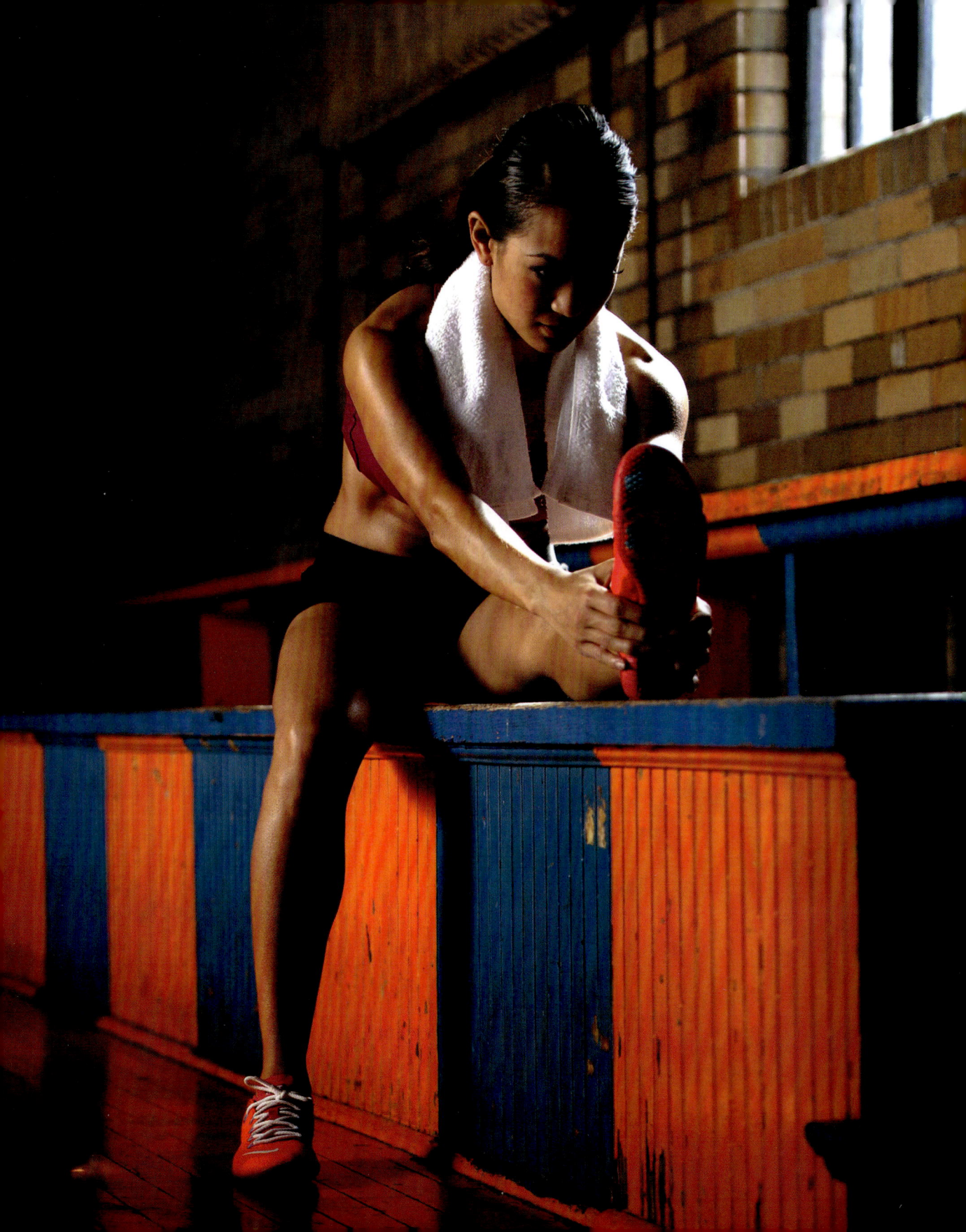

ANATOMICAL CHART

Throughout these pages, you'll find mentions of the various muscle groups strengthened and developed by bodyweight exercises. The diagrams here will help you understand musculature and general anatomy.

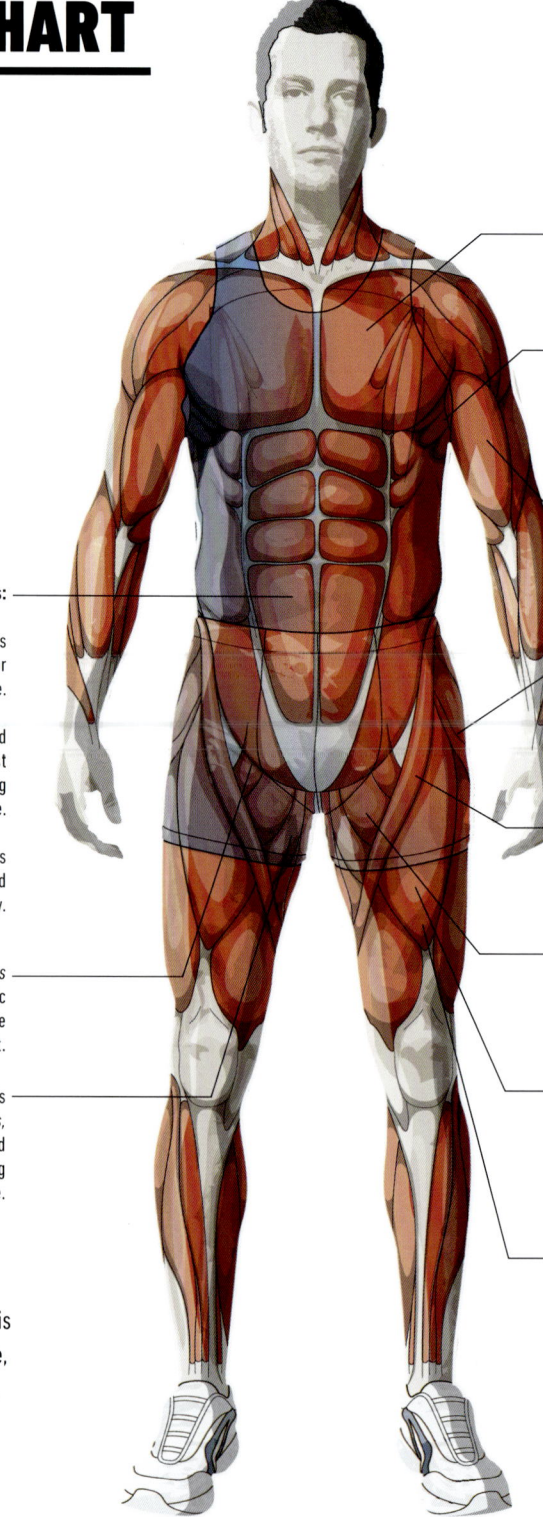

Pectorals—*Pectoralis major* and *pectoralis minor* help move the shoulder joint.

Serratus anterior—Originating between the first and ninth ribs, it inserts at the shoulder blade and moves and stabilizes it.

Biceps—This two-headed muscle is responsible for shoulder flexion, elbow flexion, and upward rotation of the palm.

Tensor fascia latae — This thigh muscle helps to stabilize the pelvis atop the femur (thigh bone) during standing.

Sartorius—The longest muscle in the body, it assists in flexion and lateral rotation of the hip, and flexion of the knee.

Pectineus—This flat, quadrangular muscle moves the thigh toward the body and rotates it toward the center.

Quadriceps—Comprised of the *rectus femoris, vastus lateralis, vastus intermedius,* and *vastus medialis,* which extend the knee.

Rectus femoris—See *quadriceps.*

The abdominals consist of the following three groups:

Rectus abdominis—Also known as the "six-pack," this runs the length of the front of the abdomen and is important for posture. Its primary function is flexion of the lumbar spine.

Internal and external obliques—Found on the lateral and anterior portions of the abdomen, these pull the chest downward and compress the abdominal cavity, providing strength and support for the abdomen and spine.

Transversus abdominus—The innermost of the flat muscles of the abdomen compresses the ribs, providing thoracic and pelvic stability.

Iliopsoas (hip flexor)—A combination of the *psoas major* and *iliacus,* and essential to athletic activities such as running because they're the strongest flexors of the thigh at the hip joint.

Adductors—Commonly called the inner thigh, this group of muscles includes the *adductor brevis, adductor longus, adductor magnus, pectineus,* and *gracilis.* They function to contract and pull the leg to the body's midline.

How many muscles are in the body? This is tricky to answer because each muscle is actually made of many layers of muscle tissue, and there are three types of muscle—skeletal, cardiac, and smooth. However, the commonly accepted answer is 650 skeletal muscles (the ones attached to bone).

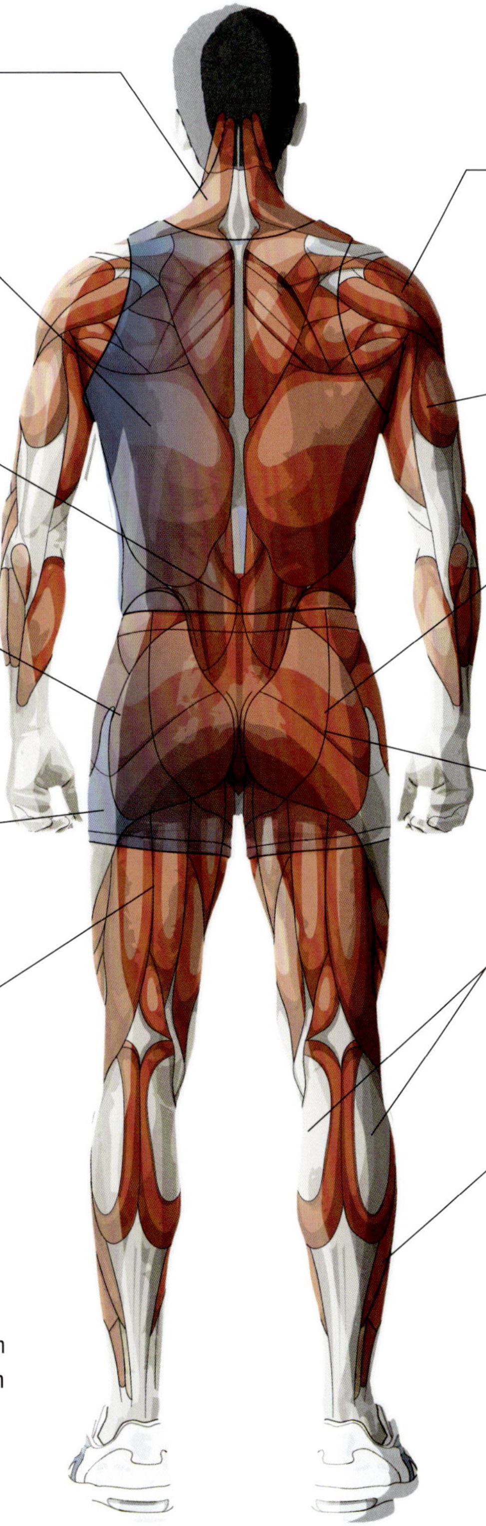

Trapezius—Resembling a trapezoid, it functions to move the scapula and support the arm.

Latissimus dorsi—The primary function of the broadest muscle of the back, also known as the "lat," is the adduction of the arm. It's often used when performing a pull-up or a chin-up.

Erector spinae—This bundle of muscles and tendons extends the length of the vertebral column. It functions to straighten the back and provide side-to-side rotation.

Abductors—Located in the buttocks and lateral hip region on both sides of the body, the abductors consist of the *gluteus maximus, gluteus medius, gluteus minimus,* and *tensor fascia latae.*

Iliotibial band—This is a longitudinal fibrous reinforcement of the *tensor fascia latae.* The action of the ITB and its associated muscles is to extend, abduct, and laterally rotate the hip.

Hamstrings—Consisting of three posterior thigh muscles, the semitendinosus, semimembranosus, and biceps femoris, hamstrings are responsible for knee flexion and hip extension.

Deltoids—The posterior, anterior, and lateral deltoid are primarily responsible for abduction of the arm on the frontal plane (lifting the arm up and out to the side).

Triceps brachii—This large muscle on the rear of the upper arm is principally responsible for extension of the elbow joint and straightening of the arm.

Gluteals—The *gluteus maximus, gluteus medius,* and *gluteus minimus* make up the buttocks. They're responsible for movement of the hip and thigh.

Piriformis—A pear-shaped muscle in the glute region that aids in external rotation of the hip. The *piriformis* laterally rotates the femur with hip extension and abducts the femur with hip flexion.

Gastrocnemius—These two heads of muscle run from just above the knee to the heel. Commonly called the calf, the *gastrocnemius* is essential for running and jumping.

Soleus—This powerful muscle in the rear portion of the lower leg works with the *gastrocnemius* to perform plantarflexion of the foot (pulling toes toward shins).

The 650 skeletal muscles are all named in Latin after their location, shape, function, or insertion and origin points. The hardest-working muscle in the body isn't shown here. It's the cardiac muscle—the heart—which beats once per second, or even faster during exercise or duress.

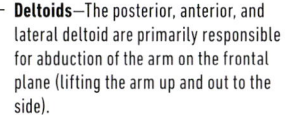

MUST-HAVES AND USEFUL EXTRAS

The best part about bodyweight resistance training is you need little more than your body and determination to have an incredible workout.

Ingenuity will allow you to use your surroundings, park benches, climbing frames, or chairs to replace the free weights and cardio equipment that keep you mentally and financially chained to your gym membership.

However, there are a few optional items I strongly suggest you invest in for optimal performance during the exercises and workouts.

THE MUST-HAVES

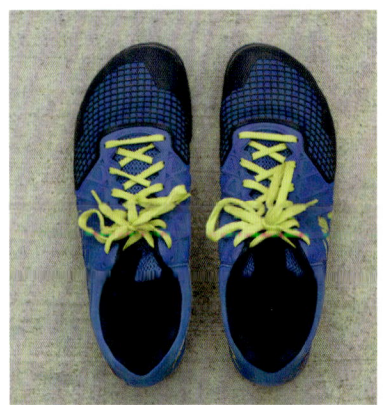

SHOES To make sure you can feel your connection to the floor, I advocate wearing a minimalist-style shoe when training. If you're new to minimalist footwear, I strongly recommend alternating between your old shoes and the minimalist style for two to four weeks to allow your body to adjust to the decrease in support and cushioning.

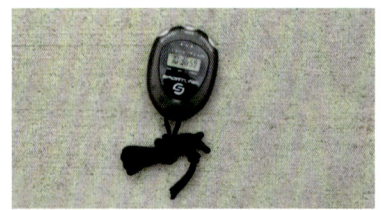

WATCH OR TIMER A watch or timer is essential for keeping track of the work and rest intervals in some workouts.

USEFUL EXTRAS

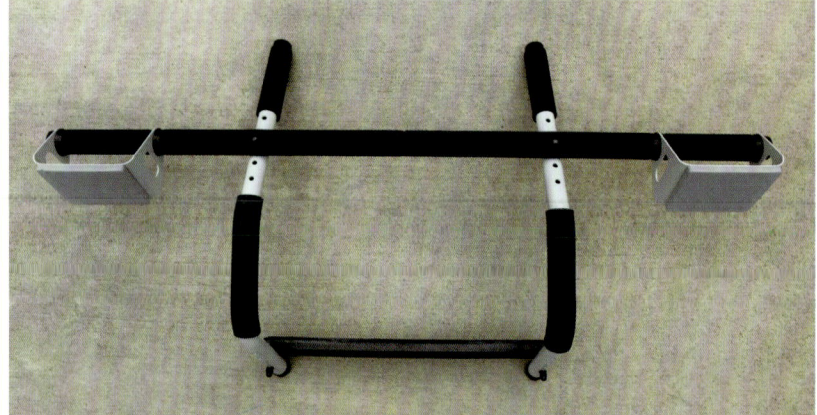

PULL-UP BAR A pull-up bar is not essential, as you can find a number of alternatives for bar-oriented exercises. However, to maximize training performance, I strongly suggest you invest in a door-mounted bar or freestanding pull/dip station.

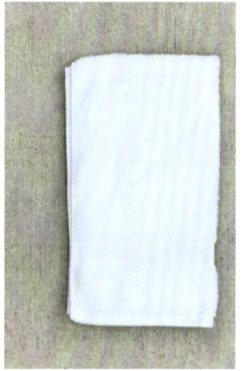

TOWEL In addition to mopping your brow, a towel can also be used to help assist with some exercises.

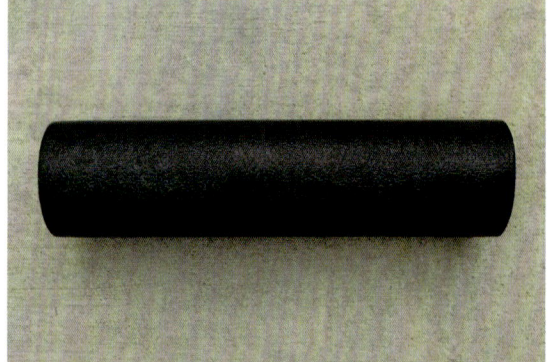

FOAM ROLLER Using a foam roller to provide pre- and/or post-workout myofascial release will increase your performance and decrease your risk of injury.

HOW TO USE THIS BOOK

This book begins with the pertinent questions of what, when, where, and why bodyweight resistance training. Please read this information, as it will educate you on the foundation-building "Big Six."

It also explains how to warm up and cool down functionally and how to hydrate and fuel your body correctly. These topics will help you work out safely, improve your performance, and reduce your recovery time so you can work out more efficiently.

This book presents a plan engineered to take a beginner from Level 1 to Level 3 over a 90-day period, increasing strength, building lean muscle mass, and decreasing body fat along the way.

THE METHOD

01 Hydrate and perform functional warmups before every workout.

02 Refer to the first day of the 30-day program for Level 1 to determine which workout to perform.

03 Turn to that workout page and perform the exercises it lists, referring as necessary to the individual exercise pages for reference.

04 After every workout, foam roll for recovery, and hydrate and refuel your body. You're done for today!

05 Tomorrow, move on to the next day's workout in Level 1. Over the course of a month, complete the exercises in Level 1. Then repeat for Levels 2 and 3.

THE EXERCISES

The exercises are explained with step-by-step photos, and each has a unique more difficult and less difficult version. Review these exercises until they're familiar.

THE WORKOUTS

Workouts vary in length, style, and format to keep your body on its toes. Some have built-in finishers, short metabolic-boosting sets, and core circuits that target your abs but also your back, hips, glutes, and other stabilizing muscles.

THE PROGRAMS

The three programs are an easy-to-follow graphical guide for each level. Each one provides a comprehensive 30-day plan. Combined across all levels, they create a 90-day bodyweight evolution.

Q&A

What if I can't perform every exercise or every rep at the end of the 28-day period?
You can either repeat the level and extend your overall commitment, or move on to the next level and continue to substitute any exercise from the previous level until you have it mastered.

What do I do after 90 days?
Start again, but this time perform all the more challenging progressions for each exercise, or create your own workouts.

What should I do on my rest day?
Enjoy it—it has been hard earned! And definitely foam roll and recover.

THE BIG SIX

In some shape or form, every exercise in this book takes its cues from the Big Six! These exercises are utilized on a nearly daily basis as you progress through the workouts in this book. The next few pages teach the benefits of each exercise, but above all provide tips and tricks for mastering form.

SQUATS

The squat doesn't work only the legs—it's a full-body exercise. Your hamstrings, quads, and glutes are indeed the prime movers when you squat, but your core muscles also work to stabilize you.

CORRECT FORM

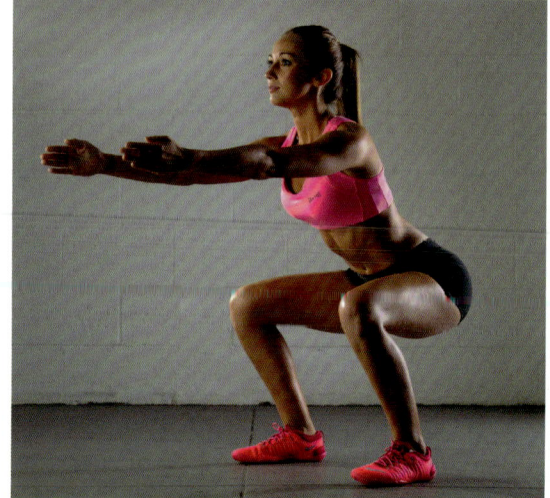

Keep your chest up, your glutes back, and your feet flat on the floor. Your back will arch slightly. The shins are close to vertical and the knees line up with the toes.

WHY SQUATS RULE

They boost HGH and testosterone.
Squats increase muscle-building hormones throughout the entire body, causing a stimulus for growth.

They improve core strength and posture.
Abdominals, back, and obliques must work to stabilize your spine and maintain an upright posture throughout the motion.

They improve hip mobility.
Deep squats work the hip through a larger range of motion, increasing hip mobility and flexibility, which may prevent back pain.

They decrease the risk of injury.
Building strength in the quads, glutes, hamstrings, lower back, and abs reduces your risk of injury when running, jumping, or changing direction.

They increase efficiency.
Squats are a supercharger for the metabolic benefits of your workout.

They increase athletic performance.
Squats generate power, which will make you explosive on and off the field or court.

EVALUATING A SAFE DEPTH

Some people are unable to perform deep squats due to hip dysfunction or weak or tight muscles. Here's how to establish the safe depth of your squats.

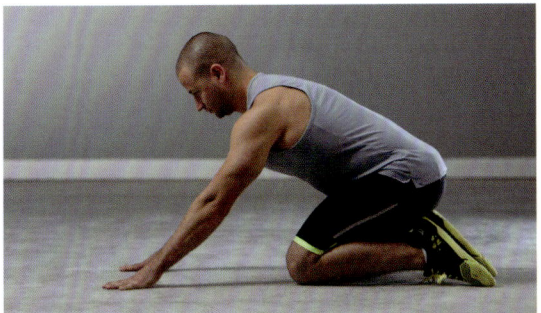

Face sideways on all fours in front of a mirror, core engaged and knees just wider than your shoulders. Drop your bottom down toward your feet and observe yourself.

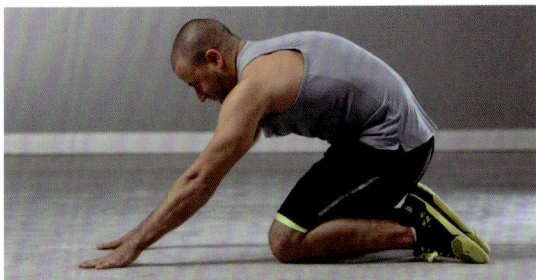

If your back looks rounded, you may have a weak or tight adductor magnus or glutes. When performing a squat, stop before your back gets round. It's okay to go shallow. As you progress through the book, your muscles will strengthen and hip mobility will increase. You can then squat more deeply.

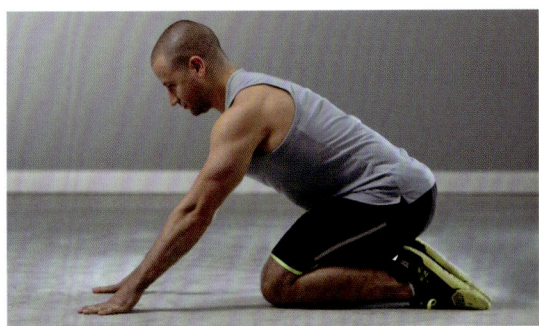

If your back looks flat, you will be able to perform a good, deep squat with moderate depth.

HIP DYSFUNCTION

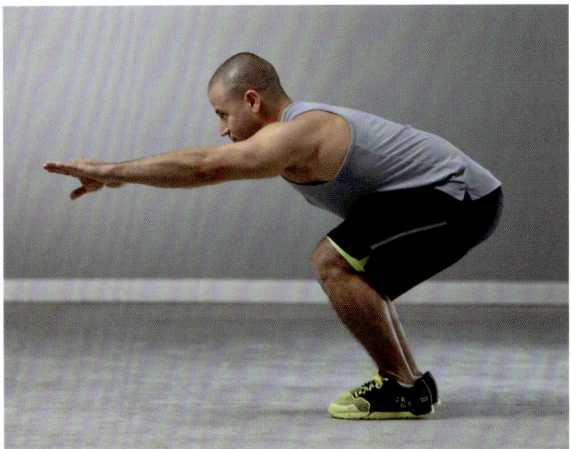

If you tip forward while squatting, you have weak glutes, which are the primary muscles used in hip extension. You're tipping because your lower back is switching on to compensate. Squat less deeply. Progress through the book and your muscles will strengthen so you can squat lower.

ANKLE DORSIFLEXION

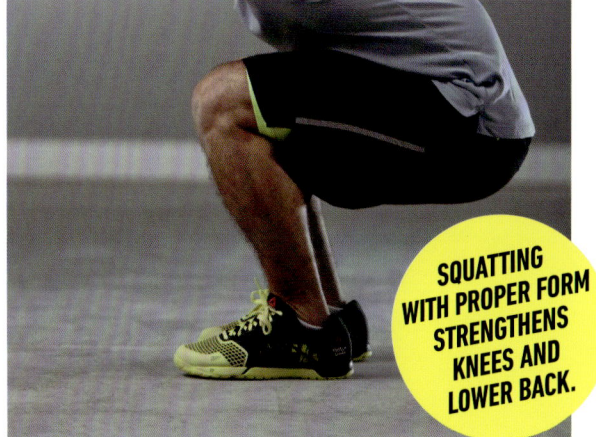

SQUATTING WITH PROPER FORM STRENGTHENS KNEES AND LOWER BACK.

Keep your feet flat on the floor: As shown above, correct ankle dorsiflexion (pulling the feet and toes back toward the shin) is about 15 degrees. Lack of flexibility in the calves and soleus, or wearing bulky training shoes, can cause lost mobility in the ankles. Lack of dorsiflexion can lead to several issues when you squat; the easiest to spot and correct is the heels lifting off the floor. You'll improve flexibility by progressing through the book; more flexibility will also enhance any athletic move that involves landing and decelerating the body.

LUNGES

Lunges prepare the body for deceleration and change of direction. Any weaknesses could lead to overcompensation, decreased performance, and possibly injury.

As you perform a lunge, focus on moving your torso only up and down, not pushing it forward. This keeps your weight balanced evenly through the front foot, allowing you to dig the front heel down and back to perform the movement. Press into the floor with your heel, which tones more lower-body muscle.

These key points ensure perfect, pain-free lunges.

CORRECT FORM

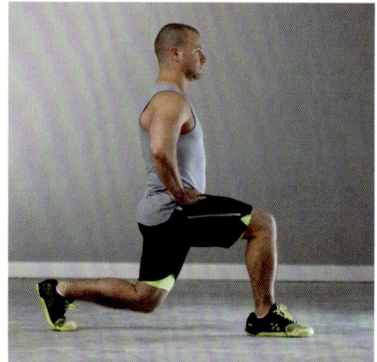

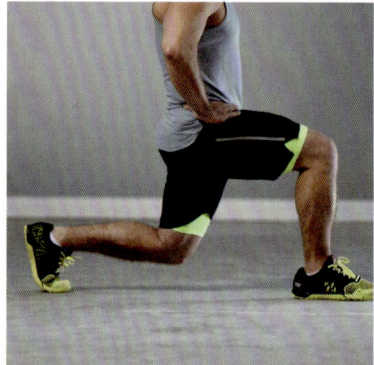

Stack the feet, ankles, knees, and hips on top of each other, and step straight back, keeping them in line. Keep the chest up, and the shin of the front leg relatively vertical.

Keep the trailing knee underneath the hips to load the hip, utilizing the front leg glute to perform the majority of the work.

WATCH OUT FOR THESE FLAWS

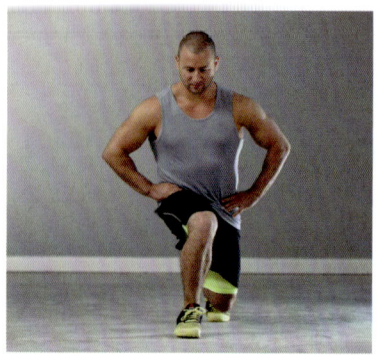

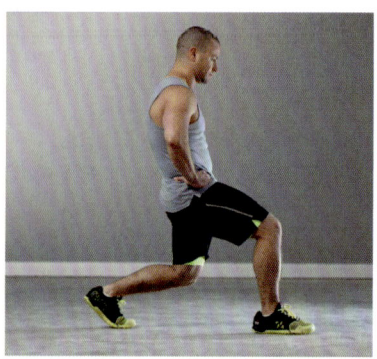

Don't let the knees cave in, and keep the hips forward at all times.

The trailing hip should not sink or dip.

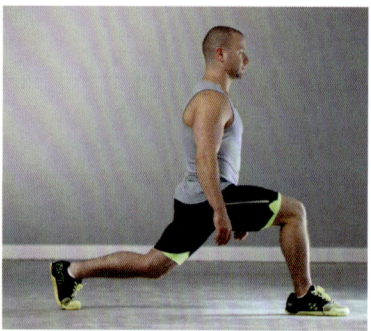

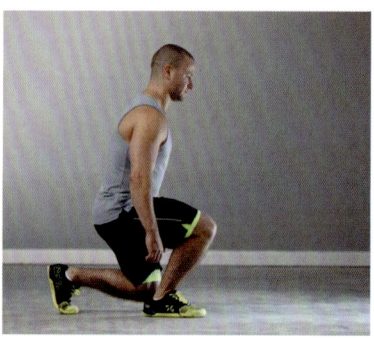

Don't over-stride ...

... or under-stride.

PUSH-UPS

The push-up may be the perfect multi-muscle (compound) exercise, effective at building strength and stability and burning body fat.

Most people associate push-ups with the chest, arms, and/or back, which is correct since the primary movers are the triceps, pectorals, serratus anterior, and lats. What most people forget, though, is that the push-up is a "moving plank," and abdominal muscles dominate when it comes to spinal stability during push-ups. The rectus abdominis is the primary stabilizer for preventing your hips from sagging, while the obliques prevent lateral shifting and twisting.

CORRECT FORM

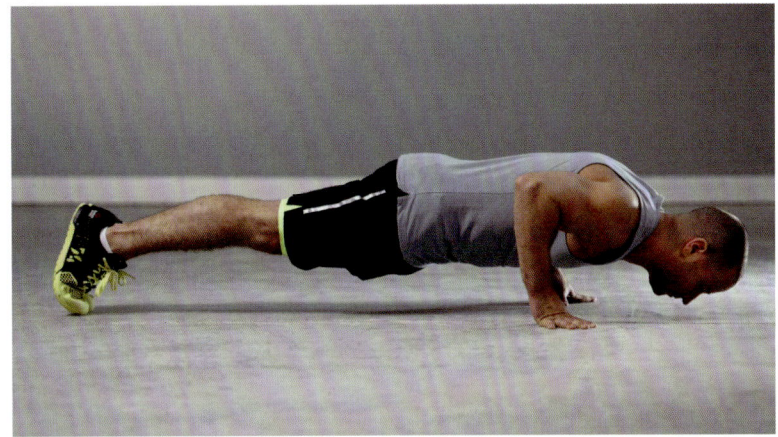

Keep elbows above wrists, hands rotated outward roughly 45 degrees. Tighten your core, and keep the pelvis in a posterior pelvic tilt—imagine wearing a belt and pulling the buckle up toward your navel.

STARTING POSITION

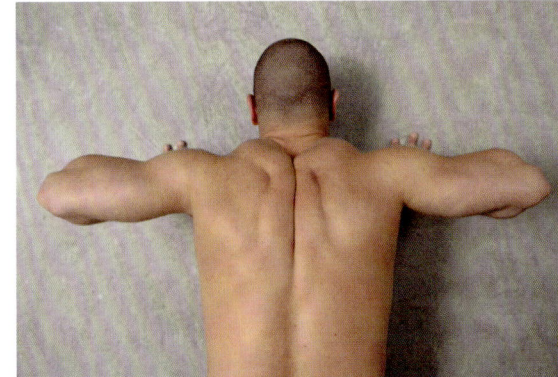

Incorrect starting position: People often set up with their hand position shoulder high and elbow width to make the exercise easier. Viewed from above, this looks like the letter T.

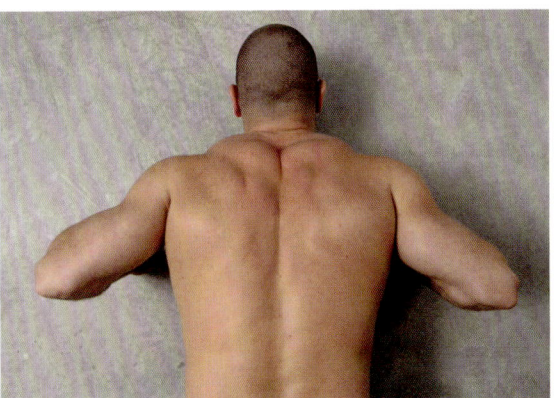

Correct starting position: The arms should form an angle of 20 to 40 degrees from the body. Viewed from above, you'll look like an arrow. This is easier on the shoulder joint and leads to higher activation of the pectorals and triceps.

BURPEES

Done correctly, the burpee might be the best metabolic-boosting exercise on the planet, an incredible total body strength and cardiovascular exercise.

The burpee has four athletic components: a squat, a martial arts or wrestling-style sprawl as the legs hop back, a push-up, and a vertical leap. The key to successfully completing a burpee is to break it down into these parts.

START SLOW. PERFECT EACH STAGE, THEN ADD SPEED AND REPS.

CORRECT FORM

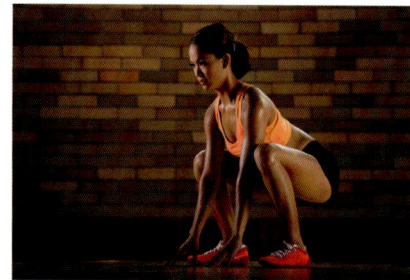

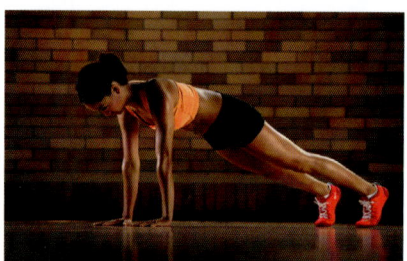

01 Squat: The final phase of the squat should look like a sitting frog. You'll also return to this position before the vertical jump. Hip mobility often inhibits jumping the feet far enough forward to have heels on the floor. Make sure to rock your weight back into your heels and lift your chest.

02 Sprawl: This extends the legs and positions you in a plank. Don't jump too far—keep arms at 90 degrees and shoulders over wrists. Don't sag—engage your core and use a posterior pelvic tilt to lock it in.

03 Push-up: This is where I see the greatest number of flaws during burpees. You should not sprawl all the way to the floor with no control, "bounce" your chest off the floor, or lift your chest and arch like a cobra.

04 Leap: Always start the leap from the squat position. This stable platform allows you to drive through the lower body and propel yourself into the air. While in the air, make sure to achieve "triple extension," which means you've fully extended not just the arms, but the ankles, the knees, and the hips. Getting into triple extension requires starting from a bent position, in which all joints are primed for movement.

INVERTED ROWS

Think of inverted rows as the counterpunch to the push-up. They utilize all the pulling muscles, opposite those used during a push-up.

Inverted rows work biceps, lats, traps, and deltoids. They're essential for creating balance and symmetry in the body.

CORRECT FORM

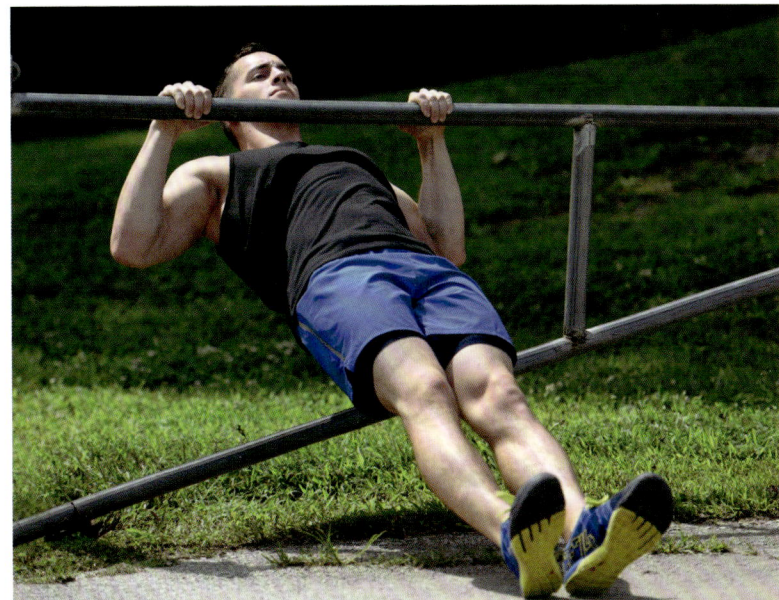

All inverted row variations require you to keep your body in an elevated horizontal inverted plank. Maintaining elevated hips in this way fires the glutes and hamstrings, and your abdominals stabilize the spine. Your key focus is to squeeze the shoulder blades and lift the chest to the bar.

FIXING FLAWS

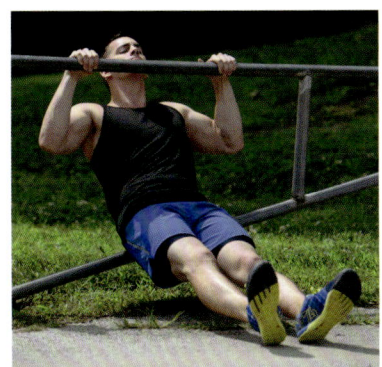

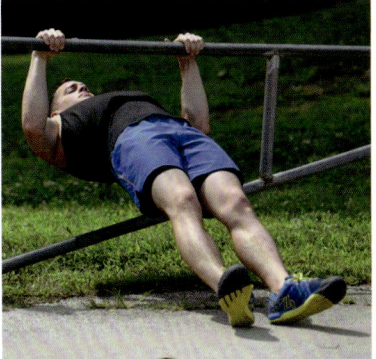

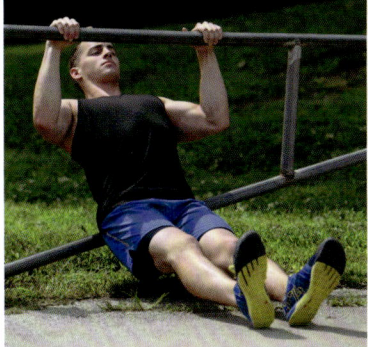

The head bob: Don't jut out the chin to find an extra inch or two of motion. A failure to retract the shoulder blades misses the entire purpose of an inverted row. Instead, keep the chin slightly forward and down, and the neck aligned with the cervical vertebrae.

The hip thrust: Don't fail to retract the scapulae, let the elbows drift behind the body, or jerk your forearm to get halfway up and thrust your crotch to the heavens. Instead, squeeze the glutes, engage the core, and use a posterior pelvic tilt to help lock in the core.

The sag: Don't let hips sag or glutes drop. This indicates a lack of strength in the glutes, hamstrings, pelvic floor, and core. To build strength and work up to a horizontal inverted plank, bend legs, place feet flat on the ground, and engage the glutes and core for stability.

PULL-UPS

Most of us spend large amounts of time sitting at a desk, and this leads to the devolution of the body. Pull-ups build incredible strength and posture, and also decompress the spine.

CORRECT FORM

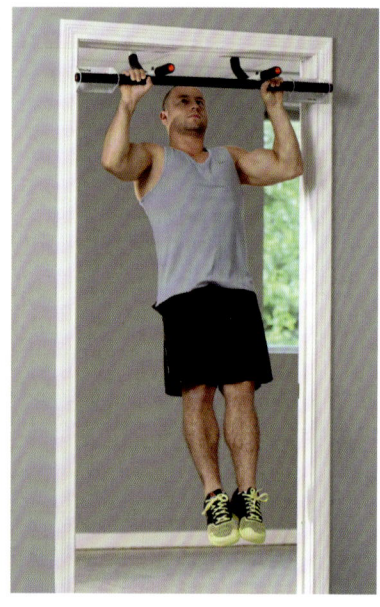

Despite popular belief, pull-ups aren't vertical; you should move up and back.

Pack the shoulders and brace the core by assuming a hollow body hold position with your feet slightly forward of your hips. Tighten the glutes to unload the spine. Look at the bar, keeping the chin up. Pull backward, squeezing the shoulder blades and engaging the lats, lifting as if trying to touch your chest to the bar. Lower slowly, with control.

These points apply to both overhand pull-ups and underhand chin-ups.

ACHIEVING MORE MOBILITY

Correct mobility is absolutely critical when undertaking pull-ups. Before performing pull-ups, begin with a drill to open the shoulders and chest, creating mobility to hang correctly. You'll need a foam roller and a towel.

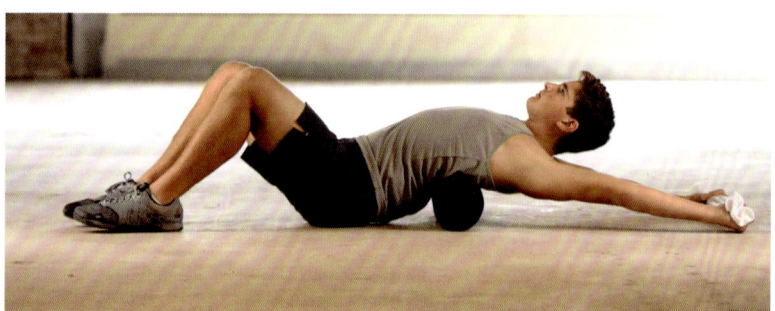

01 Place the foam roller directly below the shoulder blades, lift the hips, and extend the arms, keeping the towel taut, the backs of your hands on the floor, shoulders packed, and elbows locked.

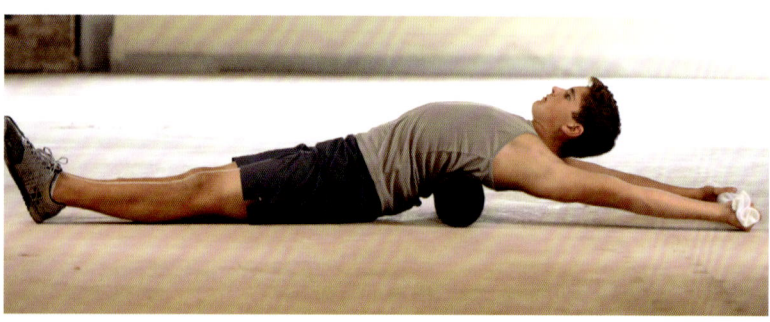

02 When ready, extend your legs and your lower back to the floor without elevating hands or bending arms.

DEAD HANG

Now that you're mobile, the next step is to get comfortable hanging. The genesis of any pull-up is the dead hang. A strong grip equals a strong upper body. Get comfortable hanging from the bar but make sure you keep correct form with your shoulders packed.

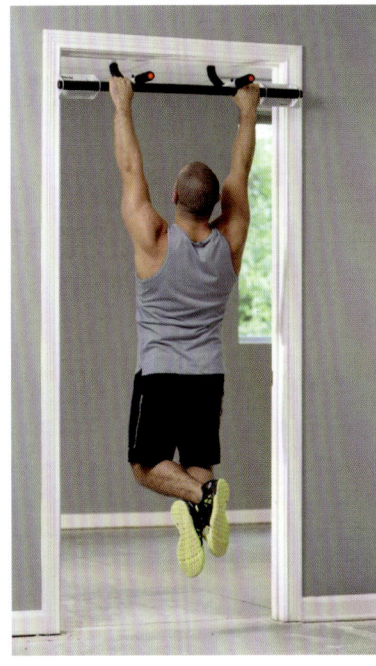

Shoulders packed: Think of the dead hang as a hanging plank! Just like a plank, it's all about keeping your shoulders down, rib cage down and in, core engaged, and glutes tight.

FIXING FLAWS

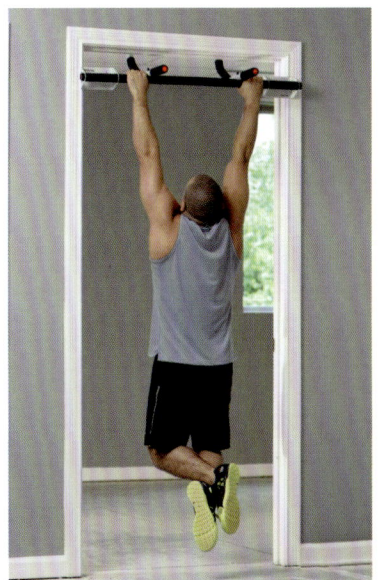

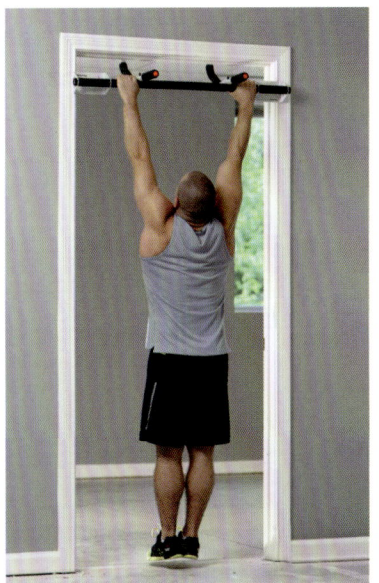

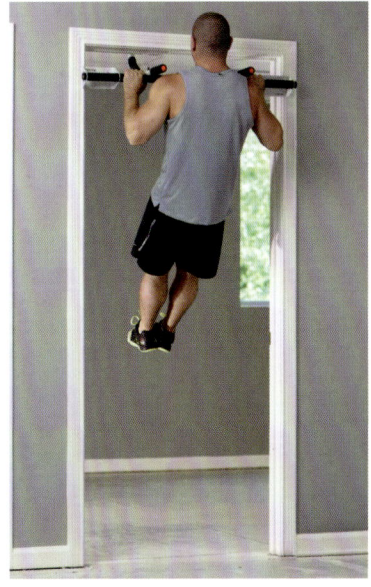

Shoulders by ears: If your shoulders look like this, practice the hanging scapula retraction found in Level 1 until this position becomes comfortable for you.

Chin up: The simplest trick for great pull-ups is keeping your chin up. By so doing, you'll lengthen your body and position it to maximize your results on the bar.

Lean back: Squeeze and engage the back muscles, and at the top of the motion lean slightly back as if touching chest to bar. This allows the large back muscles to activate.

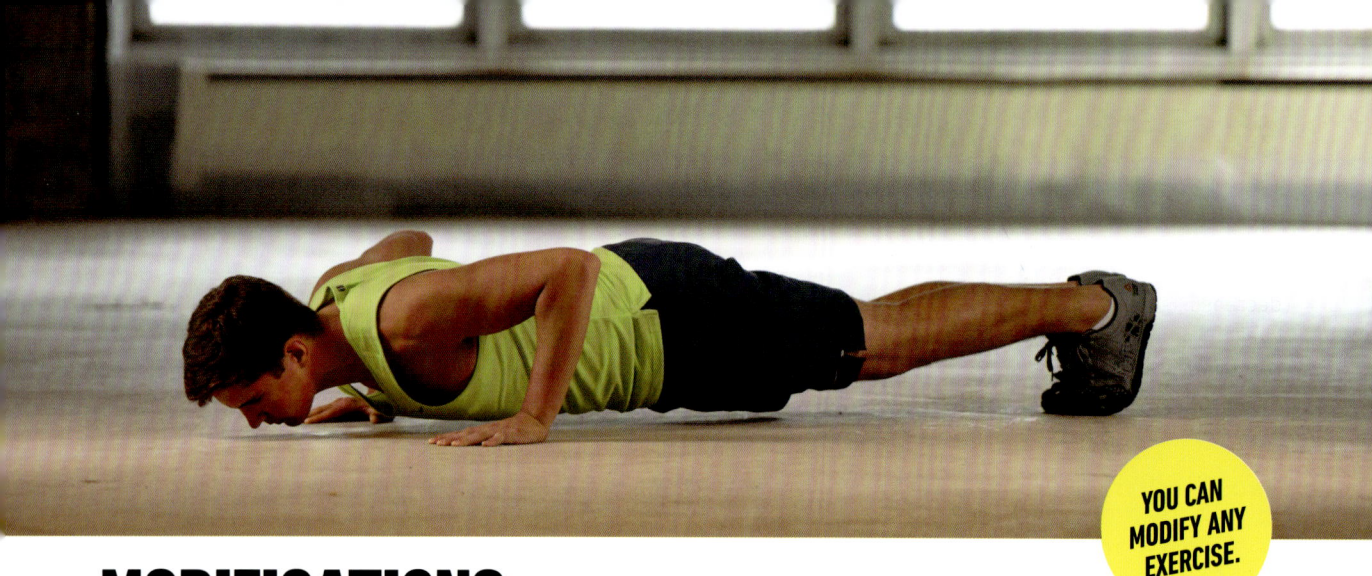

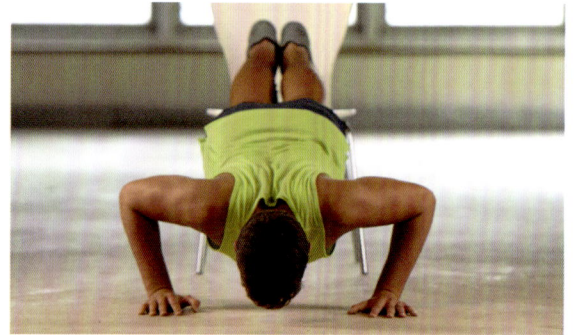

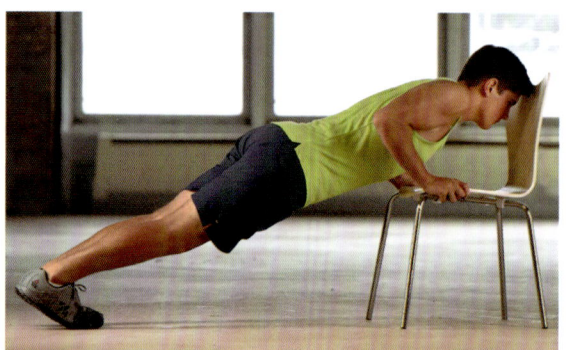

YOU CAN MODIFY ANY EXERCISE.

MODIFICATIONS

Almost every exercise can be made more or less challenging with some fundamental modifications. This allows you to quickly and easily adapt an exercise to meet your ability level. These pages show how to apply each modification to a push-up, but it's possible to perform them on any exercise.

BODY ANGLE

Adjusting the angle between your body and the floor allows you to shift more or less weight onto the working muscles.

MORE DIFFICULT ⁞⁞⁞⁞⁞⁞⁞⁞⁞⁞⁞⁞⁞⁞⁞⁞
Elevating the feet makes the exercise more challenging by transferring weight to the upper body, which then has to work harder.

LESS DIFFICULT ⁞⁞⁞⁞⁞⁞⁞⁞⁞⁞⁞⁞⁞⁞⁞⁞
The work of a push-up is performed by the chest, back, and shoulders. With the hands elevated on a chair, bench, or other prop, your weight shifts from the upper body to the lower body.

STABILITY

Stability is the constant fight between your body's center of gravity and its contact with the floor—its base of support. Simply raising one foot off the floor decreases stability and makes an exercise more challenging. Stability-based modifications improve core and joint strength, making you more athletic and decreasing the risk of injury.

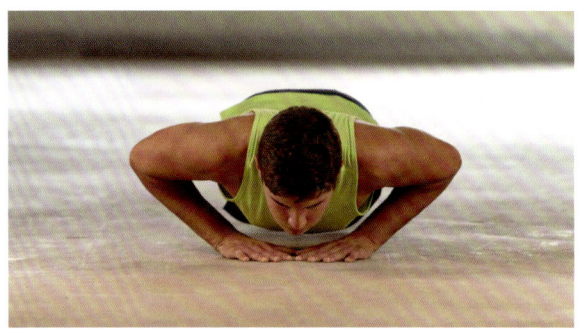

MORE DIFFICULT ||||||||||||||||||||||
Touching fingers and thumbs in the shape of a diamond directly under your chest narrows the base of support and decreases stability.

LESS DIFFICULT ||||||||||||||||||||||
By opening either the feet or hands, you widen the base of support and make the exercise easier because your weight is distributed over a larger area.

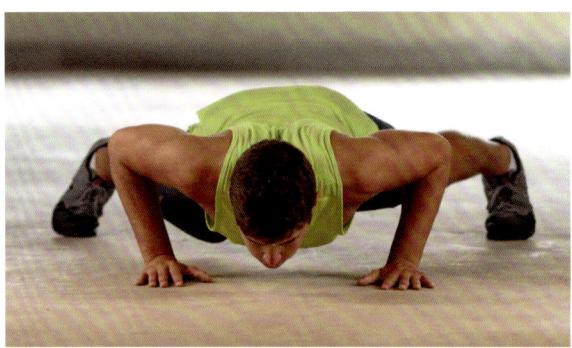

RANGE OF MOTION

In a full range of motion (ROM), you perform an exercise from the absolute top point to the absolute bottom point and back again. Changing the ROM by shortening, lengthening, or even stopping can make the exercise easier or harder.

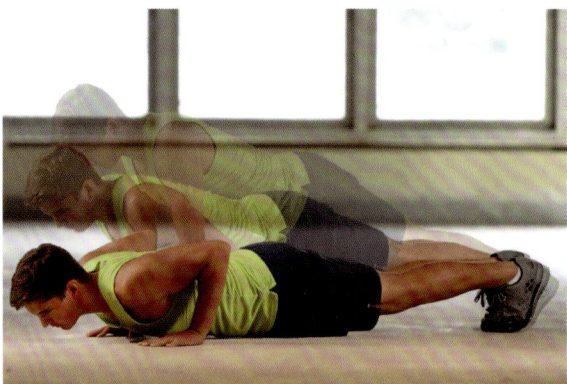

MORE DIFFICULT ||||||||||||||||||||||
Performing a greater amount of work on each rep during the toughest part of the exercise increases the challenge. Lower; then come up only halfway, lower fully again, and go fully up. You've performed 1.5 reps.

LESS DIFFICULT ||||||||||||||||||||||
Half push-ups, in which you lower your body only halfway, decrease the ROM—a good way to build confidence in the early stages of practicing a new exercise.

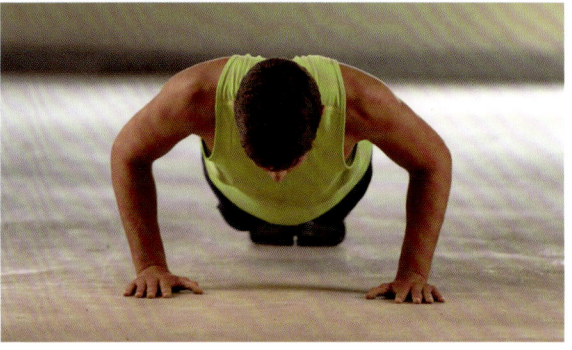

POINTS OF CONTACT

The more points of contact you have with the floor, the easier the exercise. With fewer contact points, you have to move the same mass with fewer joints.

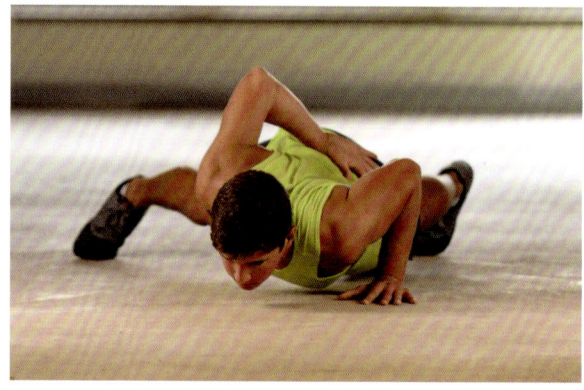

MORE DIFFICULT ||||||||||||||||||||
Raising an arm off the floor decreases the number of joints from four to three, increases the load on the working arm, and decreases stability.

EVEN MORE DIFFICULT ||||||||||||
The surface area of the points of contact also plays a role in modifying the exercise. Going from the entire palm on the floor to a two-finger push-up decreases the surface area.

LESS DIFFICULT ||||||||||||||||||||||
Dropping the knees to the floor inclines and shortens the body, increasing stability and decreasing the amount of mass moved during the push-up.

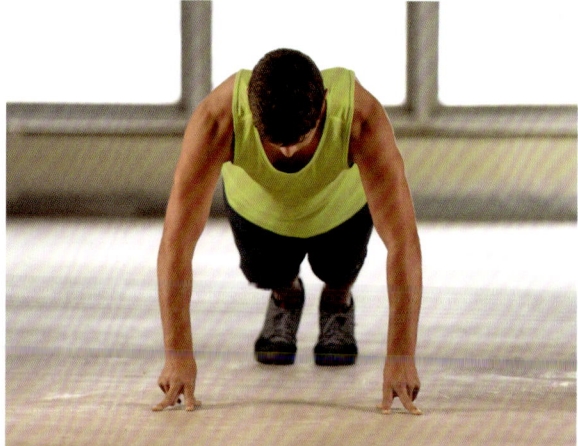

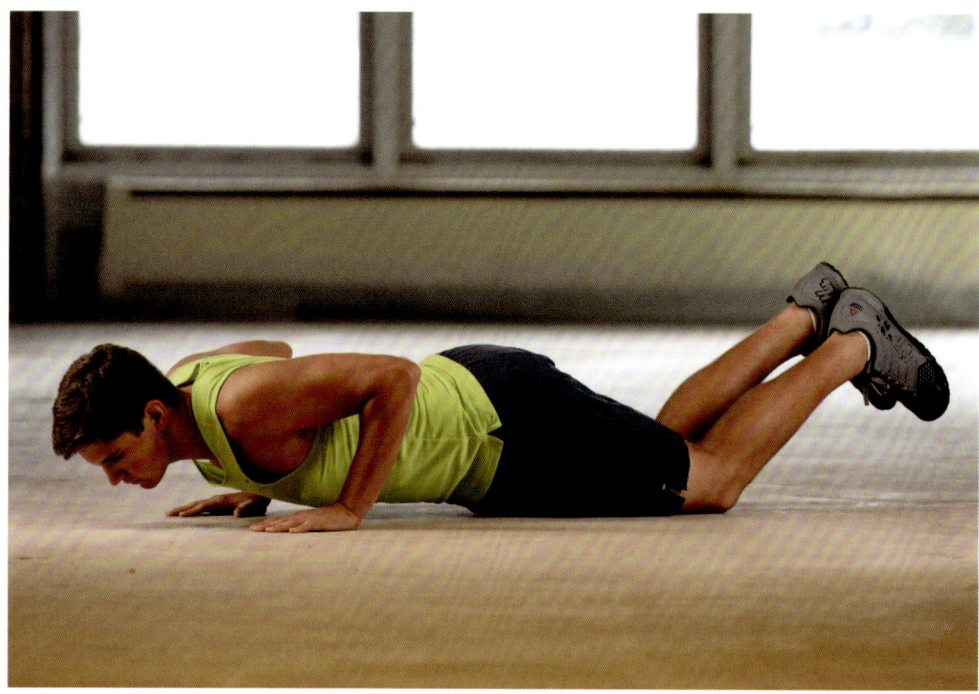

SPEED

Altering the speed of an exercise can make it easier or harder. To know the speed of an exercise, though, you must understand the different types of muscle contraction, as each relates to the speed.

TYPES OF MUSCLE CONTRACTION

Concentric contractions: When a muscle is activated and required to lift a load, it begins to shorten. Contractions that permit the muscle to shorten are called concentric contractions. Bicep curls are a concentric contraction, but for the speed modification, think of them as acceleration.

Eccentric contractions: An eccentric contraction increases tension on a muscle as it lengthens. Eccentric contractions usually occur when the muscle opposes a stronger force, causing it to lengthen as it contracts. An example is the lowering phase of a squat. Think of eccentric contractions as controlled movements similar to decelerating or braking while at high speed.

Isometric contractions: In this type of contraction, the muscle is activated, but instead of being shortened or lengthened, it's held. Think of it as a racecar driver with the engine at peak revs but clutch balanced waiting for the green light. Isometric contractions can also form a pause at the mid-point of an exercise.

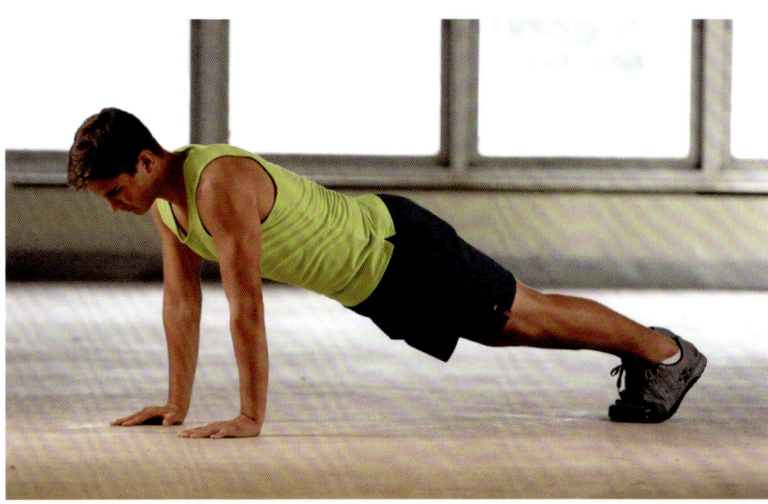

MORE DIFFICULT ||||||||||||||||||||||
Hold the start position: This forces you to defy gravity and hold an isometric contraction while you build strength in your core and shoulders.

LESS DIFFICULT ||||||||||||||||||||||
Slow the lowering phase: Take 4 seconds to lower to the deepest part of the push-up and then press back up to the starting position, making the chest, shoulders, and triceps contract eccentrically.

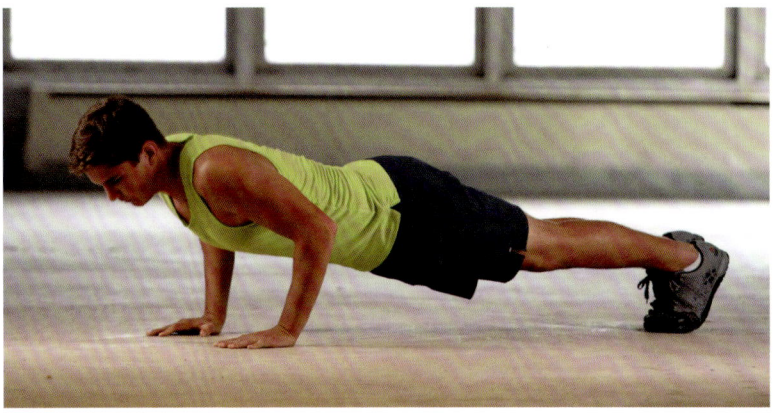

FUNCTIONAL WARM-UPS

Functional training is a classification of exercise that involves training the body for activities performed in daily life.

For example, squats equate to getting in and out of a chair, and pull-ups hark back to the survival skills necessary for early humans, who had to pull themselves into the higher branches of trees to evade predators.

It's not that exercise such as powerlifting isn't functional per se, but unless you're in an occupation that requires lifting or moving heavy objects, an NFL lineman, or a sumo wrestler, you probably won't be moving large amounts of mass on a daily basis.

A functional exercise should prepare us for a daily activity or mimic a movement used in everyday life. Functional training should make you more stable, balanced, and confident in performing these motions.

The next five exercises can be performed independently or chained together to form a cyclical yoga-inspired flow. The goal of each is to increase mobility, improve balance, and prepare your body for the challenges ahead.

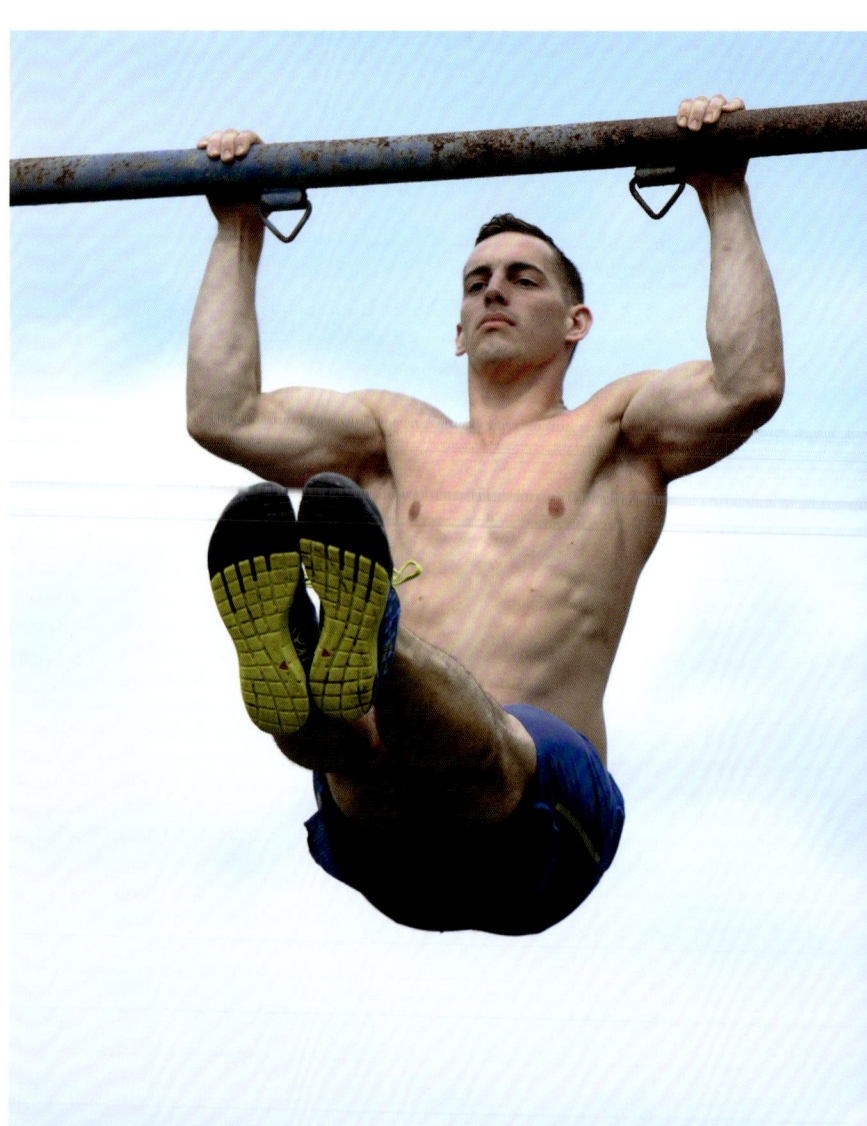

Performing an exercise like the L-sit chin-up requires core and shoulder strength and mobility—especially hip mobility. Performing the functional warm-ups will not only help you move better, it will also increase performance and help prevent injury.

INLINE LUNGE

As a functional warm-up, the inline lunge activates the glutes, quads, and hamstrings. It also forces you to engage your core and challenges your proprioception—your unconscious ability to perceive movement and spatial orientation, which arises from stimuli within the body.

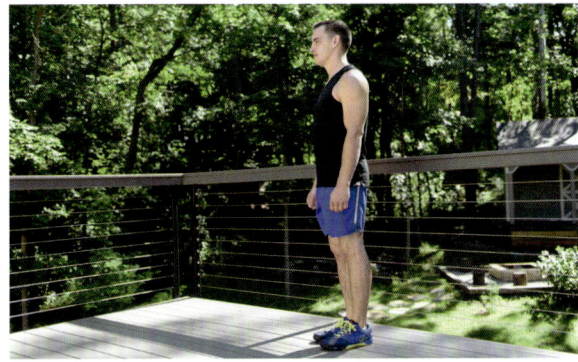

01 Stand tall with arms at your sides. Activate your core and glutes.

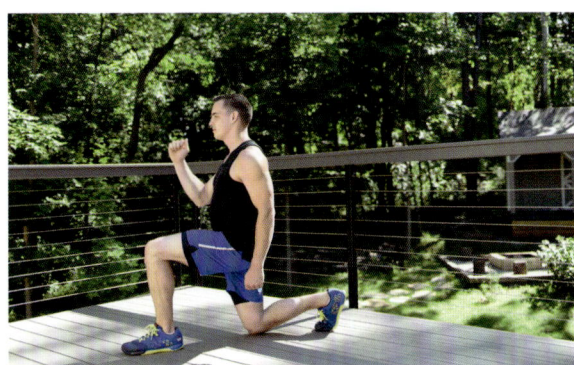

02 Take a step forward with one leg, bend both legs, and lower into a lunge position. Attempt to place the toes of the rear foot in line with the front heel and knee, as if standing on an invisible tightrope.

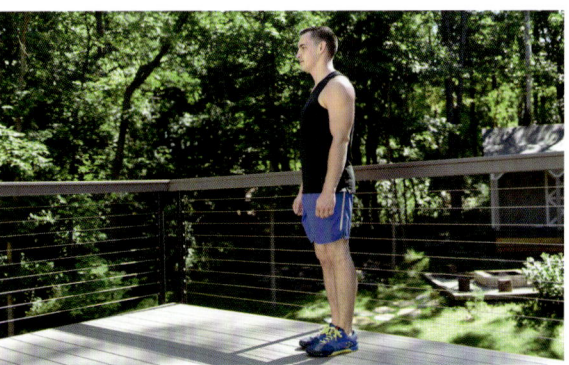

03 Straighten both legs, pressing them firmly into the floor. Alternate legs. Perform five lunges per leg, for 10 reps total.

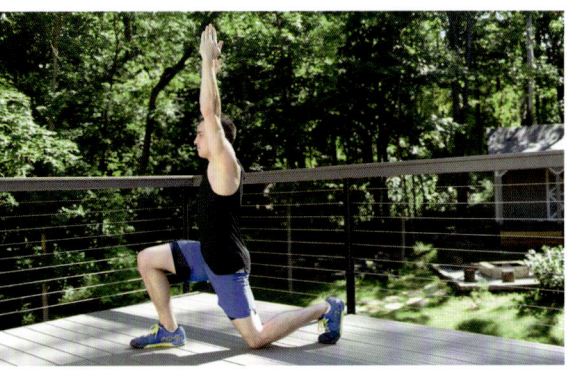

Variation
For an added balance challenge, try extending the arms overhead during the lunge. This will require, and in turn result in, greater trunk stability.

RESTING SQUAT

Since the dawn of time, our ancestors knew the power of resting squats. Human beings have crouched all the way down into these to perform activities like relaxing, working, and cooking over a fire. The sitting squat will help to open your hips and provide dorsiflexion in the ankles and feet, preparing you for squats.

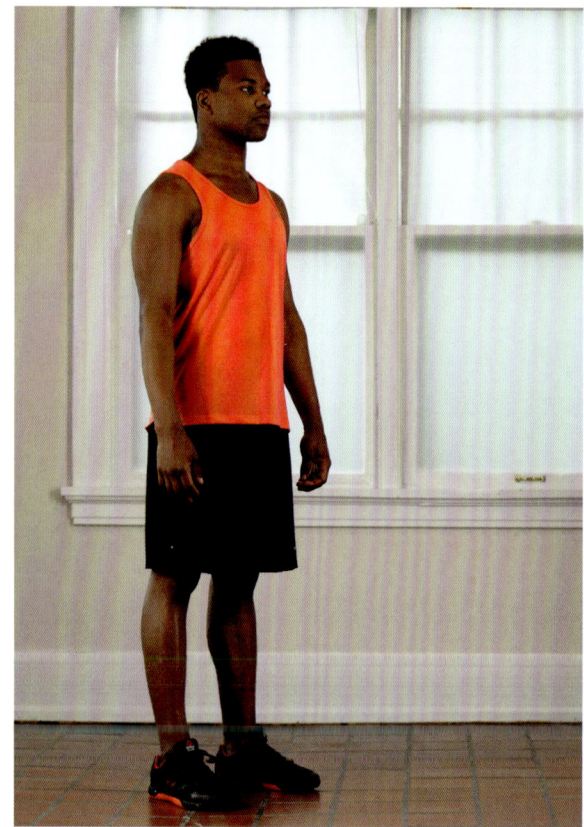

01 Stand tall with feet roughly shoulder width and arms hanging by your sides.

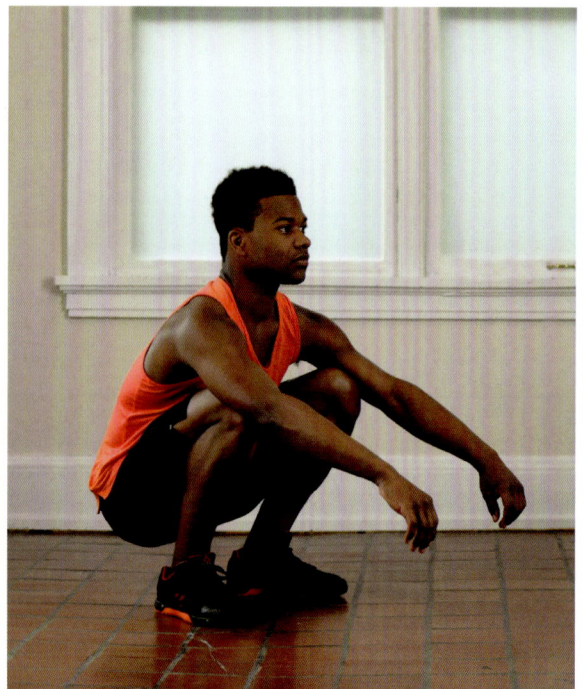

02 Bend at the knees and lower until your glutes are resting on the back of your calves. Do not let your heels lift off of the floor. Keep your chest up and hold this position for 30 seconds before standing. Repeat 3 to 5 times.

TRUNK STABILITY PUSH-UP

Without adequate stability in the trunk, you waste energy, resulting in poor performance and increasing your risk of injury. The trunk stability push-up helps strengthen and stabilize the spine and trunk during a closed-chain upper-body movement—one where the upper body is fixed in place against an immobile surface.

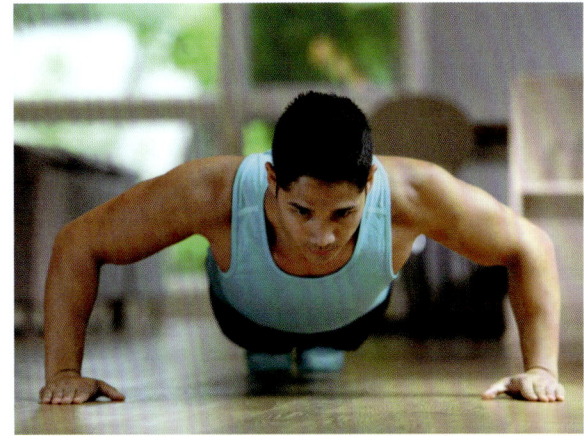

01 Lie on your stomach with your hands slightly wider than shoulder-width apart and thumbs level with your forehead. Raise onto your toes and lift your torso from the ground.

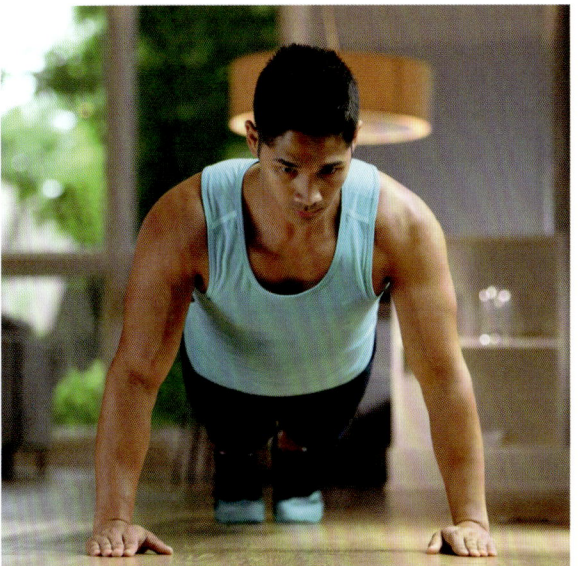

02 Maintaining a rigid torso, lift yourself as a unit into a push-up position, making sure the lumbar spine does not dip down.

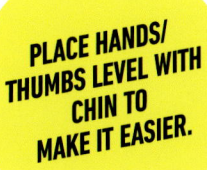

PLACE HANDS/ THUMBS LEVEL WITH CHIN TO MAKE IT EASIER.

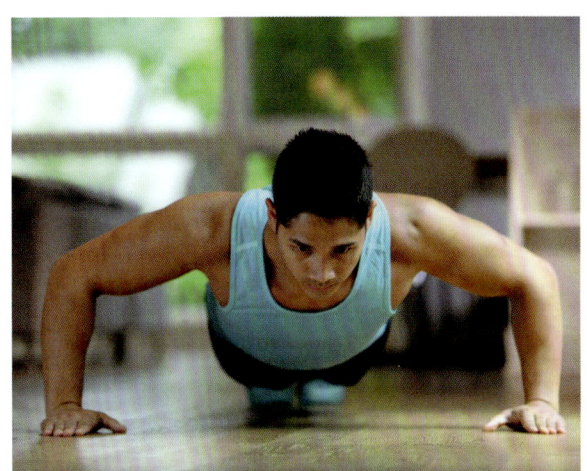

03 Lower back down into the same position as in step 1. Perform 3 to 5 reps with correct form.

INNER THIGH MOBILITY

Performance is compromised by poor joint mobility. The greater your joint mobility, the greater your ROM, and the more kinetic energy/tension—and therefore power—you'll be able to generate. Warm up the hips and groin with this simple yet incredibly effective inner thigh mobility stretch.

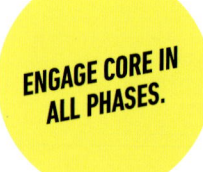

ENGAGE CORE IN ALL PHASES.

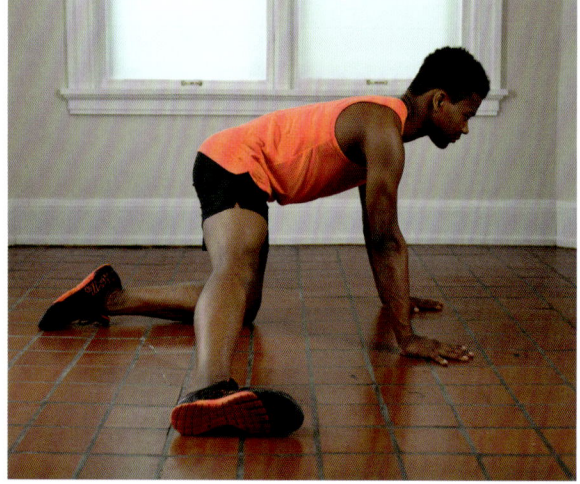

01 Begin on your hands and knees with your back flat, and straighten your right leg out to the side until it is perpendicular to your torso.

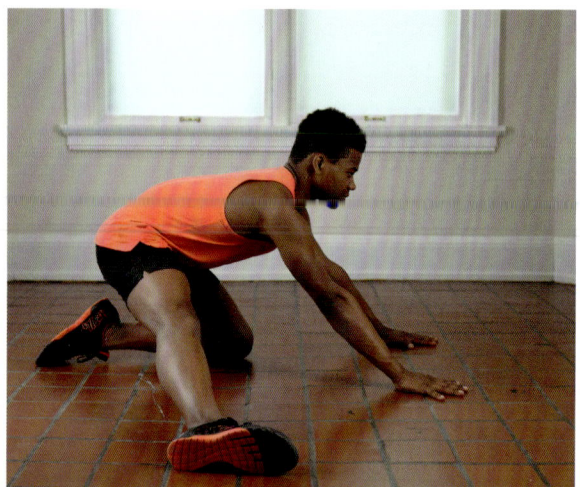

02 Keep your back flat and push your hips back as far as possible.

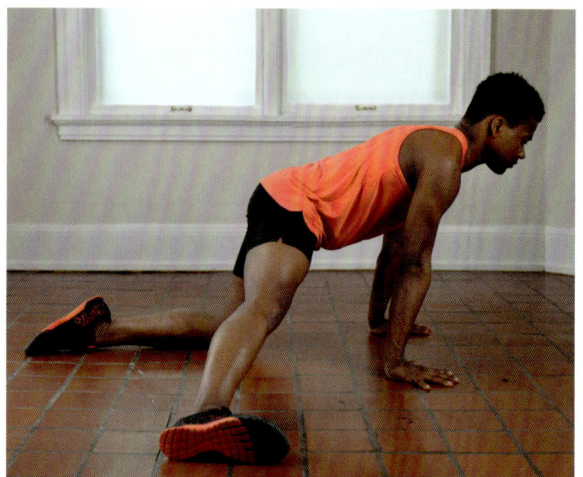

03 Push your hips forward as far as you can, keeping your back flat and arms straight. Return to the starting position to complete 1 rep. Perform 8 reps on each leg.

THORACIC ROTATION

Improve your posture by increasing the mobility in your thoracic spine. It's especially beneficial for those who spend a lot of time at a desk or keyboard or spend too much time bench pressing at the gym.

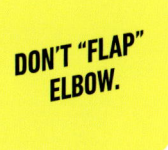

DON'T "FLAP" ELBOW.

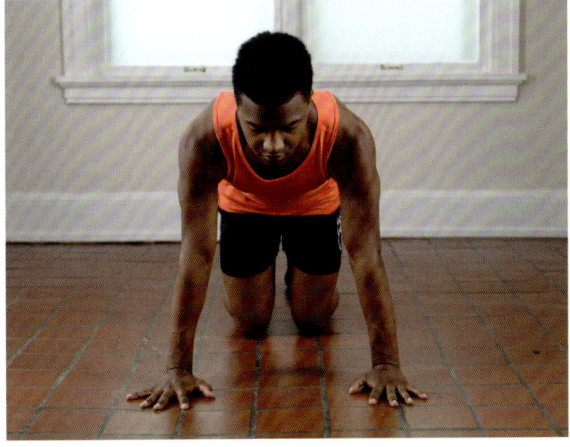

01 Begin on your hands and knees, with a flat back and straight arms.

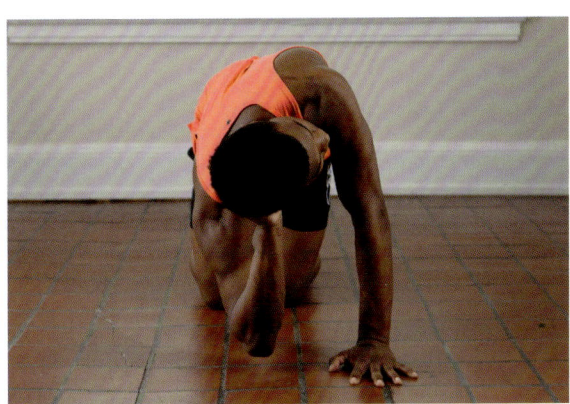

02 Bring your right hand behind your head and rotate your right elbow in toward the floor. Make sure to rotate through the thoracic spine and trunk rather than through the arm.

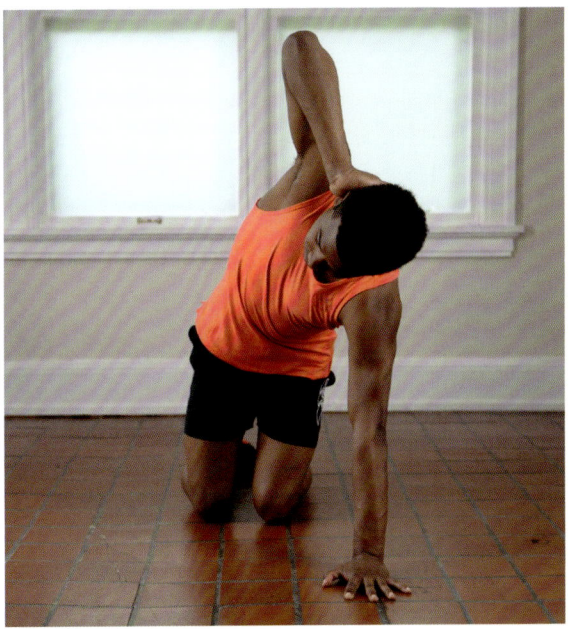

03 Rotate the right elbow outward to the ceiling, opening the chest and rotating your head and upper back as far as you can. Rotate back inward and repeat for 8 reps, then switch sides.

RECOVERY

Bodyweight workouts require you to exert great stress on your body. Afterward, your muscles will be tired and sore. Recovery practices are critical for injury prevention and consistent training, and they enable you to give maximum effort for maximum results. Make these four simple practices part of your regular post-workout routine.

STRETCH

Stretching isn't sexy, but it's the most underrated aspect of athletic development.

Without the necessary flexibility and muscle pliability, you'll struggle to find the depth required to maximize your ability to burn calories and build new muscle.

❯ Run through all of the exercises found in the Functional Warm-Ups pages post-workout as well as pre-workout to increase your flexibility and mobility.

FOAM ROLL

The fascia is connective tissue that wraps around the muscles in the body. It can become tense or constricted while working out, causing pain.

You can massage yourself with a foam roller to relieve muscle tightness. This is called self-myofascial release.

❯ Perform foam rolling, a key component of recovery. See Foam Rolling Technique.

FOAM ROLLING TECHNIQUE

Use a foam roller as a warm-up, after working out, or whenever you feel pain, to "roll out" the muscles. This alleviates soreness and stiffness, promotes circulation of oxygenated blood, and even breaks up scar tissue and restrictions in the fascia.

A foam roller also allows you to apply targeted pressure to specific spots in the muscle that may be causing pain.

Look for a high-density foam roller that's about 3 inches (7.5cm) in diameter. You can find them at sporting goods stores or online.

The basic technique is the same, regardless of whether you use it on the legs, back, or arms. There's a lot of freedom for experimentation when using the roller. See what works well and feels best for you, and manipulate the roller to the correct position. You can create your own techniques to meet your needs.

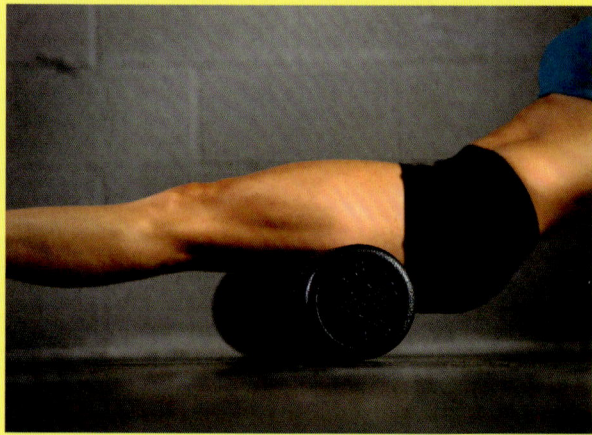

01 Position your body on the roller. The weight of your body will apply pressure on your muscles. Roll back and forth slowly. When you find a tender spot in the area you're working, pause and wait for the discomfort to diminish. This could take up to one minute and may be uncomfortable.

SLEEP

Sleep is the necessary downtime your body needs to restore itself.

Other mammals don't willingly delay sleep the way we humans do. Sacrificing hours of sleep over a long period of time can negatively impact your mental strength and commitment to training sessions. Another drawback of not getting enough rest at night is that you'll want to eat more than you need to. Leptin is a hormone that regulates appetite, and its levels fall in the bodies of people who haven't gotten enough rest, causing an increase in food craving.

If you find it difficult to get to sleep, make sure to cut out caffeinated beverages. One of the many benefits of regular exercise is that it can help you fall asleep faster, and it contributes to sounder, deeper sleep. But don't exercise right before you go to bed, because that may have the opposite effect. It could get you wired and make it harder to get to sleep.

> Sleep at least 7 hours; note that many athletes may need up to 9 hours.

ICE

Intense exercise causes microtrauma, or tiny tears, in muscle fibers.

This sounds scary, but it's a good thing because micro tears stimulate muscle cell activity, helping repair the damage and actually strengthening the muscles. Icing helps the body recover faster and reduces muscle pain and soreness after intense training sessions.

It constricts blood vessels and flushes waste products out of the affected tissue. It decreases metabolic activity and slows down physiological processes. And it reduces swelling and tissue breakdown. Afterward, the body has to warm itself, resulting in increased blood flow that improves the healing process.

> Fill your tub with water 53 to 59° (12 to 15°C) and submerge your body for between 10 and 15 minutes for maximum benefit.
> Or instead of an ice bath, apply localized ice (for example bags of frozen peas) to specific areas of the body for 10 to 15 minutes. Don't apply these directly to the skin; wrap them in a towel first.

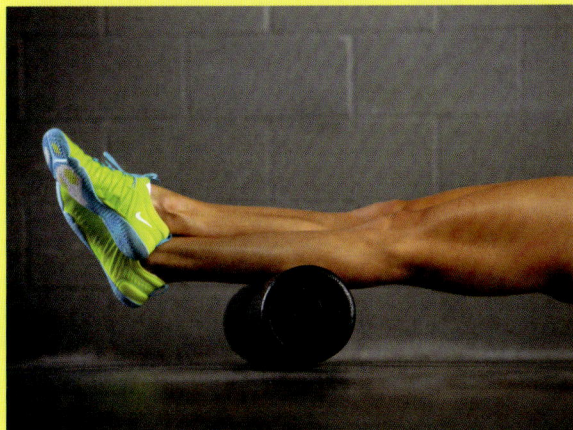

02 When the area is no longer sensitive, roll up or down the muscle on the roller. When you identify any other sensitive spots, again pause and wait for the discomfort to diminish.

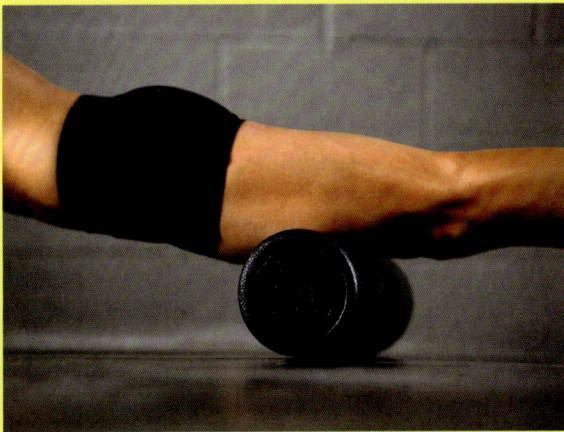

03 When tender areas can be rolled over without pain, continue rolling regularly to keep the area relaxed.

PRE- AND POST-WORKOUT STRETCHES

FORWARD FOLD TO FLAT BACK FOLD

A staple in yoga classes, the forward fold, or *uttanasana*, stretches the hamstrings and calves and releases the lower back. By developing the forward fold into flat back fold, or *ardha uttanasana*, you can increase the stretch to include the hips. This stretch will increase flexibility and prevent injury.

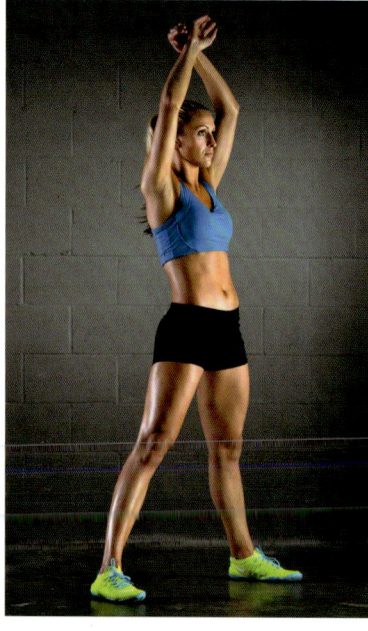

01 Stand tall with arms loosely by your sides. Inhale and lift arms overhead.

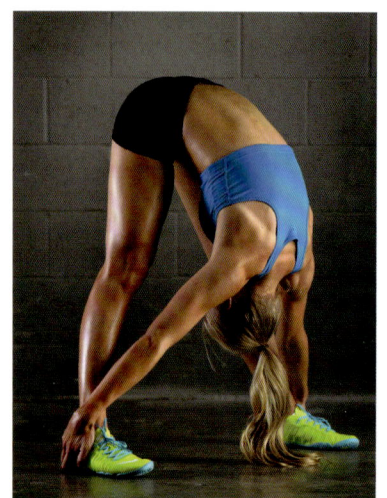

02 Exhale and release arms down either side of your body. Bend forward from the hips and roll down your spine, bringing your nose toward your shins.

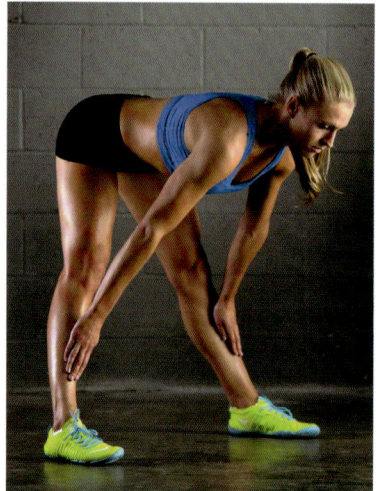

03 Inhale and lift your head as you flatten your back and shift your weight back, lifting your butt. Place hands as far up on the legs as needed to comfortably flatten your back.

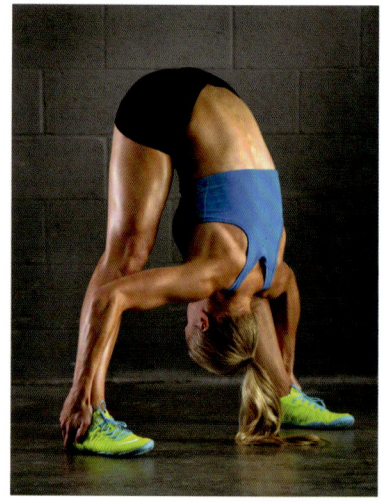

04 Exhale and return to your forward fold. Repeat 3 times.

SIDE LUNGE

The side lunge is a dynamic stretch that tones and stretches the lower body, building strength at the same time. The side lunge opens the hips, creating stability and balance. It also stretches the hips, calves, Achilles tendons, hamstrings, and groin. It combines the components and benefits of three popular yoga poses: low crescent lunge, chair pose, and side angle pose.

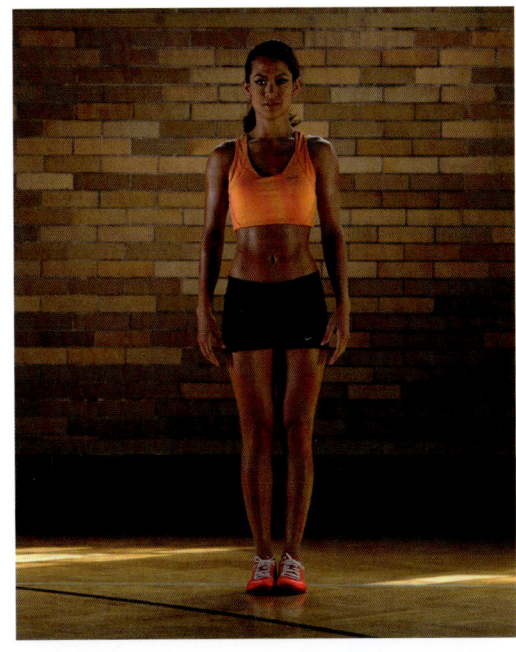

01 Stand tall, feet together, and hands hanging loosely at your sides.

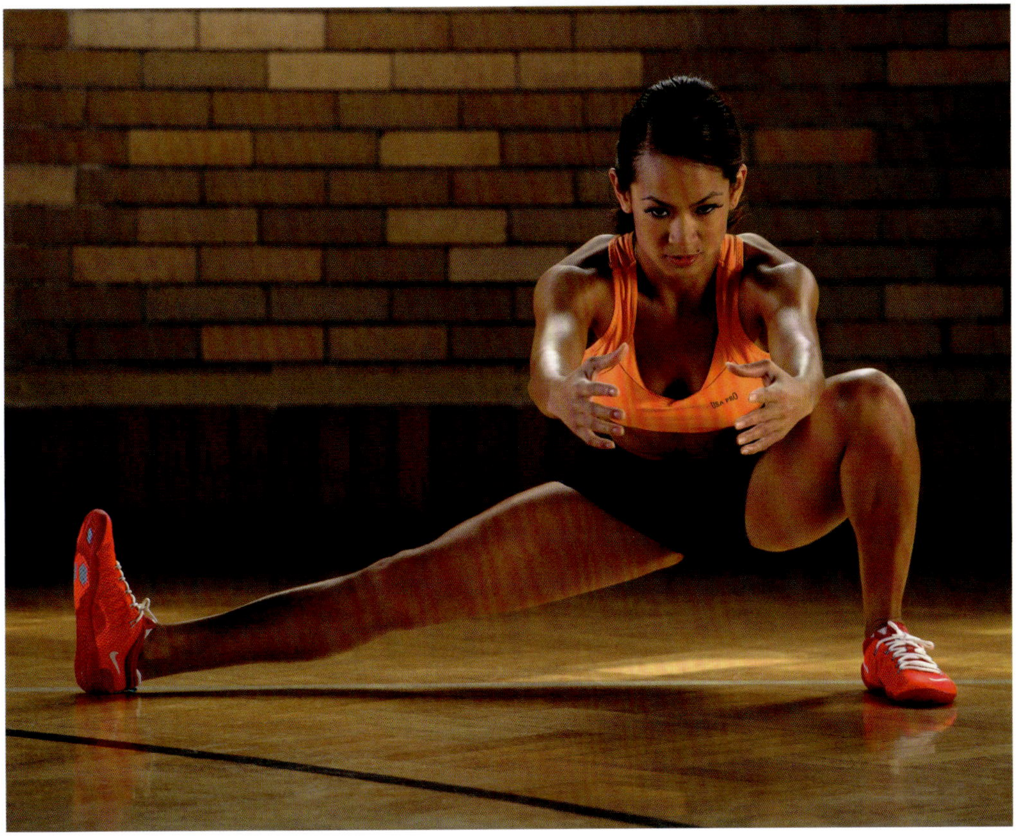

02 Take a giant step to your left. Bend your left knee to at least 90 degrees, but lower if possible. Extend your arms in front of you for balance. Hold for 30 seconds before returning to center. Repeat 3 times on each side.

DEEP LUNGE STRETCH

Tight hip flexors can inhibit your abs, glutes, and inner thighs from getting the results you want from your workouts. They can also cause injuries, including lower back pain, IT band syndrome, and even patellar tendonitis. The deep lunge is an activation stretch that will wake up and stretch the hip flexors, making your workouts more efficient and preventing injury.

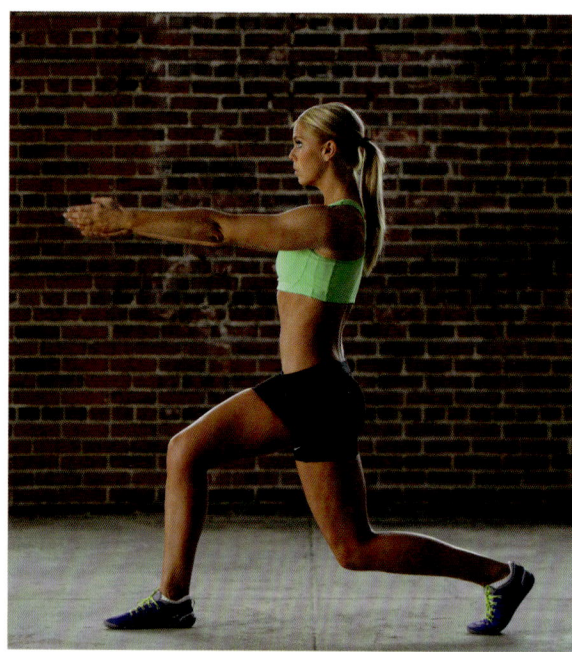

01 Lunge forward with your right leg, keeping your right knee above your ankle and your weight in your heel. Your left knee should be bent under your hip. Raise your arms until they are parallel to the floor and make sure your toes are pointing forward.

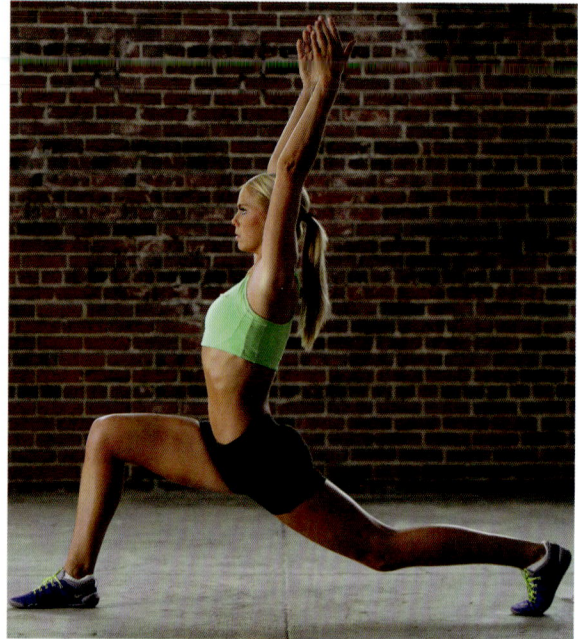

02 Reach your hands toward the ceiling, keeping your arms in line with your ears. Extend the back leg and sink your hips down slightly. Hold for two to three deep breaths. Return to start and repeat 5 times before switching to the left leg.

EXTENDED SIDE ANGLE POSE

Extended side angle pose is a popular yoga posture that strengthens your thighs, hips, and ankles while stretching your groin, back, and hips and opening the chest. This stretch can also increase lung capacity.

[**If your hands do not comfortably reach the floor, place a yoga brick or similar object under the supporting hand.**]

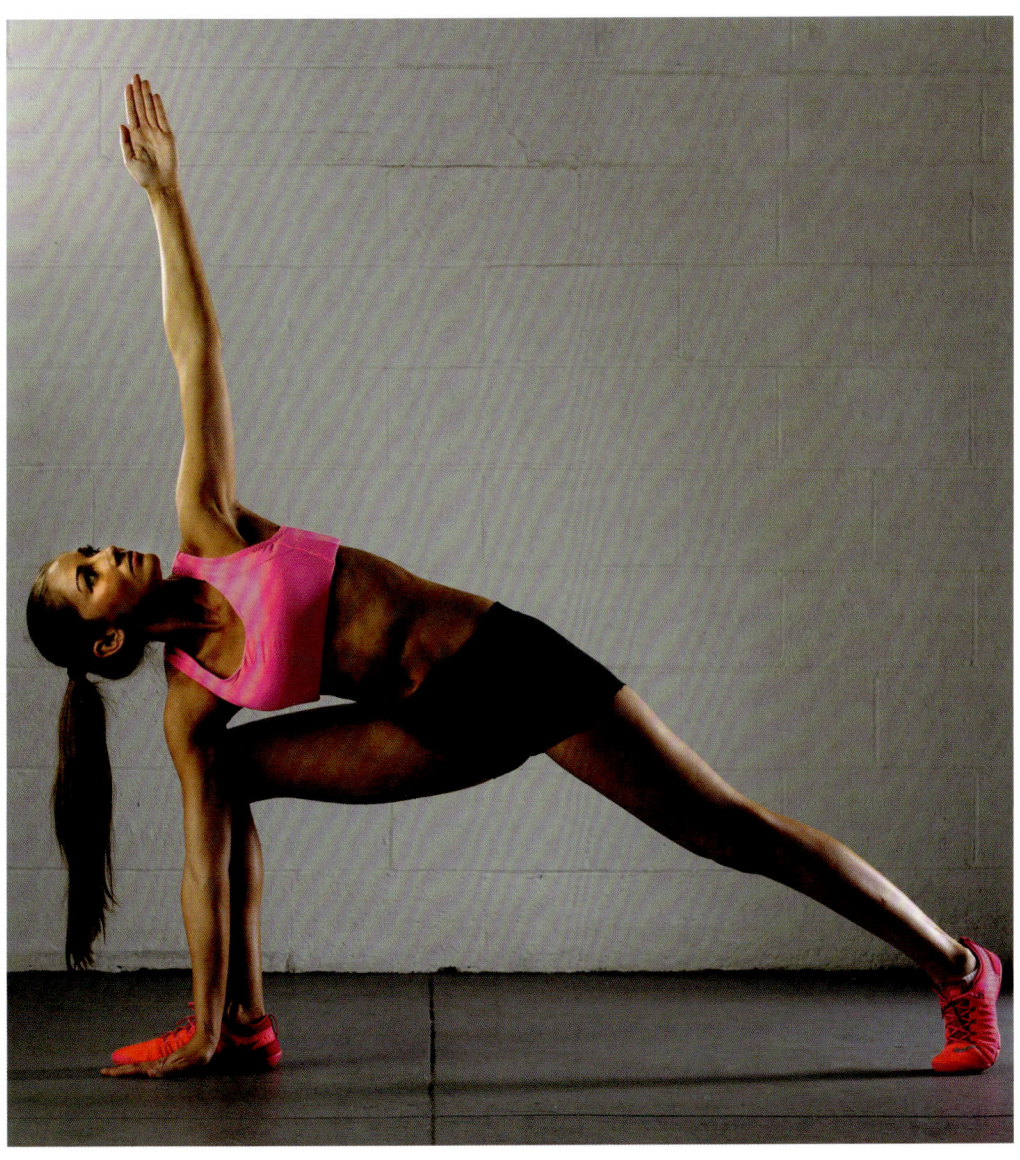

Take a giant step to the side with your left leg. Bend the right knee to 90 degrees so that the thigh is parallel to the floor. Bring the right hand to the floor and extend the left arm to the ceiling, opening your chest. Hold for 30 seconds and repeat on the opposite side.

TRIANGLE FORWARD FOLD

The triangle forward fold is an asymmetrical standing forward bend called *parsvottanasana* in yoga. It is an excellent way to stretch and activate the hamstrings while protecting the lower back.

[Keep a soft bend in the knee of the front leg to avoid unnecessary pressure on the joint and ligaments. If needed, place your hands on the shin of your front leg for added stability.]

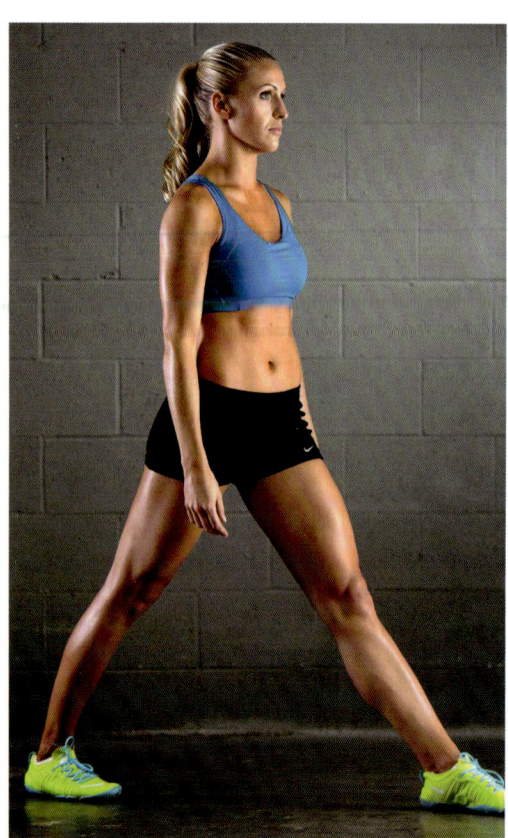

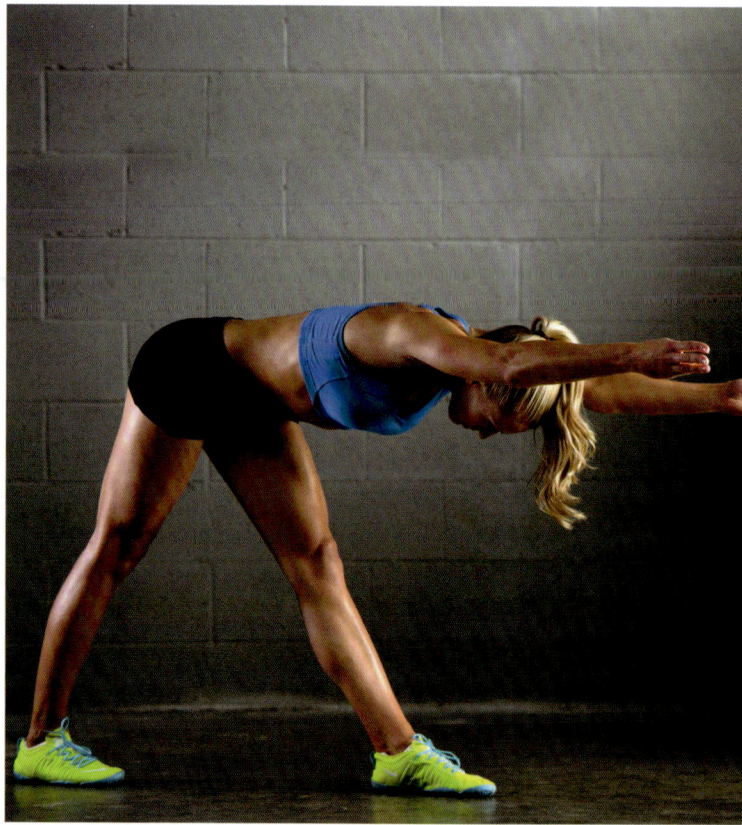

01 Stand tall, feet wider than shoulders with arms loosely hanging by sides. Take a giant step forward with the left foot. Keep the toes of both feet pointing forward.

02 Bend slowly from the hips, keeping your spine as long as possible. Pull the right hip forward to square the pelvis and reach out with the arms, activating the hamstrings to keep the torso horizontal. Hold for 30 seconds and take 5 to 10 deep breaths. Repeat on the opposite side.

HIP OPENER

Opening the hips can have many benefits: easing back pain, improving your gait, and even improving circulation in the legs. The hip opener stretches the groin, lower back, base of the spine, and hips. By releasing the muscles of the hips (the psoas major and iliacus), you can prevent injury and boost athletic performance.

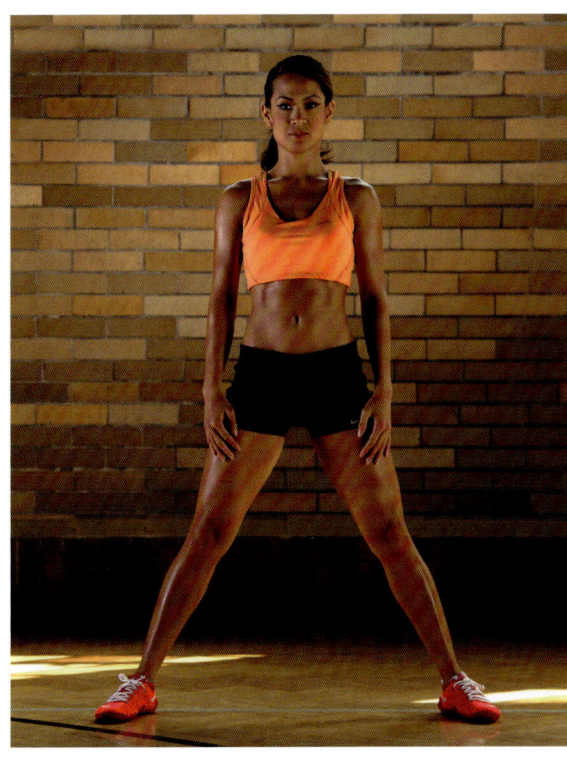

01 Stand tall, with feet wider than shoulders and arms loosely hanging by sides. Turn your feet out, opening your hips.

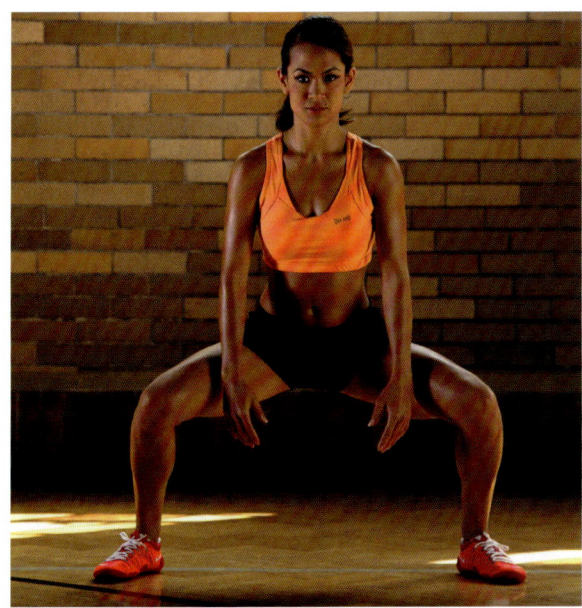

02 Bend at the knees, lowering hips toward the floor. Try to get as deep as you can while maintaining a long spine. Keep your knees directly over your toes; don't allow them to buckle inward.

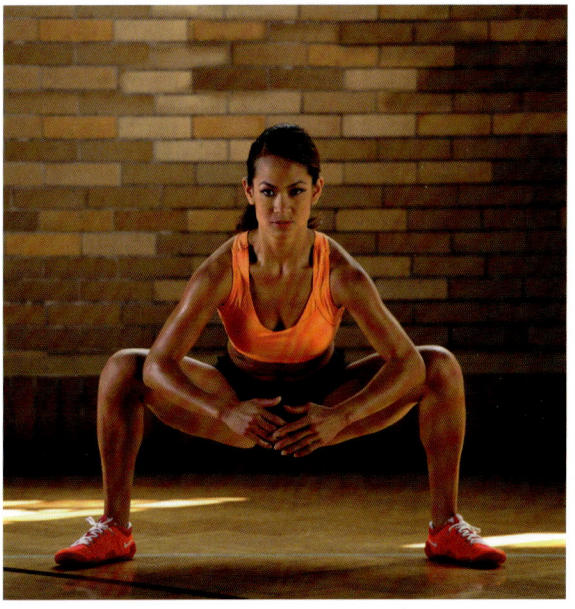

03 Bring your elbows to the insides of your thighs and gently press them out. Hold for approximately 30 seconds while you take long, deep breaths. Repeat 3 times.

NUTRITION

Bodyweight exercises are all about moving your own mass; the heavier you are, the harder it will be! So it's essential to prioritize nutrition to become a lean, mean performance machine.

Exercise effectively tears and breaks apart muscle fibers. Protein is essential for exercise because it contains amino acids, the building block of new muscle. Since it repairs muscle, you must provide the body a constant supply of protein throughout the entire day for optimum muscle growth. Having a body with lean muscle mass fueled by protein has another benefit: It decreases body fat percentage.

What about carbs? Aren't they the devil? The key is to save them for post-workout meals, when your body uses the simple sugars and starches to replace those energy stores. Whole grains, fruits, and vegetables are the best carbohydrates to consume while following the programs in this book—keep it to around 100 grams per day.

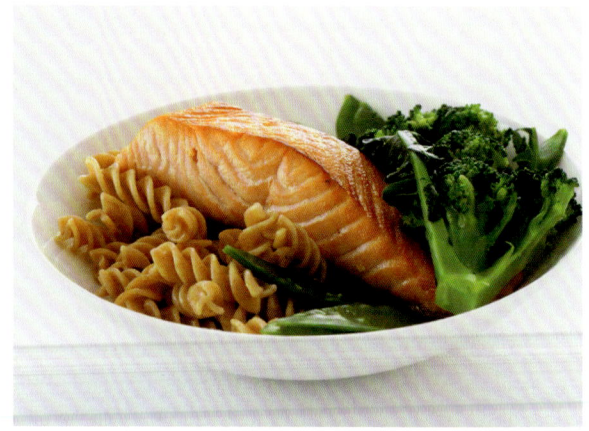

An excellent post-workout meal: With about 23 grams of protein per serving, salmon paired with whole wheat pasta or quinoa and nutrient-packed veggies helps repair and replenish the body.

PROTEIN: HOW MUCH DO YOU NEED, AND HOW CAN YOU GET IT?

To calculate how much protein to eat while on a bodyweight exercise regimen, multiply your weight in pounds by 0.9 to 1.1. The resulting range is the approximate number of grams of protein to consume daily.

Daily protein requirement for a 140-lb (63.5kg) adult	126–154g	Daily protein requirement for a 180-lb (82kg) adult	162–198g	Daily protein requirement for a 220-lb (100kg) adult	198–242g
Sample meal plan	**Protein**	**Sample meal plan**	**Protein**	**Sample meal plan**	**Protein**
Extra-large egg	7g	All of the protein for a 140-pound adult plus:		All of the protein for a 180-pound adult plus:	
2 tbsp peanut butter	7g	85g bacon	10g	170g top round steak	52g
170g tuna	52g	85g cottage cheese	10.5g		
1 cup black beans	15g	½ cup tofu	10g		
2 slices Swiss cheese	15g				
85g chicken drumstick	23g		30.5g		52g
1 cup navy beans	20g		+		+
100g Greek yogurt	10g		149g		179.5g
	149g		**179.5g**		**231.5g**

NUTRITION BLUEPRINT

Six simple steps create a solid nutritional foundation.

- Eat 4 to 6 small meals each day: breakfast, lunch, and dinner, with high-protein mid-morning, mid-afternoon, and early-evening snacks.
- Avoid sugar and processed foods.
- Limit carbohydrates to unprocessed, complex carbs such as sweet potatoes.
- Eliminate soda, sweetened coffee beverages, and other high-calorie sugary drinks, including sports drinks.
- Cut out alcohol.
- Drink lots of water—it flushes toxins and keeps you feeling satiated.

GREAT POST-WORKOUT SNACKS AND MEALS

These small meals are perfect for anyone on a bodyweight workout regimen because they include both proteins and carbs.

- A protein shake with milk and a banana
- Half an avocado stuffed with cottage cheese
- Spinach salad topped with grilled chicken
- A banana sliced lengthwise and spread with nut butter

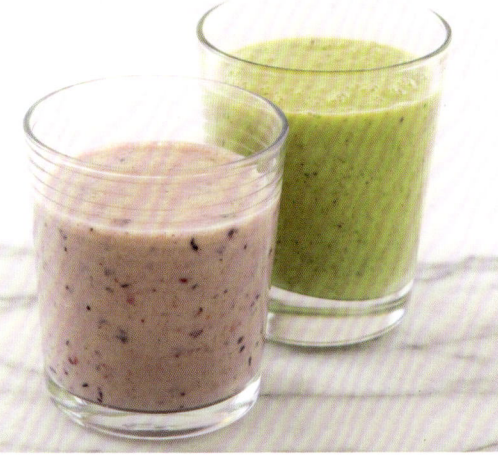

Drinking shakes that contain whey protein can make you feel less hungry later, and helps you lose body fat and better preserve muscle mass.

HYDRATION

During exercise, you may lose up to two liters of water per hour. Just a 2 percent decrease in weight caused by dehydration can lead to a 20 percent decrease in athletic performance. For every liter of fluid lost, core temperature increases, heart rate rises, glycogen stored in muscles is used more rapidly, and lactic acid increases.

HOW MUCH SHOULD YOU DRINK?

What's the ideal amount to consume when pursuing the programs in this book? The daily amount of water intake will differ from person to person and will vary based on activity.

When exercising, up your intake to 4L of water daily.

4L

The average adult needs 3L of water per day.

3L

You lose 2L of water daily through normal activities like breathing, sweating, and elimination.

2L

Make sure to drink 500ml of water—preferably mixed with an electrolyte replacement—both before and after a bodyweight workout.

500ml

LOWER-BODY EXERCISES

FORWARD HINGE

The forward hinge will help you gain awareness of the hips and correct use of the rear chain (hamstrings, glutes, and hips). It may even help alleviate knee pain and increase the depth of your squats.

01 Stand with your feet shoulder-width apart and arms relaxed, with fingertips resting on the front of your thighs.

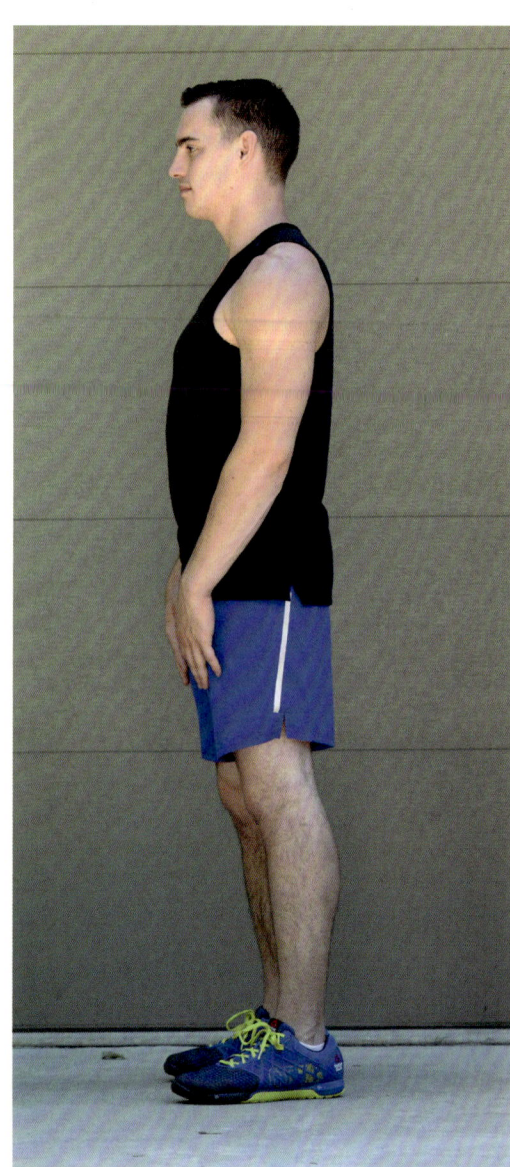

MORE DIFFICULT |||||||||||||||||||||
Modify range of motion and stability: Extend your arms in all steps. This lengthens your body, making your core work harder.

LESS DIFFICULT |||||||||||||||||||||
Modify range of motion: In step 2, decrease the angle of your hip hinge and slightly bend the knees, lessening the stress on the hamstrings.

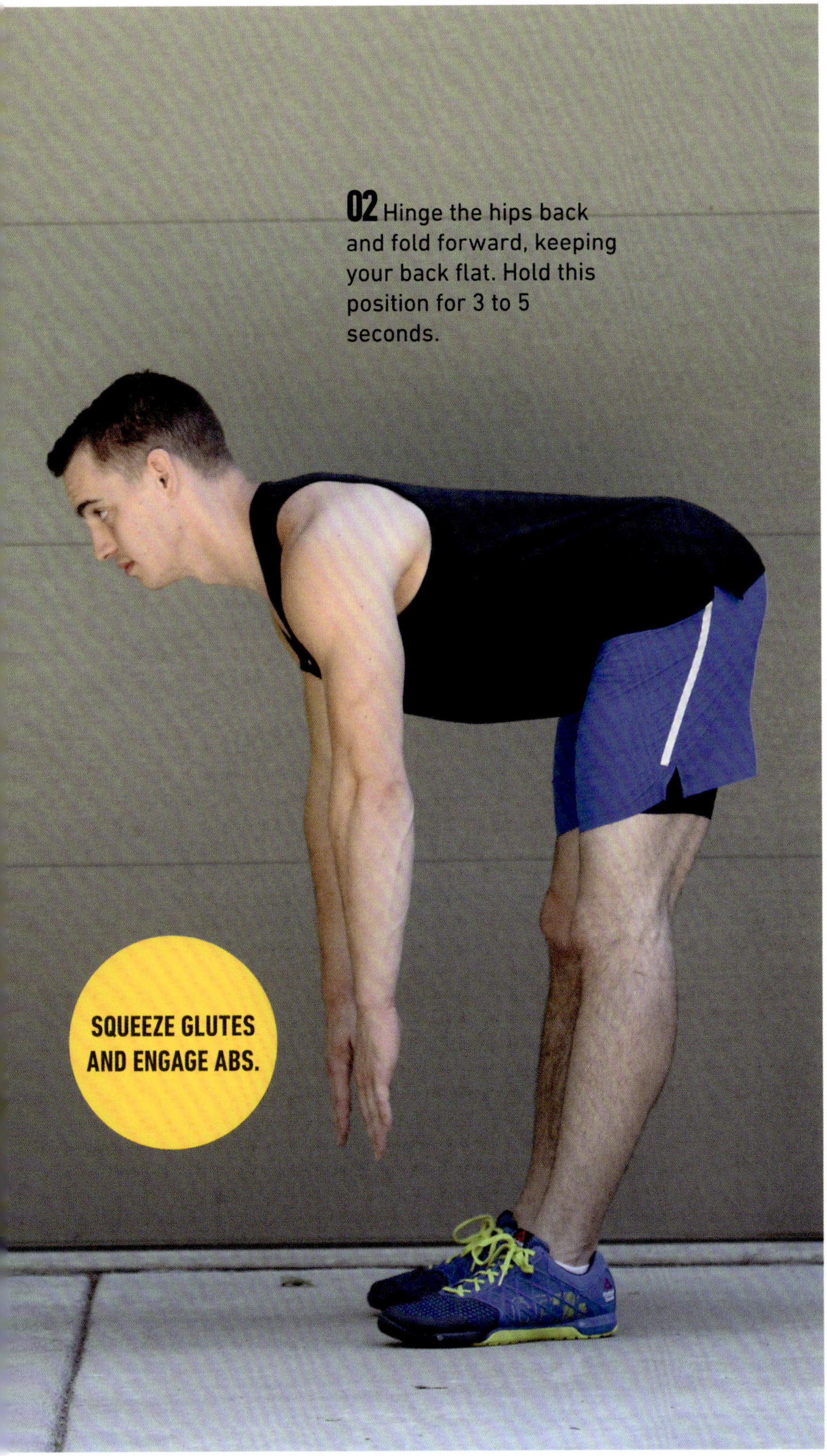

02 Hinge the hips back and fold forward, keeping your back flat. Hold this position for 3 to 5 seconds.

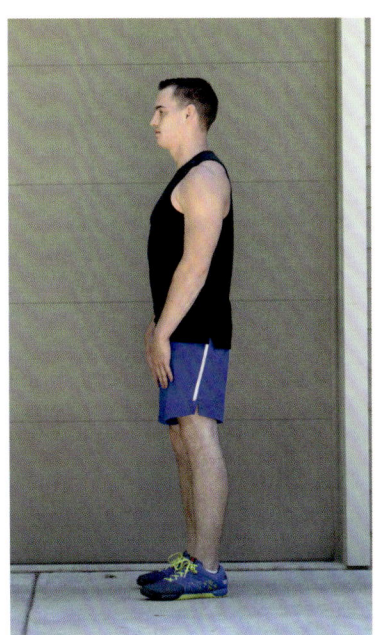

03 Return to the standing position.

SQUEEZE GLUTES AND ENGAGE ABS.

Push your hips back as far as you can until you feel a slight discomfort as you stretch your hamstrings.

IN AND OUTS

This plyometric squat engages the thighs, glutes, and hamstrings. It will challenge your balance and coordination, activate the core, and tone the lower body.

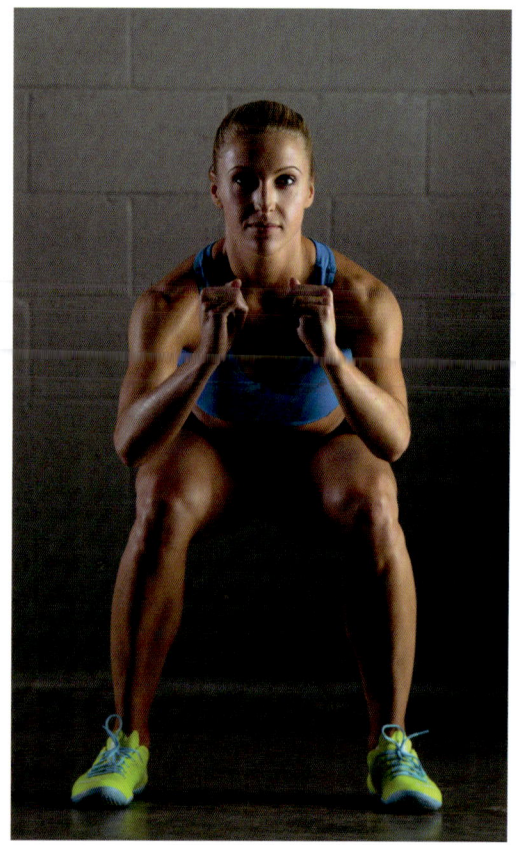

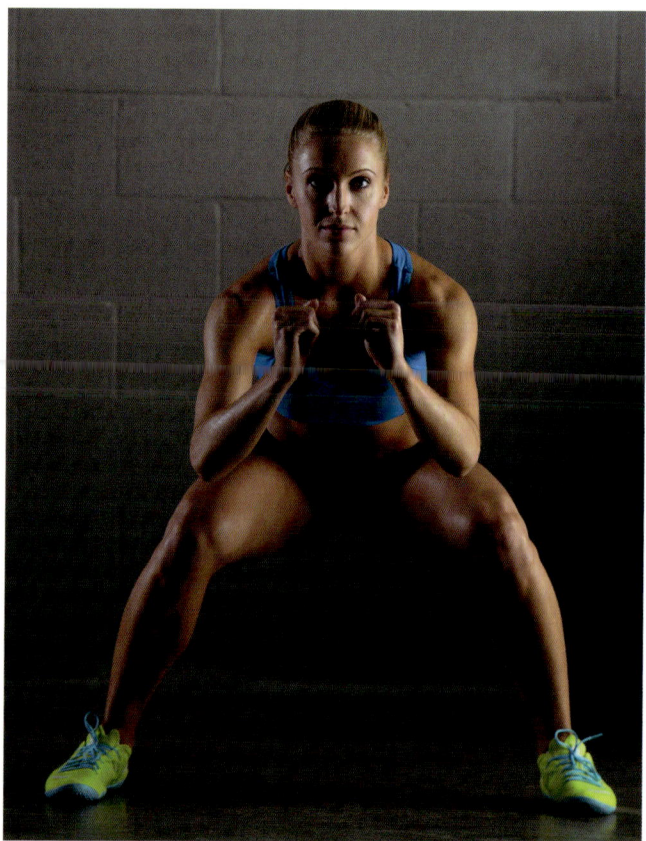

01 With your weight in your heels, inhale as you bend at the hips and knees, lowering into a squat. Try to bring your thighs parallel to the floor.

02 Make the smallest of jumps and open your feet laterally, landing with feet wider than your shoulders. Repeat, staying as low as possible in your squat position and jumping out.

SKATER JUMP

This exercise mimics the movement of a speed skater moving across the ice. Skater jumps will strengthen your legs, improve balance and coordination, and raise your heart rate.

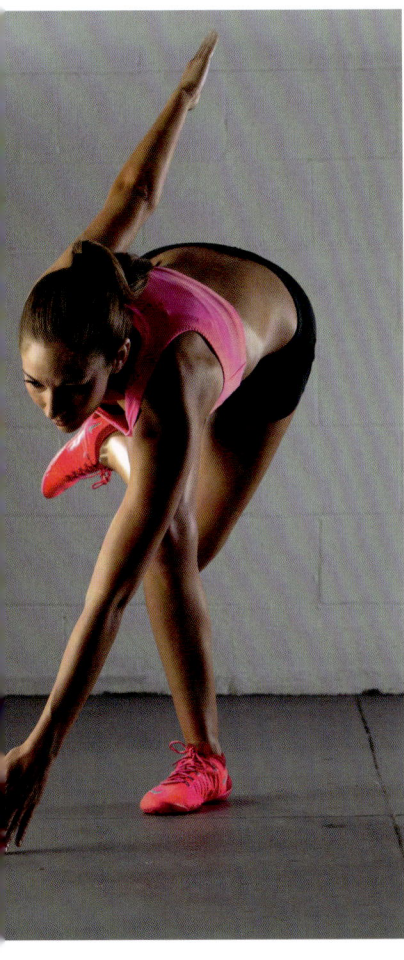

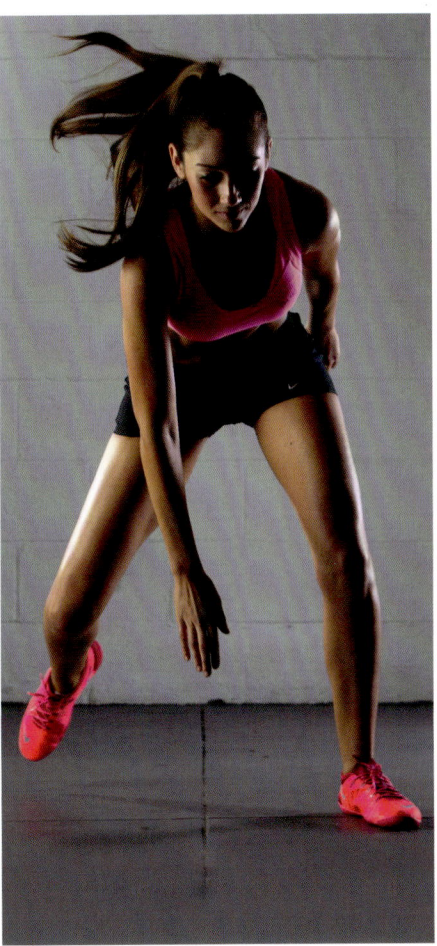

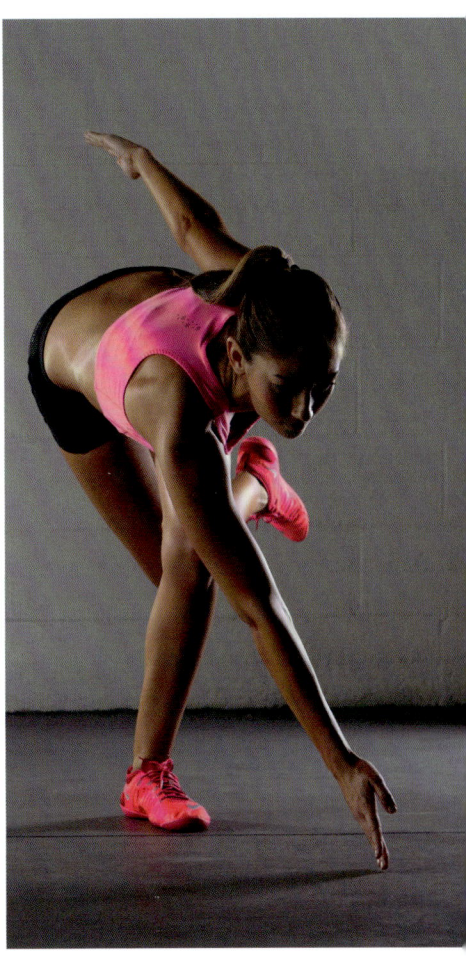

01 Stand with your weight on your right foot and a soft bend in the knee. Lift your left leg and cross it behind the right leg as you bring your left hand to the floor.

02 Bound to the left by pushing off of your right foot. Bring your right arm forward and your left arm back as you jump.

03 Land on your left foot and bring the right foot behind your left, touching your right hand to the floor. Repeat. You should be able to move from side to side in one fluid movement.

SQUAT PEDAL

This exercise combines squat jumps with jumping lunges to burn more calories than any other bodyweight resistance exercise. This metabolic booster simultaneously activates the thighs, hamstrings, glutes, and core. Keep your movements explosive, but maintain proper form.

> [If jumping is too strenuous, you can alternate bodyweight squats and reverse lunges.]

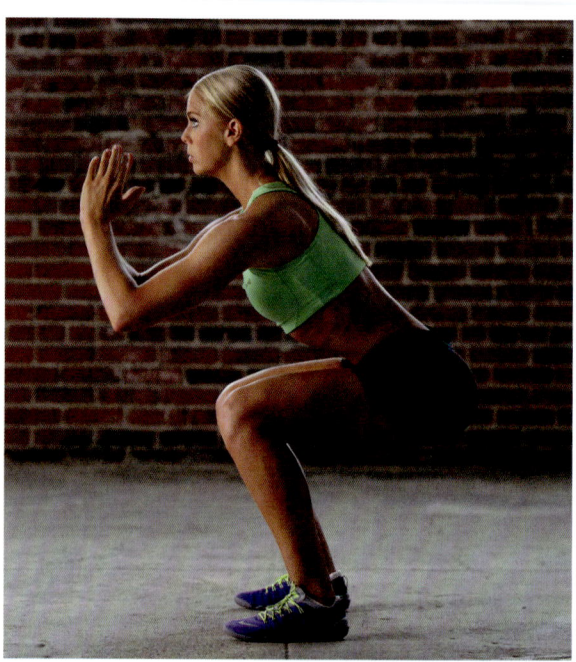

01 Stand with feet shoulder-width apart. Inhale and lower into a squat.

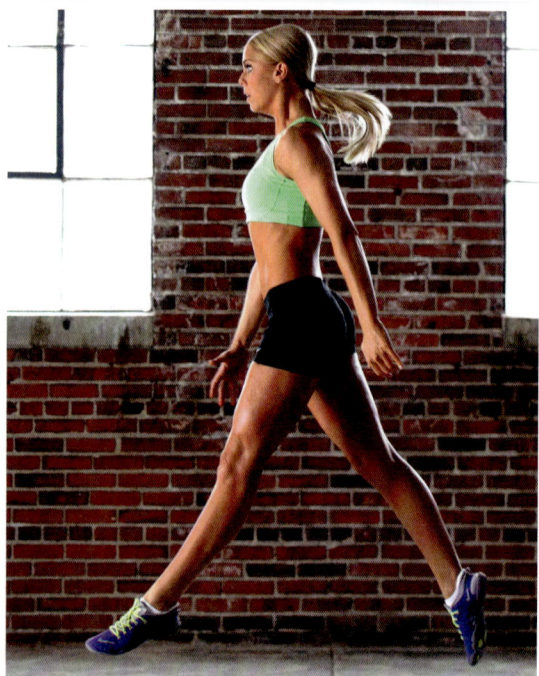

02 Engage your core and exhale as you jump up. While in the air, scissor-switch your feet.

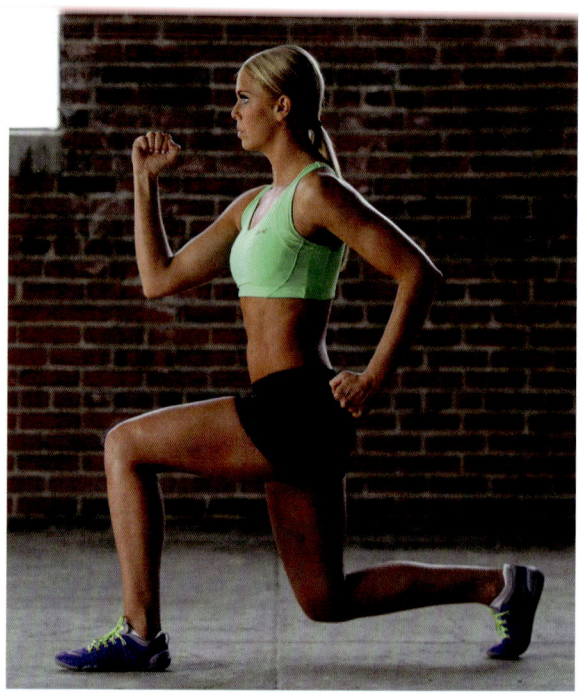

03 Land with your left foot forward and sink into a lunge.

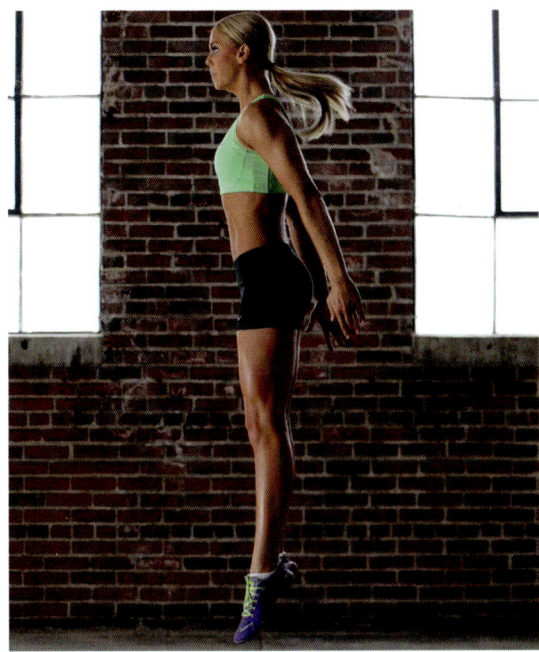

04 Explode out of the lunge, jumping up and opening your feet laterally, ready to land in the squat position.

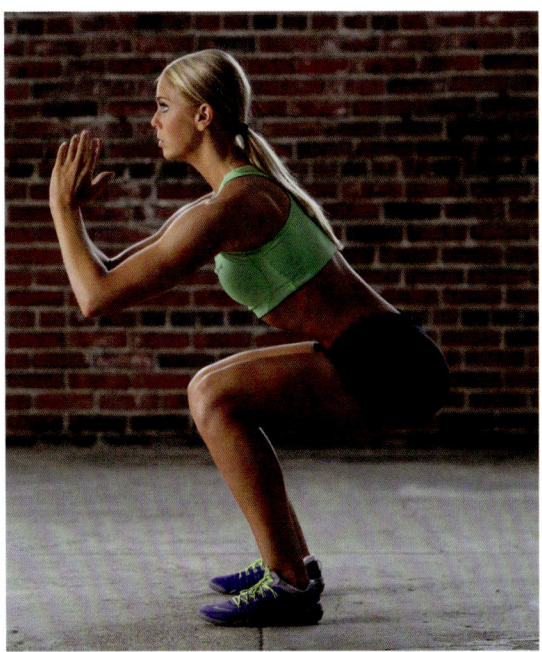

05 Engage the core and use your ankles, knees, and hips to decelerate your body, landing in a deep squat position.

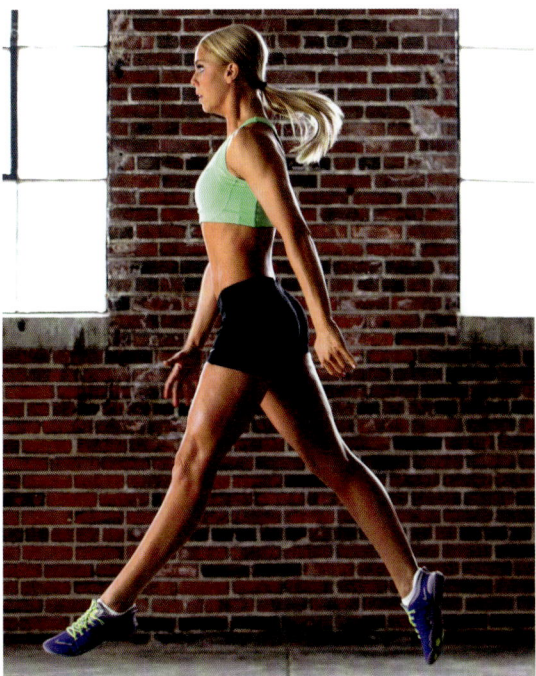

06 Accelerate through the balls of the feet, jumping with enough force to scissor-switch your feet.

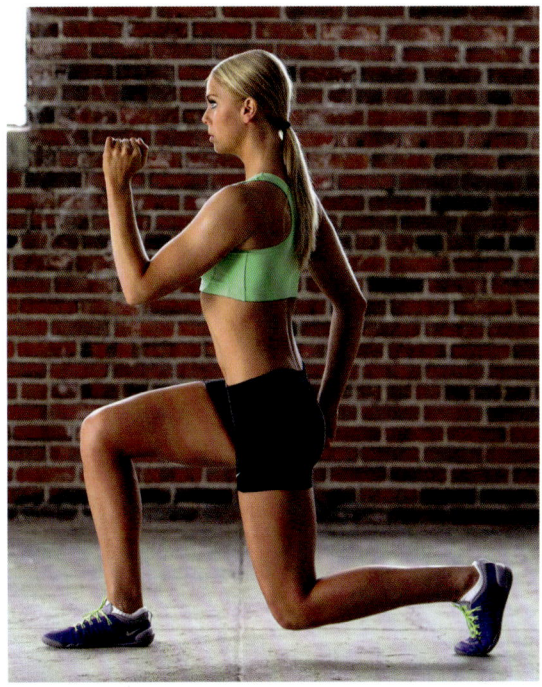

07 Land with your right foot forward and lower into a lunge. Repeat, alternating the front leg on each lunge.

ALTERNATING CROSS-OVER LUNGE

Apart from building strength in the quads and glutes, this lunge also enhances balance, coordination, and agility.

MORE DIFFICULT ||||||||||||||||||
Modify stability: In all steps, hold arms overhead to decrease balance and add load to hips, glutes, and core.

LESS DIFFICULT ||||||||||||||||||
Modify stability: Instead of taking step 4, perform all repetitions to one side to increase stability by making the exercise less dynamic.

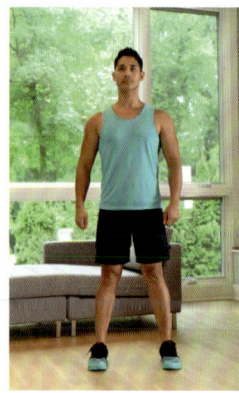

01 Stand tall with your hands by your sides and feet shoulder-width apart.

02 Cross your left leg behind your right and lunge as far as you can to the right. Landing on your heel, bend both legs and sit as low into the lunge as possible.

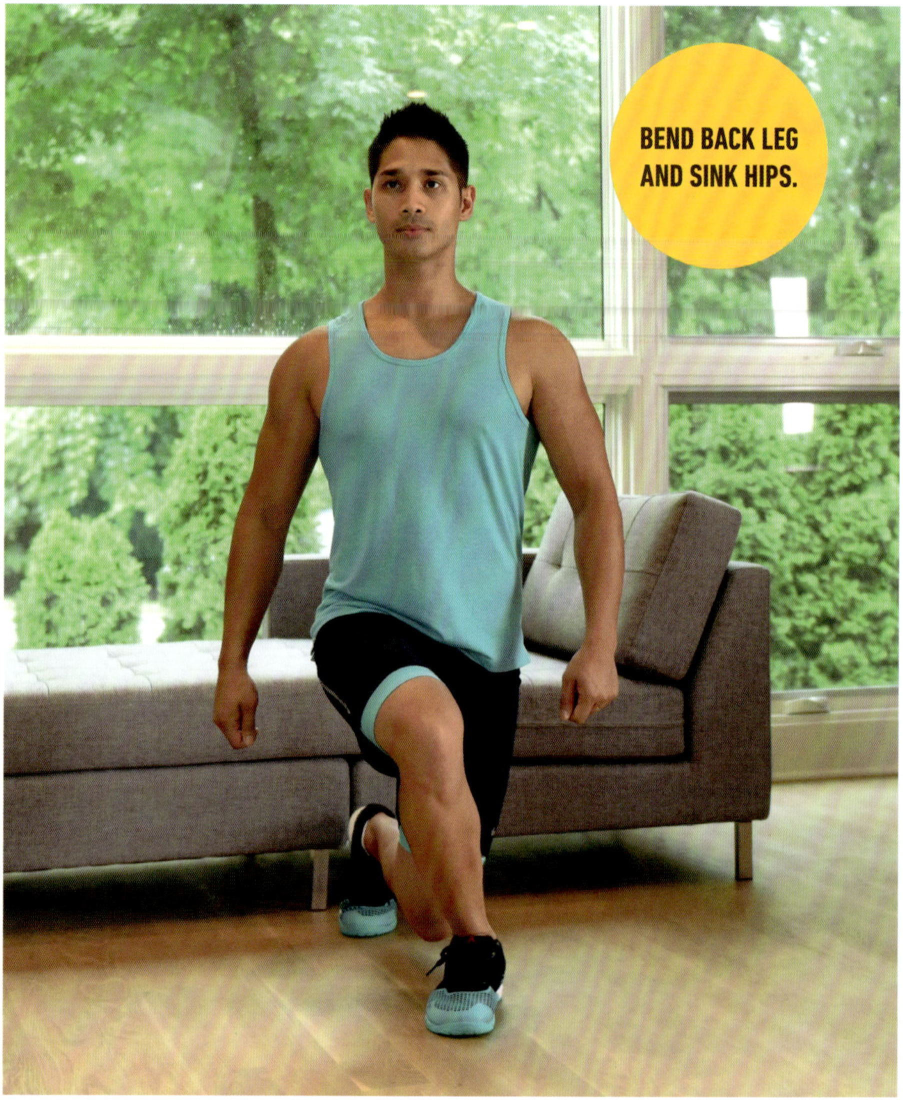

BEND BACK LEG AND SINK HIPS.

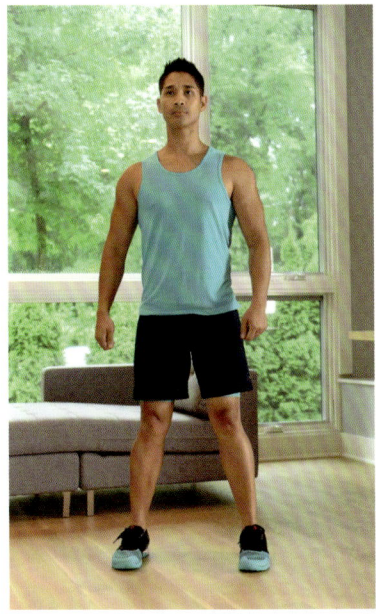

03 Press through the heel of the front foot and straighten the body back to standing position, standing tall to engage the core.

04 Repeat steps 2 and 3 with leg position reversed, crossing your right leg behind your left as you lunge.

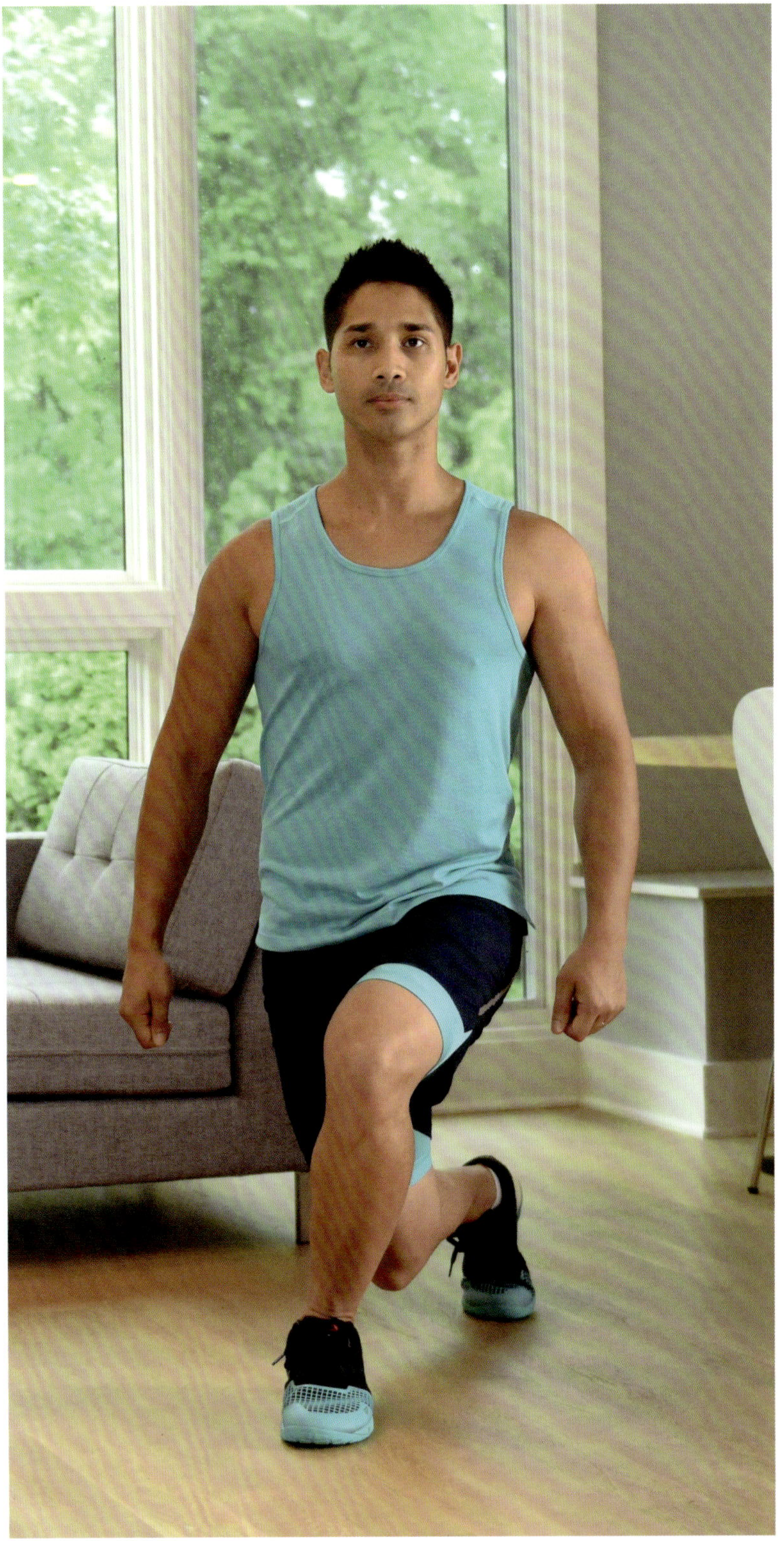

> Keep hips and shoulders facing forward. To ease pressure on the front knee, try to keep the foot pointing at approximately 45 degrees.

PIGEON PEEL

The peel in Level 1 increases strength in hips, hamstrings, glutes, and core. This version takes it further by rotating the legs, providing greater work for the gluteus medius and tensor fascia latae.

MORE DIFFICULT ⅠⅠⅠⅠⅠⅠⅠⅠⅠⅠⅠⅠⅠⅠⅠⅠⅠⅠⅠⅠ
Modify points of contact: In step 2, extend and elevate the arms to remove any leverage, increasing the load on the glutes and core.

LESS DIFFICULT ⅠⅠⅠⅠⅠⅠⅠⅠⅠⅠⅠⅠⅠⅠⅠⅠⅠⅠⅠⅠ
Modify heel placement: Move your heels away from the glutes to make the movement easier.

01 Lie flat on your back on the floor or a mat. Bend your legs and place your feet on the floor wider than your shoulders. Roll your inner thighs together and squeeze them tight.

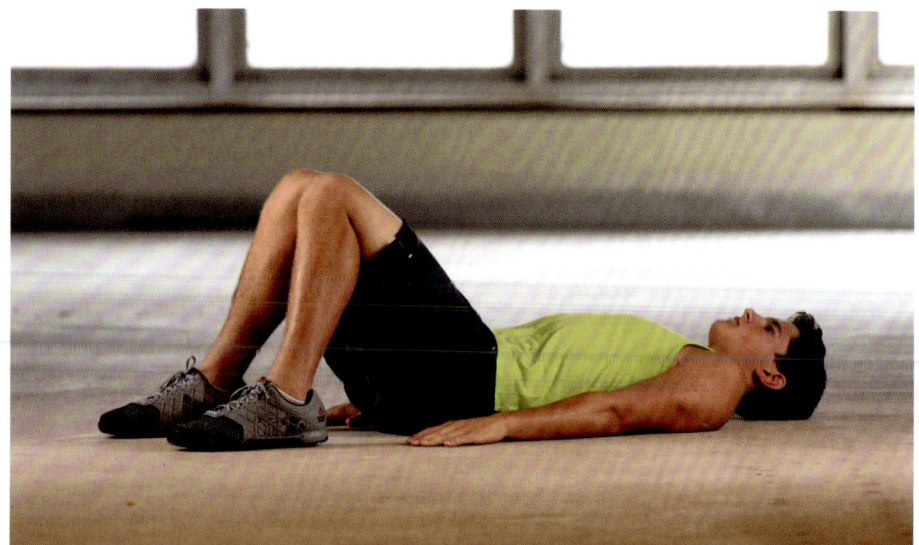

02 Press through the soles, squeeze the glutes, and lift the hips to form a straight line from shoulders to knees. Pause at the top and hold for 1 or 2 seconds before lowering back to the floor under control.

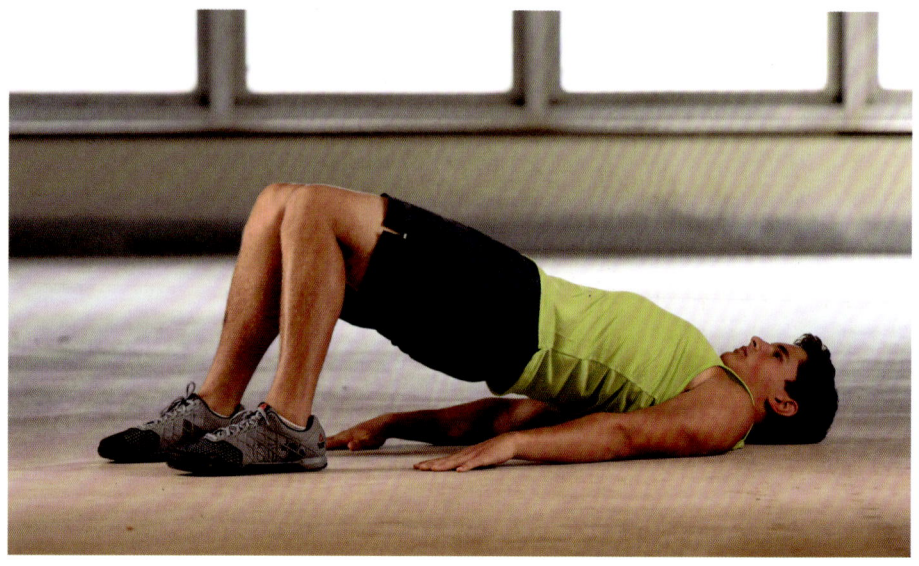

BUTTERFLY PEEL

The butterfly peel rotates the legs, providing greater work for the iliopsoas, sartorius, pectineus, and piriformis.

MORE DIFFICULT ||||||||||||||||||||||||
Modify stability: In step 2, after reaching the top of the motion, lower halfway, raise fully, then lower with control, for 1.5 reps.

LESS DIFFICULT ||||||||||||||||||||||||
Modify heel placement: Move your heels away from the glutes to make the movement easier.

01 Lie flat on your back on the ground. Bend your legs, place your feet on the ground with soles together, and open the knees as wide as possible.

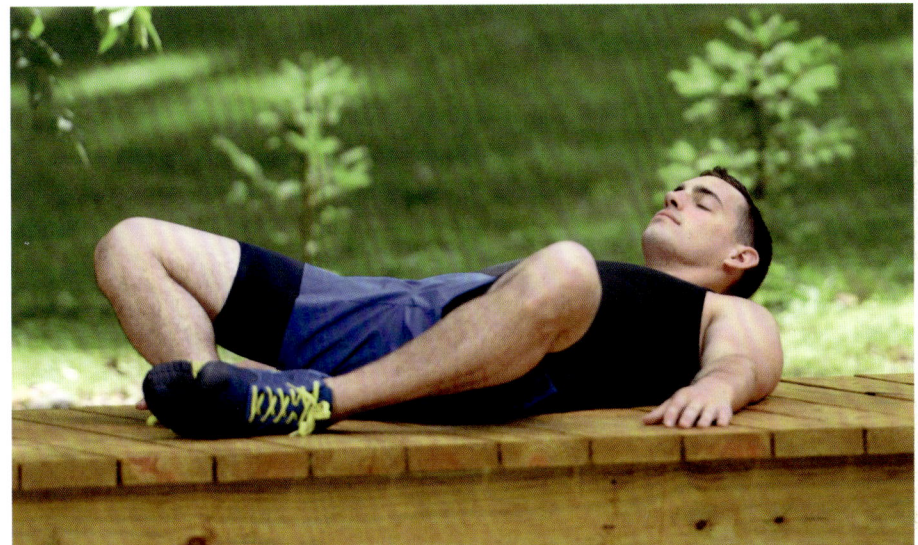

02 Press through the feet, squeeze the glutes, and lift the hips until your body forms a straight line from shoulders to open knees. Pause at the top of the motion and hold for 1 or 2 seconds before lowering back to the ground under control.

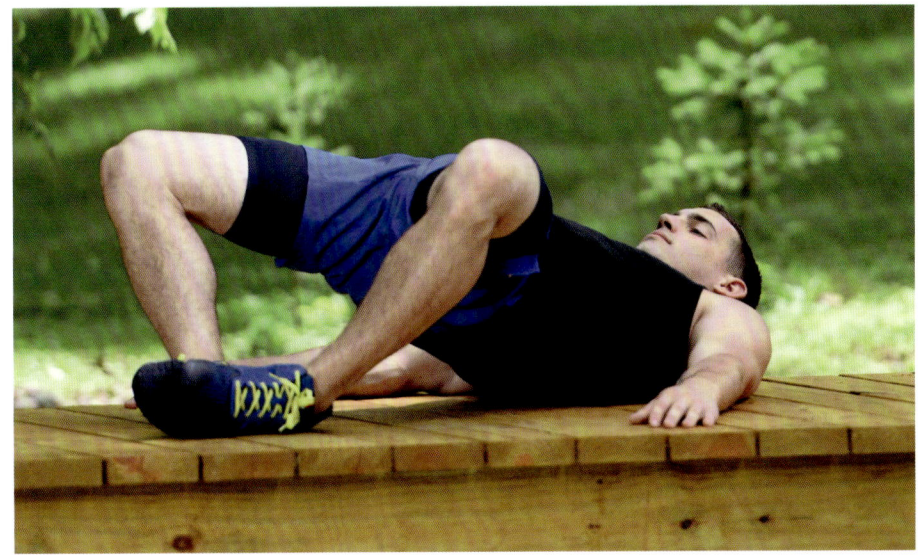

JUMP LUNGE

Jump lunges will quickly get your legs burning and your heart rate skyrocketing. This quad-killing exercise requires balance and coordination. Make sure you're maintaining proper form throughout the movement.

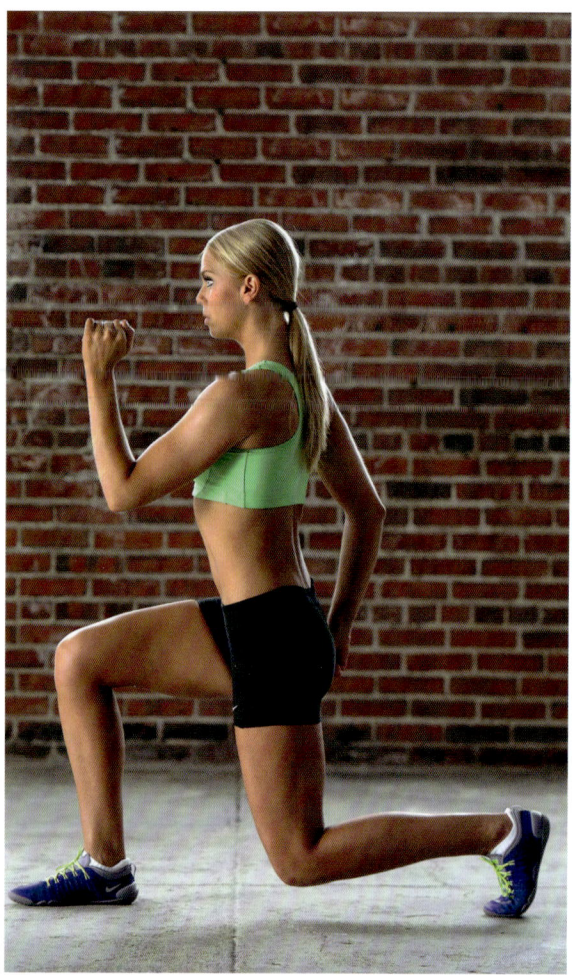

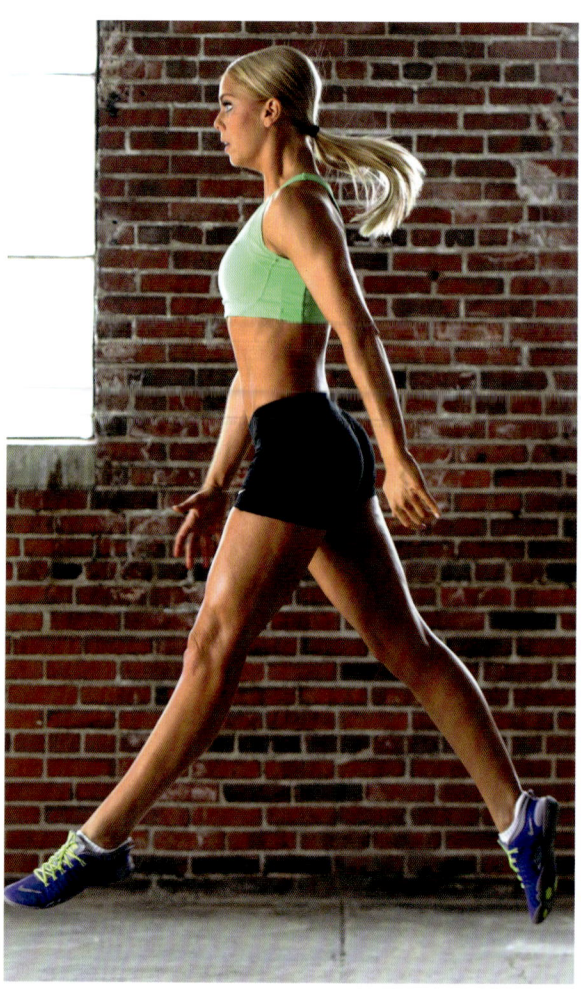

01 Stand with your right foot in front of the left. Keep your torso as tall as possible as you bend both legs to sink into a lunge position. Don't allow the front knee to go past your toes.

02 Jump up with enough force to propel both feet from the floor. While in the air, scissor-switch your feet.

> Pay particular attention to the impact imposed during the landing. Attempt to land as softly as possible so that the force of the deceleration is distributed between the knee, hip, and ankle joints.

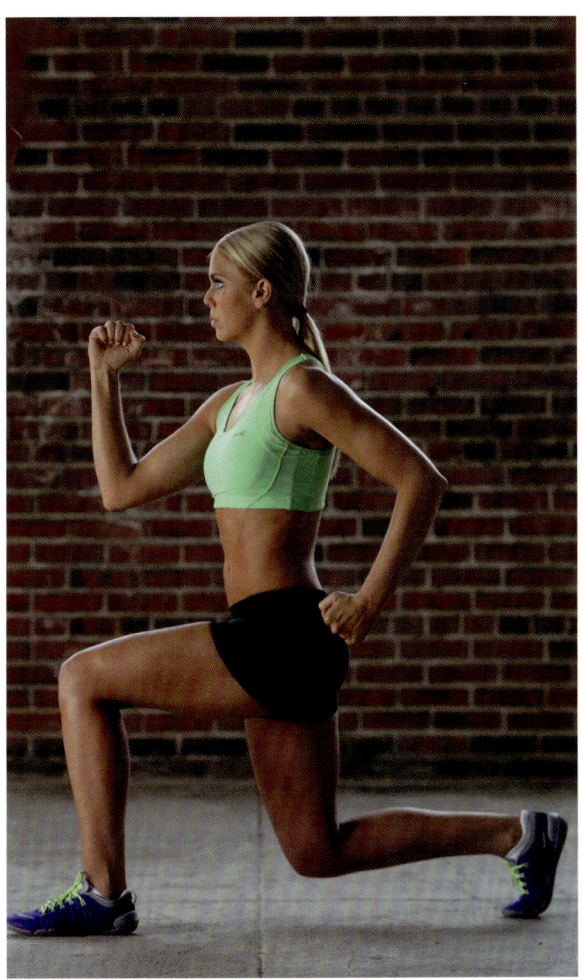

03 Land softly in a lunge position with the left foot in front.

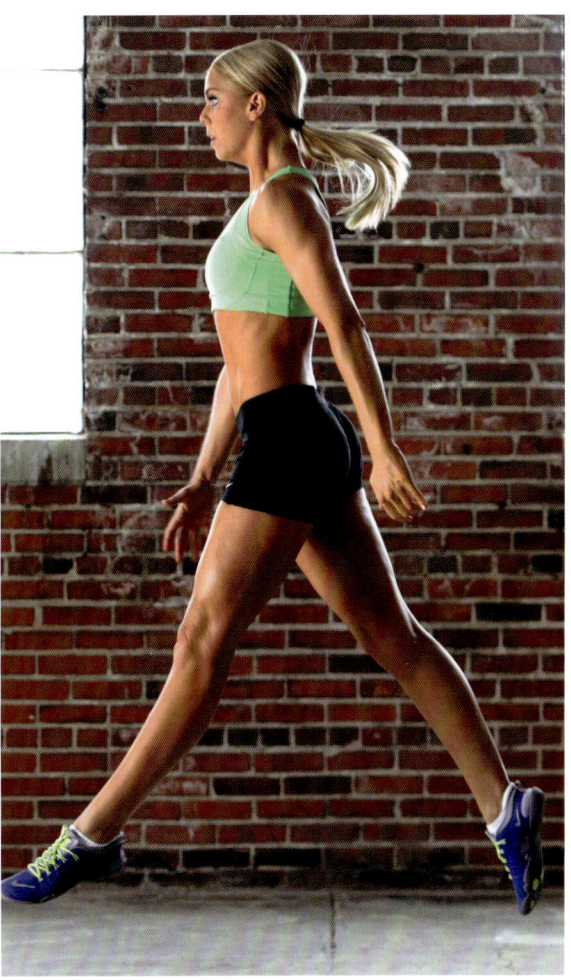

04 Jump up again, and scissor-switch your feet to land softly in a lunge position with the right leg in front.

UP DOWN

This exercise makes the simple movement of getting up off the floor fun and challenging. Build core stability and strengthen your glutes, thighs, and hamstrings as you move up and then back down.

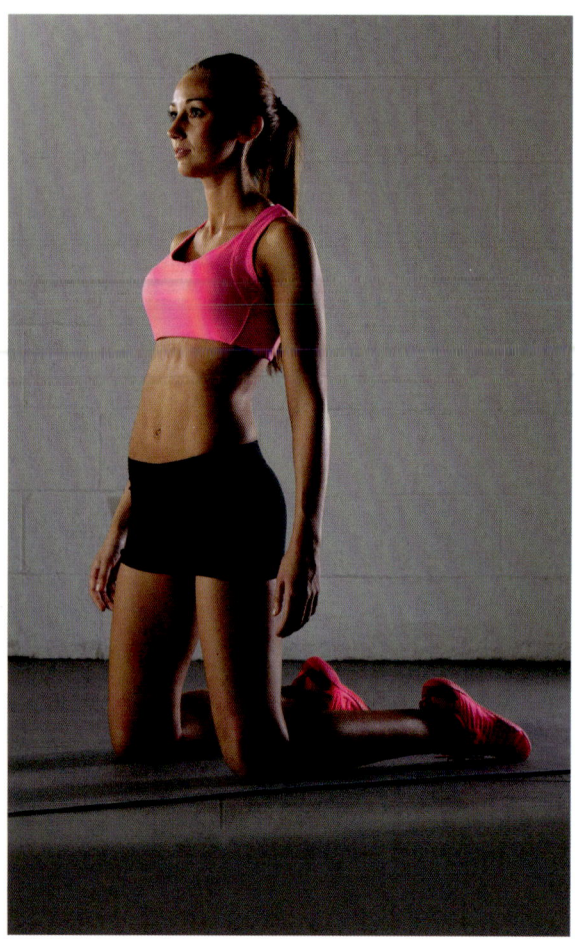

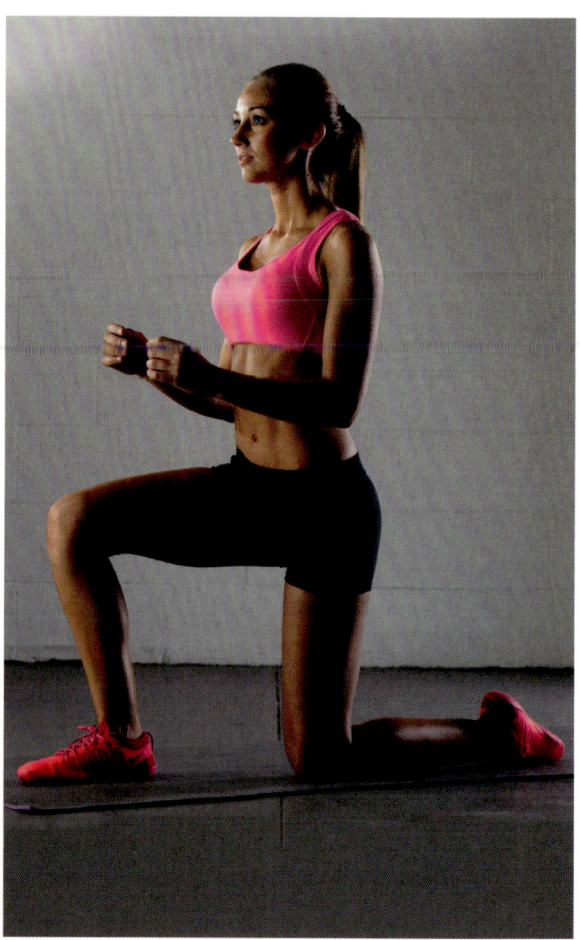

01 Begin in a kneeling position. Keep your torso tall, with your head up, shoulders back, and core engaged. If kneeling is uncomfortable, place a rolled towel under your knees.

02 Bring your right leg forward and place your foot on the floor in front of you. Your leg should be bent at 90 degrees and your thigh should be parallel to the floor.

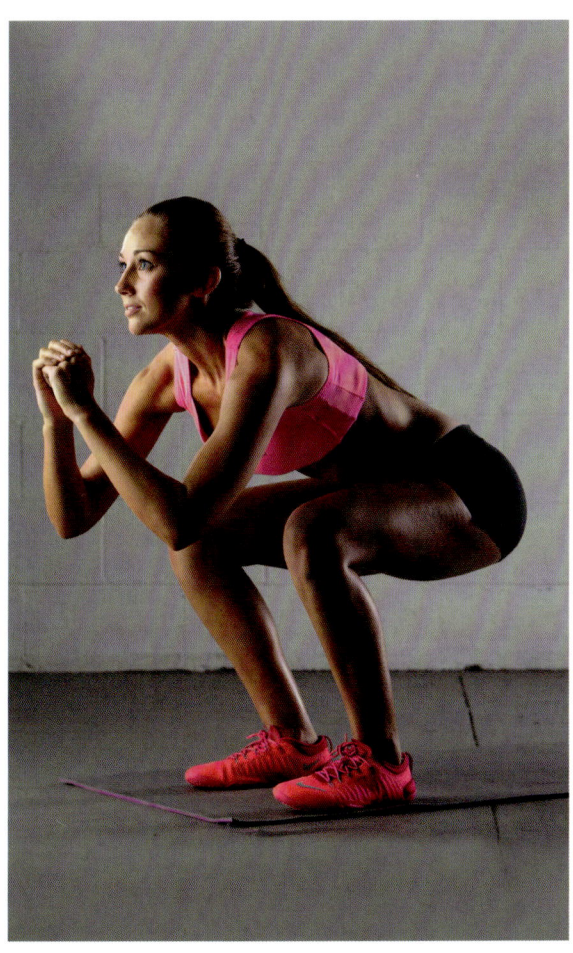

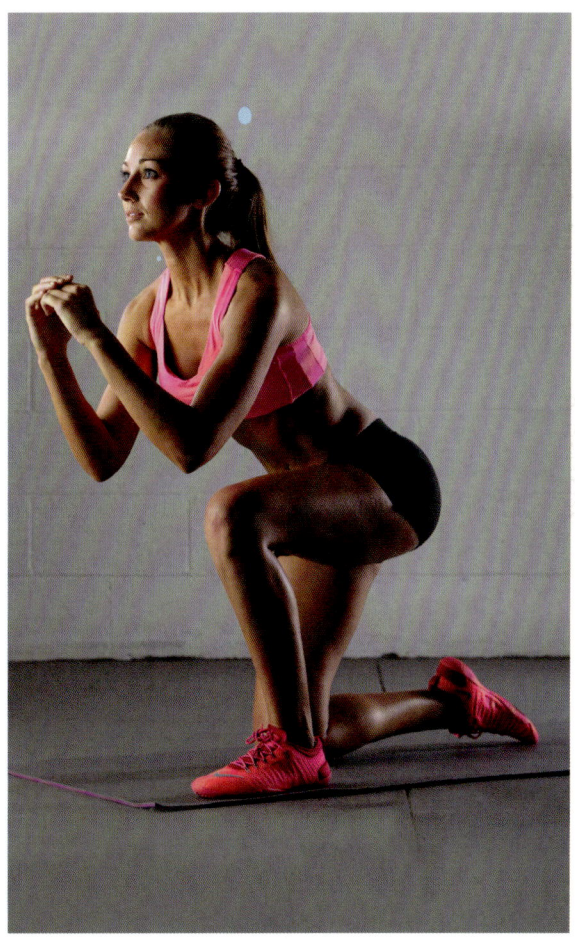

03 Bring the left leg forward and place the left foot next to the right. You should now be in a squat position with both legs bent at 90 degrees and thighs parallel to the floor.

04 Return right leg to kneeling position, followed by left leg. Repeat, alternating the lead leg.

SQUAT JUMP

A metabolic-boosting super exercise, the squat jump takes every ounce of energy and coordination while making quads, glutes, and hamstrings all beg for mercy.

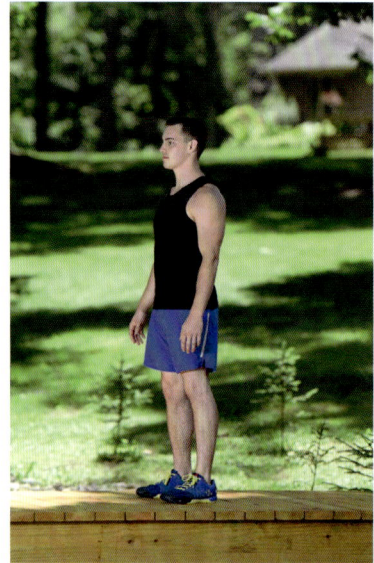

01 Stand tall with your feet shoulder-width apart and your toes pointing forward.

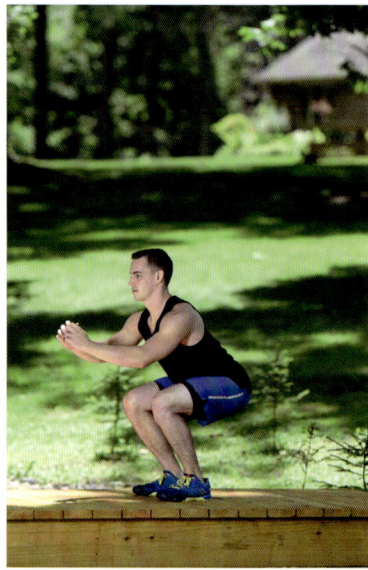

02 With your bodyweight in your heels, inhale as you bend at the knee and lower your body as if about to sit in a chair.

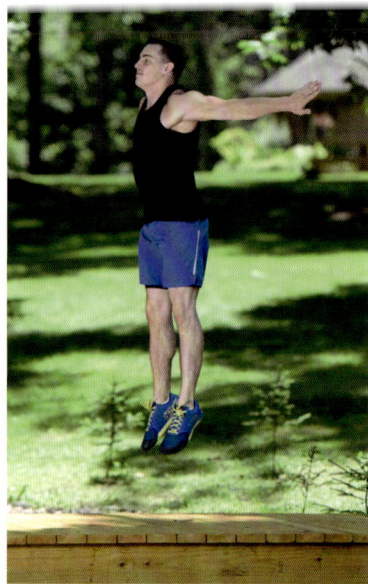

03 Engage your core and exhale as you jump up, pushing through the heels.

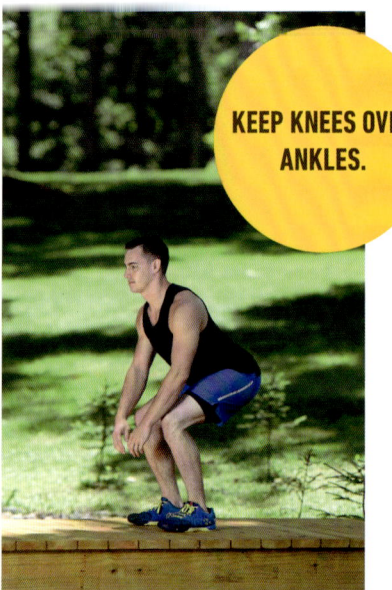

KEEP KNEES OVER ANKLES.

04 Land as softly and silently as possible, bending at the ankles, knees, and hips to decelerate the body.

MORE DIFFICULT ||||||||||||||||||||||
Modify speed: Hold the squat position in step 2 for a count of four upon landing. This removes momentum and creates an isolation hold at its deepest point.

LESS DIFFICULT ||||||||||||||||||||||
Modify range of motion: Omit steps 3 and 4. Modify step 2 by lifting arms overhead and focusing on the depth of the squat.

T-STAND

Lengthen the hamstrings and challenge your balance in this yoga-inspired, functional exercise. While it may seem simple, it will make your hamstrings burn.

[If balancing is a challenge, allow your arms to drop and your fingertips to touch the floor.]

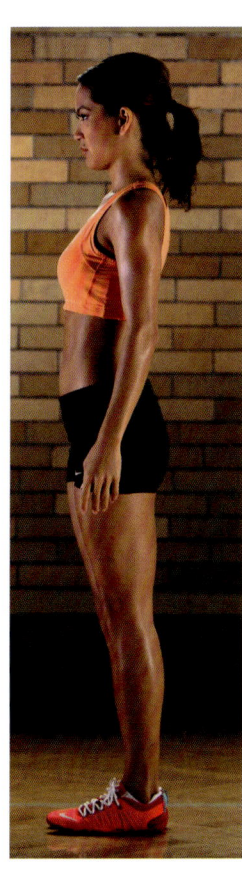

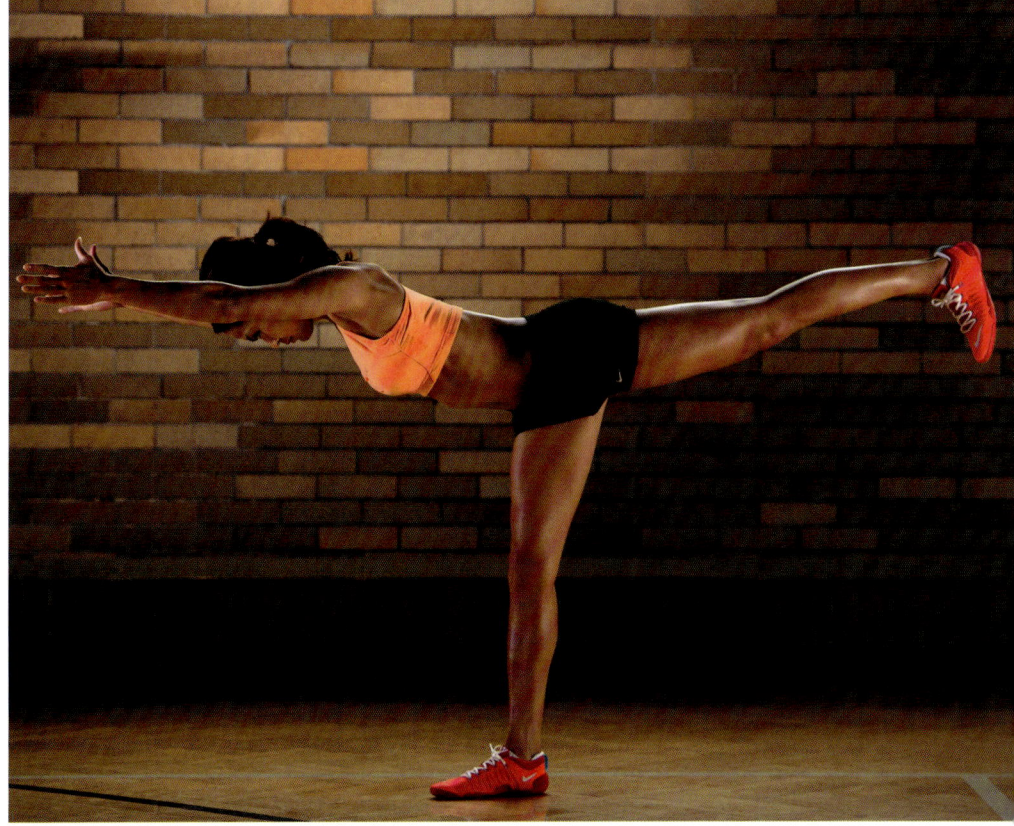

01 Stand with feet together and arms at your sides.

02 Inhale and slowly bend from the hips, lowering the torso and extending the arms. As you fold forward, raise one leg until torso, arms, and leg are parallel to the floor. Exhale as you lift the torso and lower the leg in one fluid motion. Repeat with the opposite leg.

ALTERNATING LATERAL LUNGE

Lateral lunges strengthen and tone the glutes, hamstrings, and thighs. In the process, they increase dynamic balance.

MORE DIFFICULT ||||||||||||||||||||||
Modify stability and range of motion: In all steps, elevate the bending leg to decrease your stability and require greater activation of the glutes, quads, and hamstrings.

LESS DIFFICULT ||||||||||||||||||||||
Modify stability: Throughout the exercise, perform all reps to the same side to increase stability, allowing you to build confidence and focus on depth.

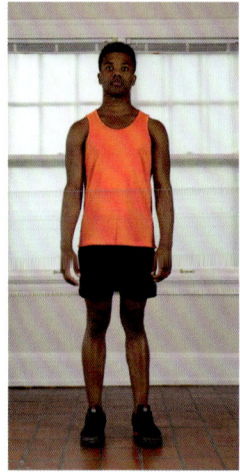

01 Stand tall with feet shoulder-width apart and toes pointing forward.

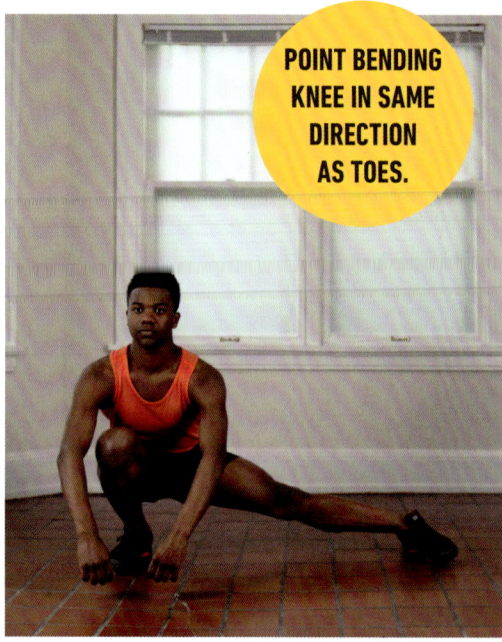

POINT BENDING KNEE IN SAME DIRECTION AS TOES.

02 Step out to the right side (laterally) away from the body. Remain tall and keep your weight in the heel as you push back your hips, lowering your body until the thigh is parallel to the floor.

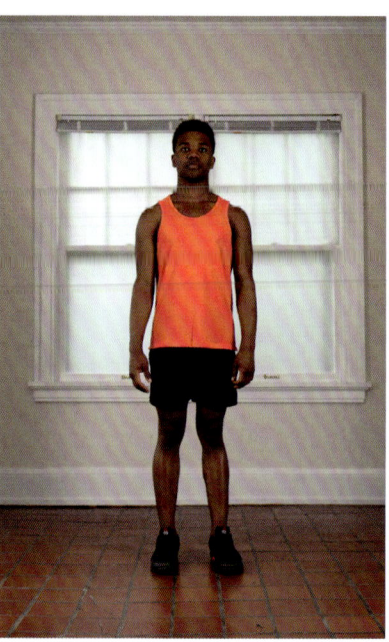

03 Push back off of the bent leg, straightening the hips and knee to return to your starting position.

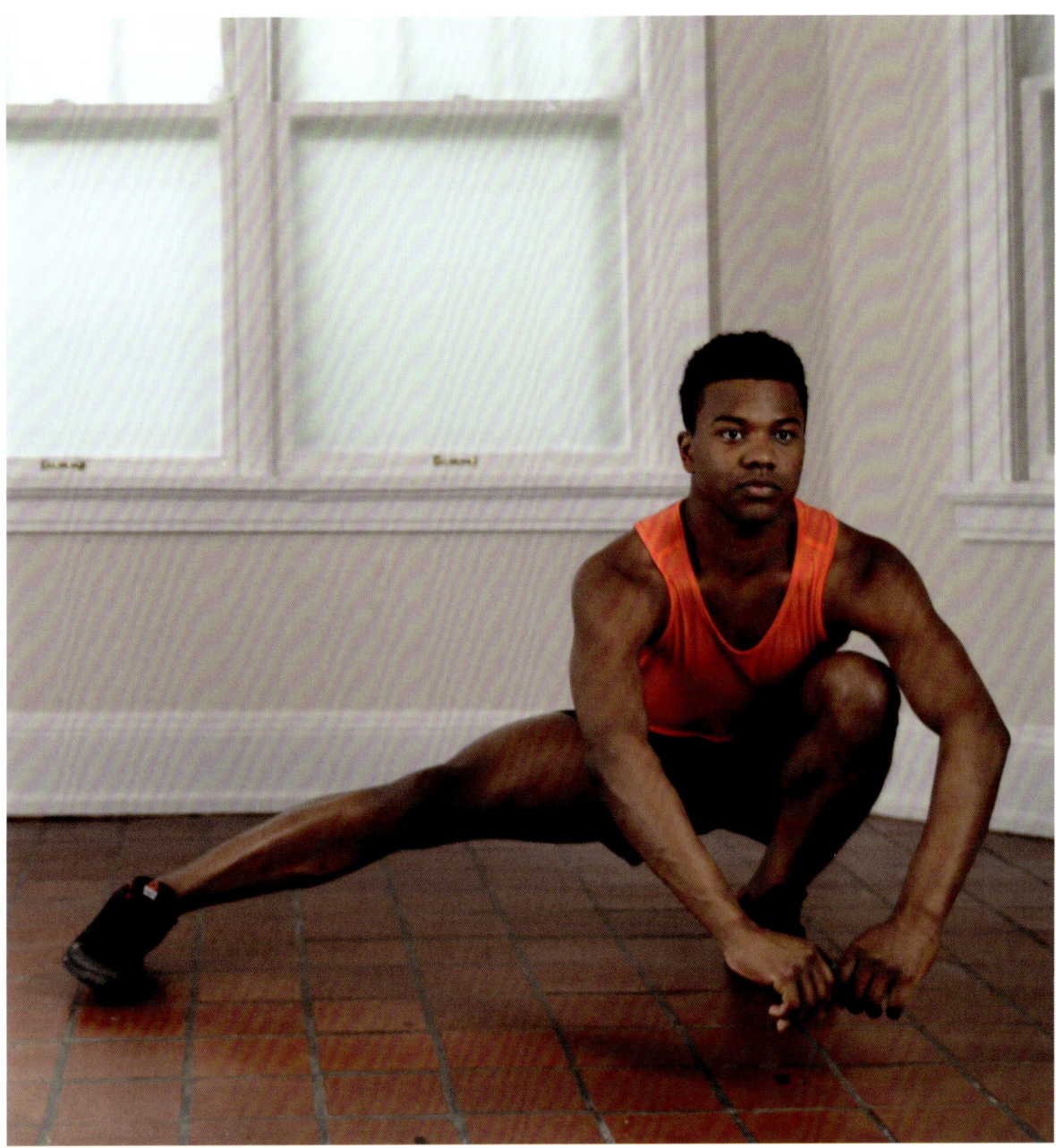

04 Repeat the lateral lunge to the opposite side.

Focus on pushing back the hips, keeping your weight in the heel of the lunging leg and glutes.

SQUAT LIFT

Develop buns of steel with this take on the traditional bodyweight squat. Adding a lateral leg lift supercharges this exercise by challenging the hips, glutes, and stabilizing leg.

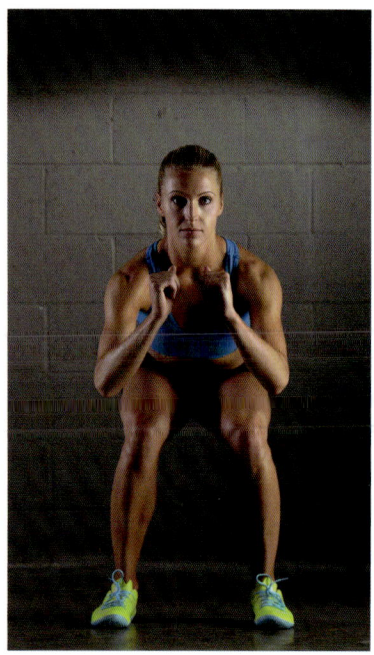

01 Stand tall, feet shoulder-width apart and toes pointing forward. With your weight in your heels, inhale as you bend at the knee and lower into a squat position.

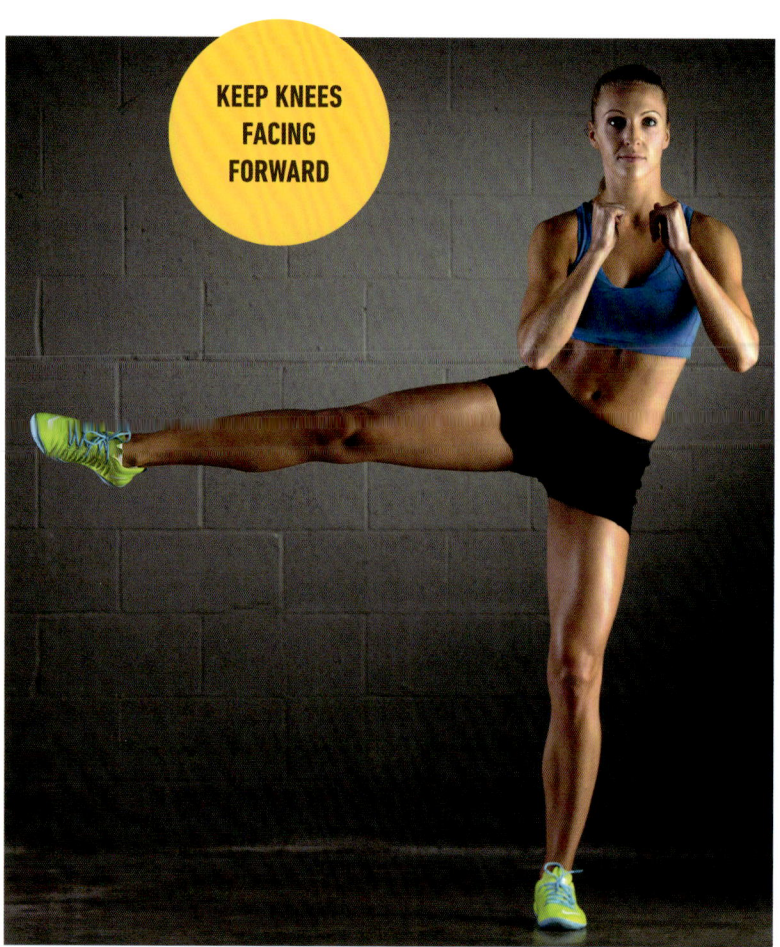

KEEP KNEES FACING FORWARD

02 Exhale as you press through your heels. Squeeze your glutes as you stand, lifting one leg to the side as high as possible and keeping your weight on the standing leg. Keep your knees facing forward.

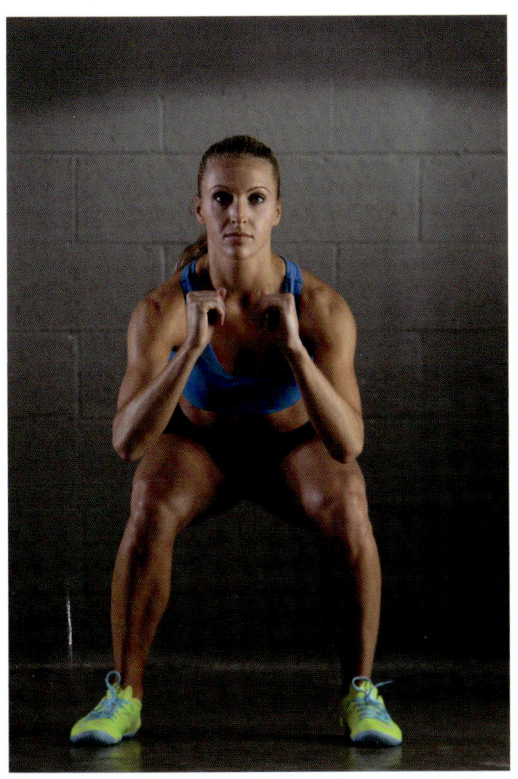

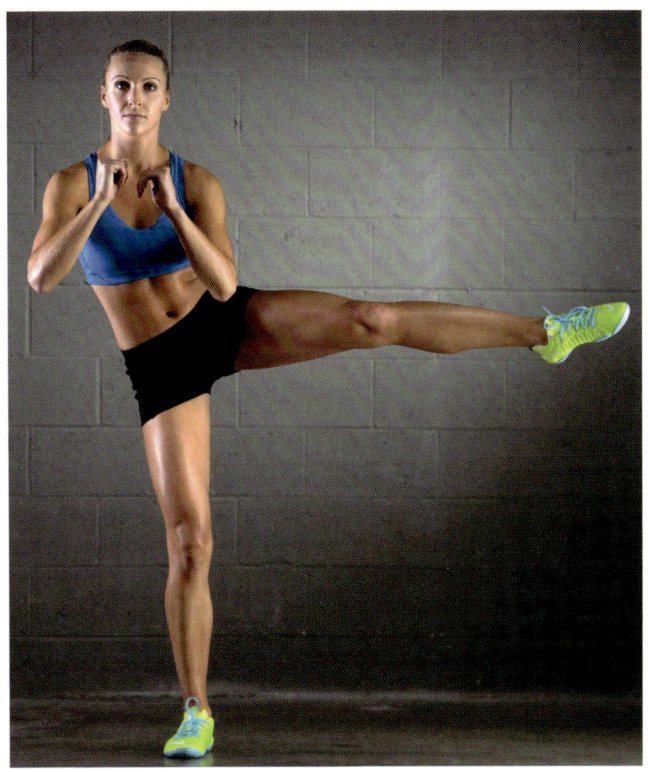

03 Lower your leg and return to the squat position.

04 Repeat, this time lifting the opposite leg.

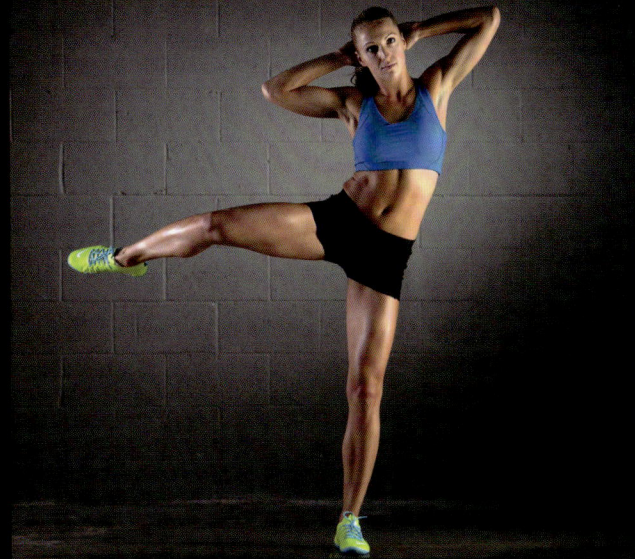

CHALLENGE

For an added challenge, bend the lifted leg at the knee and pull your shoulder and elbow toward the lifted leg, working your obliques.

SQUAT

The squat is a compound, full-body exercise that primarily engages the muscles of the thighs, hips, and glutes. It also helps to develop core strength by engaging the lower back and abdominals.

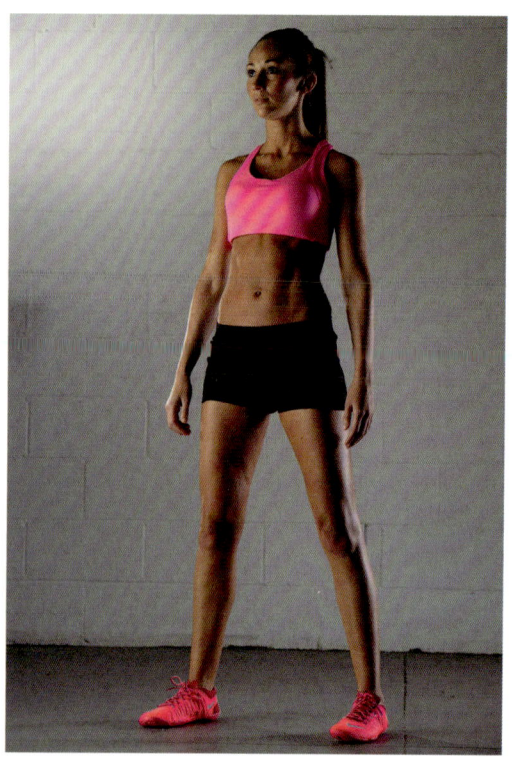

01 Stand tall, with your feet shoulder-width apart and toes pointing forward.

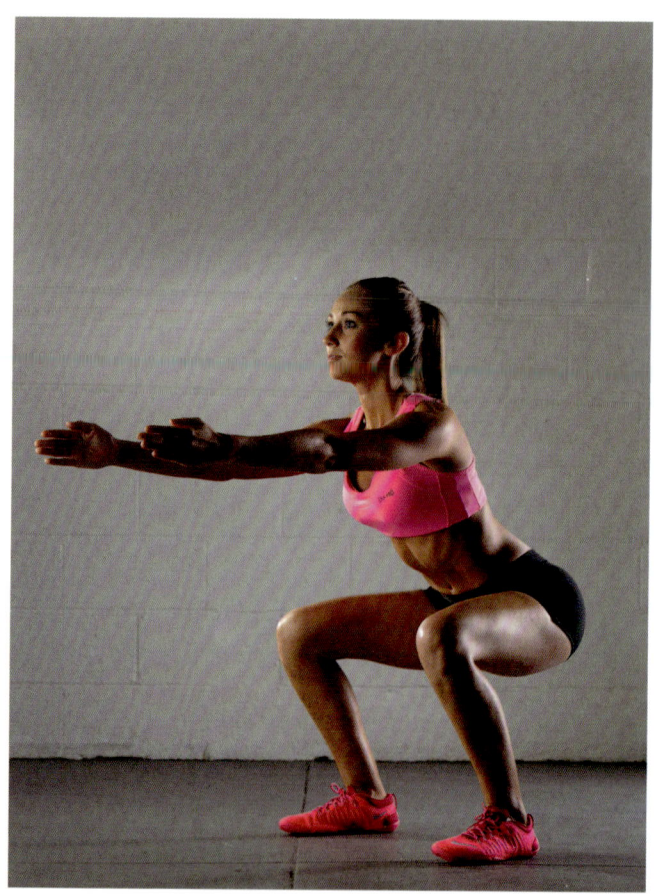

02 Inhale as you bend at the knees, lowering your body as if about to sit in a chair. At the bottom of the movement, your knees should be at a 90-degree angle and your thighs parallel to the ground. Keep your knees over your ankles and your torso tall.

X-JACK

This innovative twist on the traditional jumping jack will boost your metabolism and tone your legs, core, shoulders, and back.

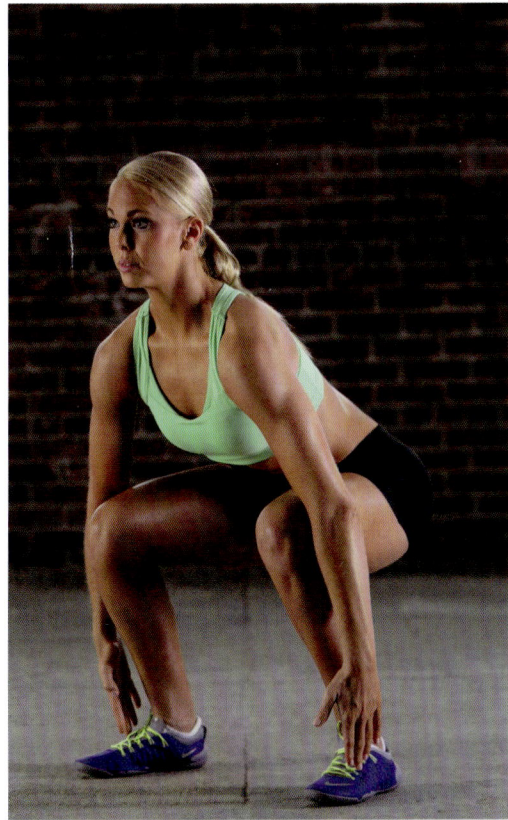

01 With feet shoulder-width apart, bend from your hips, knees, and ankles and drop into a squat position. If you can, touch your toes with your fingertips. Hold your chest up, look forward, and keep your weight in your heels.

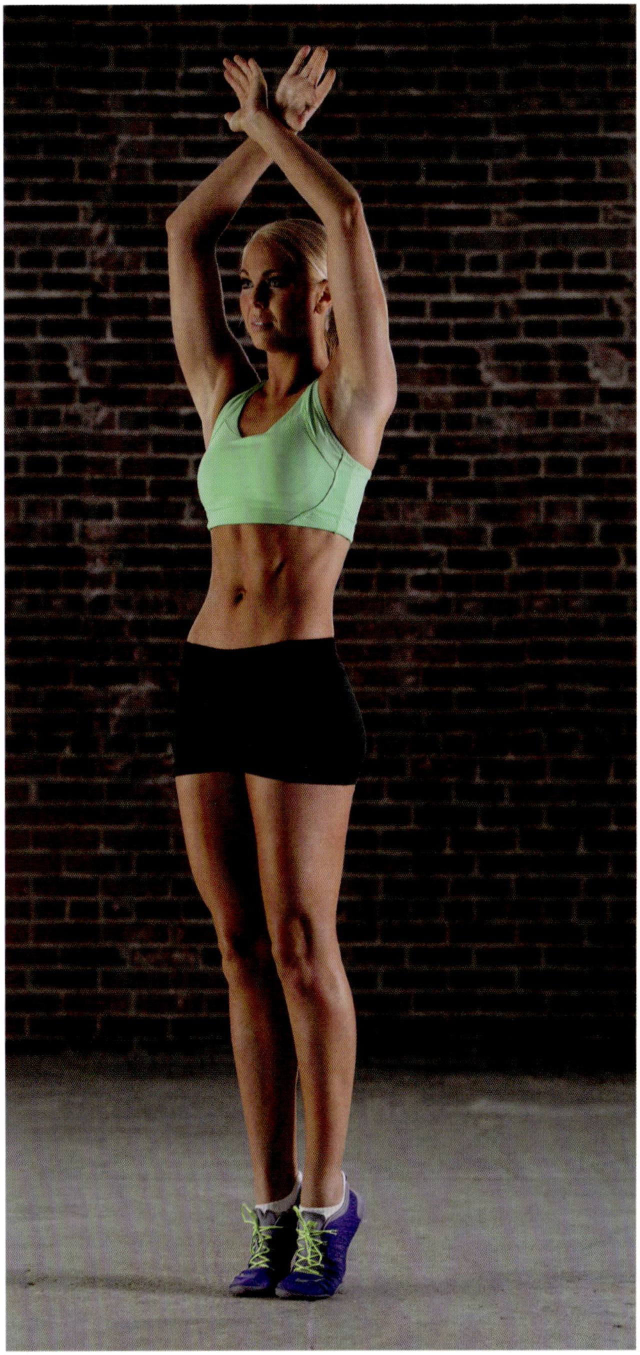

02 Jump out of the squat position. As you jump, extend your legs and raise your arms overhead, crossing your wrists to make an X. Land with your feet together, weight on balls of feet. Keep a soft bend in your knees and engage the core.

BRIDGE KICK

Part triceps dip, part pelvic peel, and part single-leg pike, this functional compound exercise requires you to activate the glutes to elevate the hips.

MORE DIFFICULT ||||||||||||||||||||||||
Modify range of motion and reps: In step 2, perform 1 full rep but lower only halfway instead of fully, then press back up to the highest point of the exercise for 1.5 reps.

LESS DIFFICULT |||||||||||||||||||||||
Modify speed: Hold the elevated kicking position in step 2 for the entire exercise to create a strength-building isometric hold.

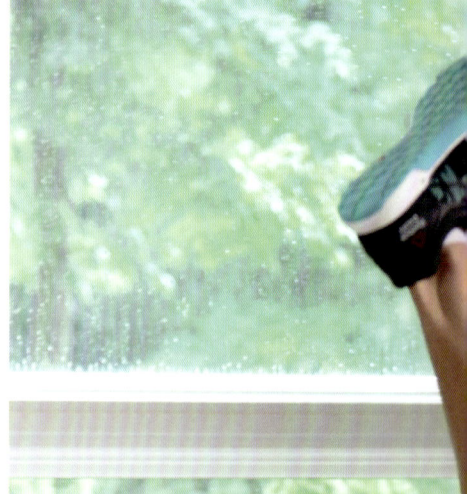

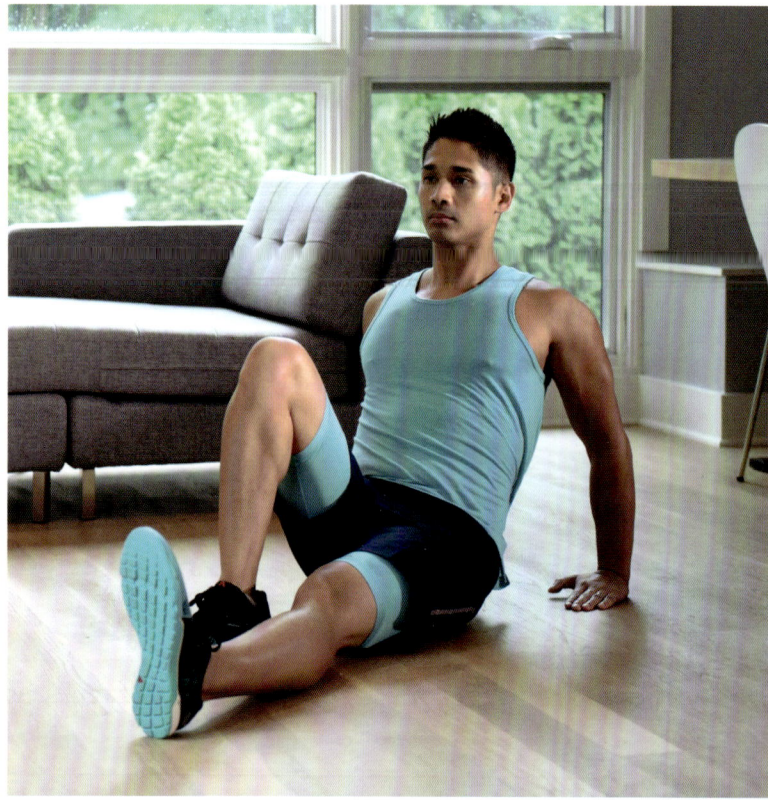

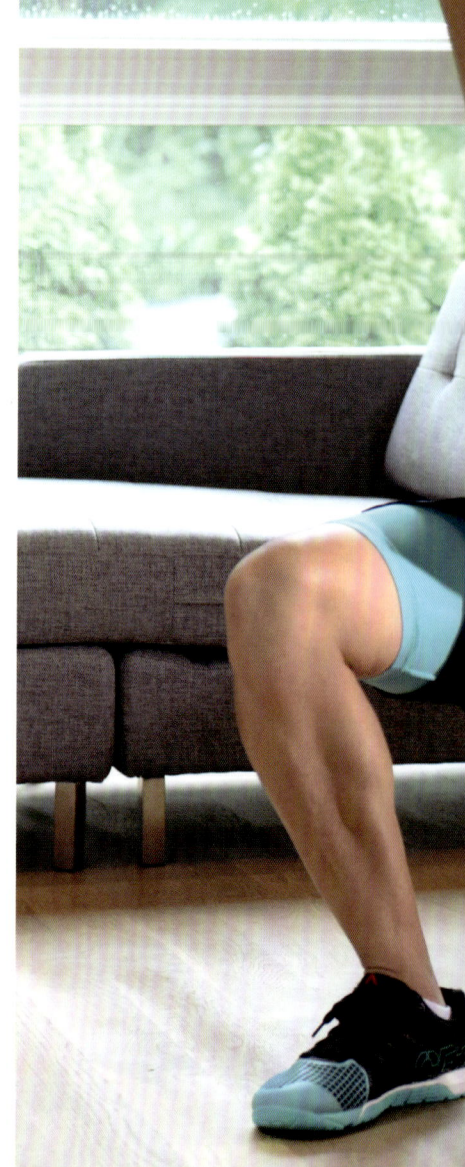

01 Sit with one foot flat on the floor, knee bent, and the other leg extended out in front. Lean back slightly and place your hands on the floor behind your hips, fingers pointing toward the toes, elbows bent.

02 Press through the palms and push through the center of the foot on the floor. Squeeze the glutes and raise the hips upward until level with the stabilizing knee. Simultaneously raise or "kick" the straight leg to 90 degrees.

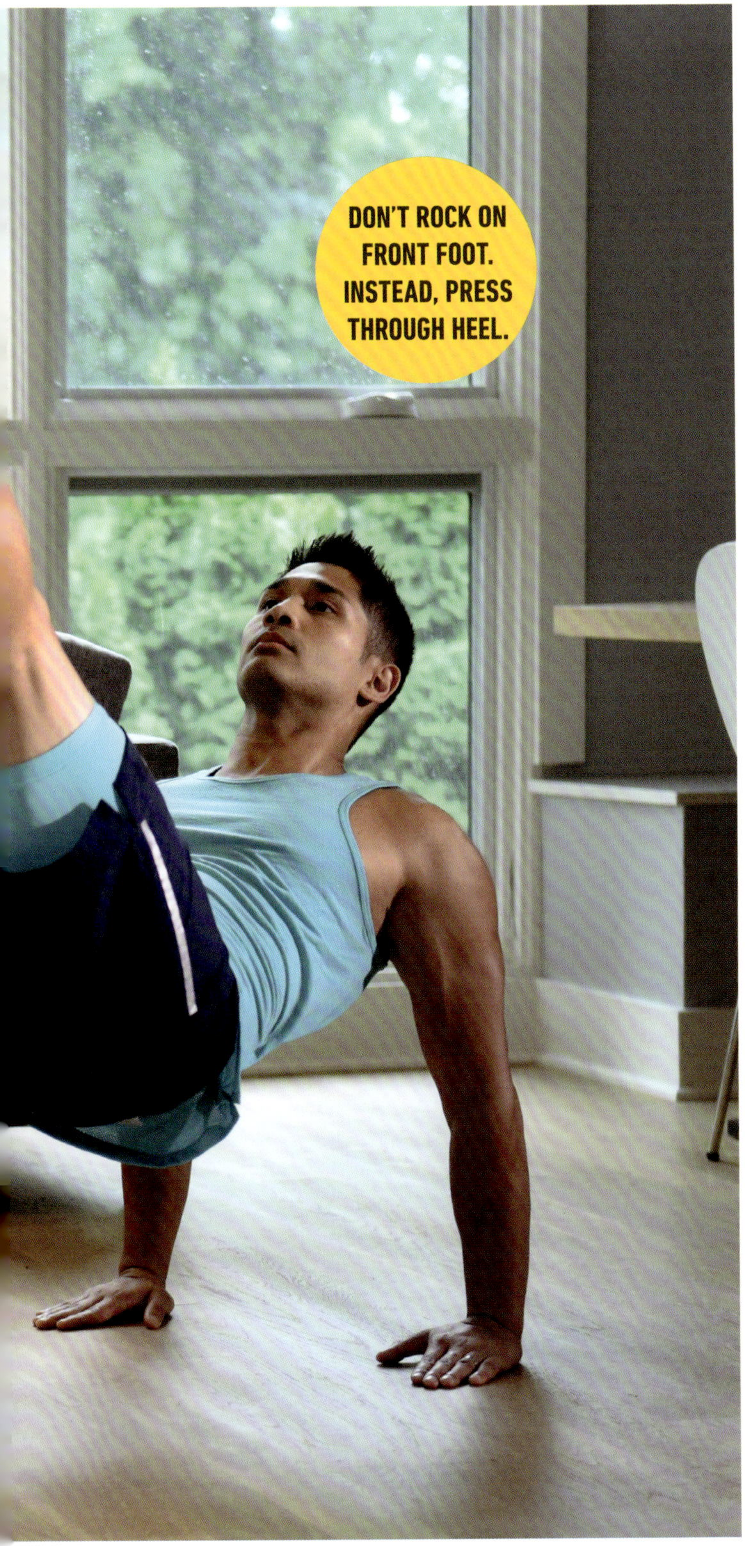

DON'T ROCK ON FRONT FOOT. INSTEAD, PRESS THROUGH HEEL.

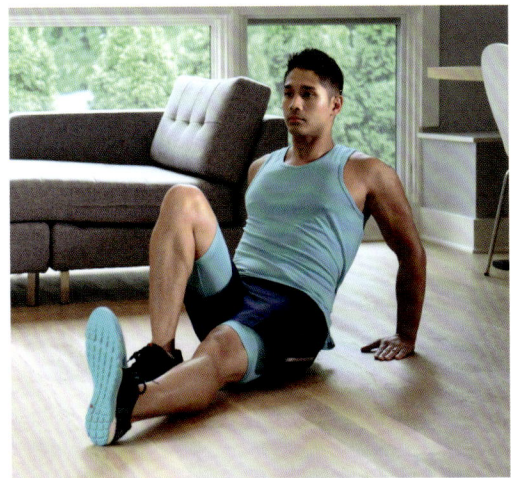

03 Bend your arms, bring your hips back to a slightly elevated starting position, and lower the extended leg back to the floor. Repeat steps 2 and 3 for the prescribed amount of reps.

[The glutes are one of the largest muscle groups in the body, so when you engage them, you burn serious calories.]

BULGARIAN SPLIT SQUAT

This unilateral leg exercise is incredibly useful as it not only builds leg strength, it also increases flexibility of hip flexors and helps create overall balance.

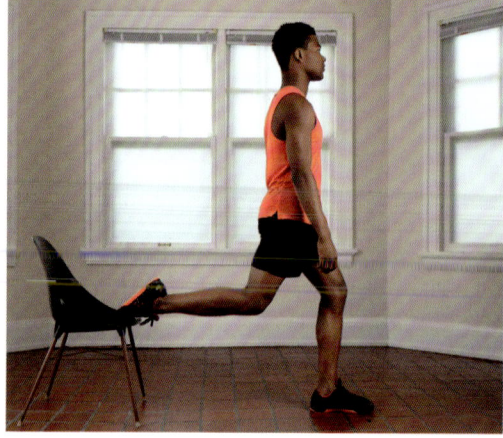

01 Stand with the top of your back foot on a bench, chair, or other elevated surface.

02 Bend your legs and lower body until the thigh of the front leg is parallel to the floor, and pause for 2 to 3 seconds.

MORE DIFFICULT ||||||||||||||||||||
Modify range of motion: In step 2, add a plyometric jump to increase the workload and create performance-enhancing power.

LESS DIFFICULT ||||||||||||||||||||
Modify speed: Hold in the deepest position of step 2 for the duration. This isolation hold will generate strength.

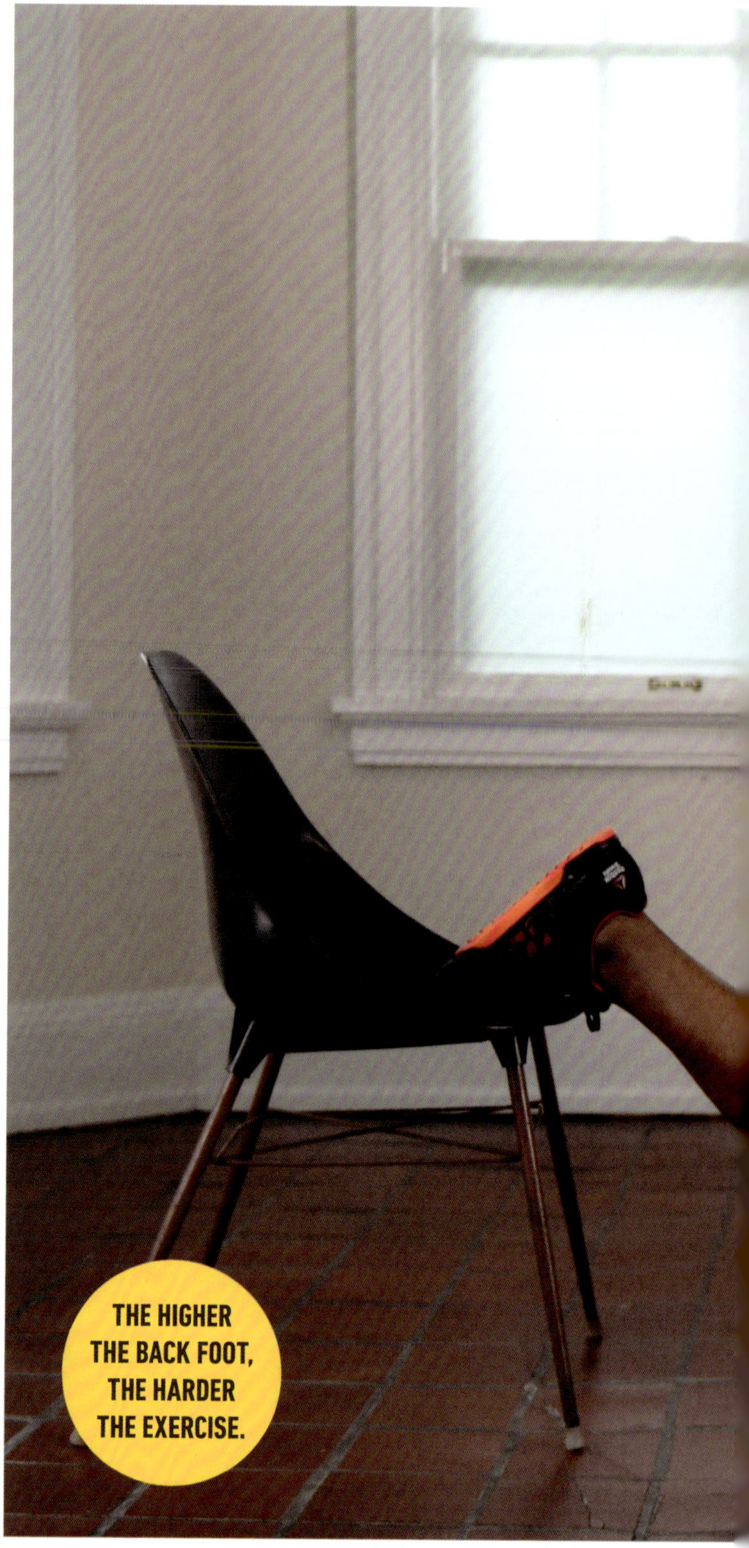

THE HIGHER THE BACK FOOT, THE HARDER THE EXERCISE.

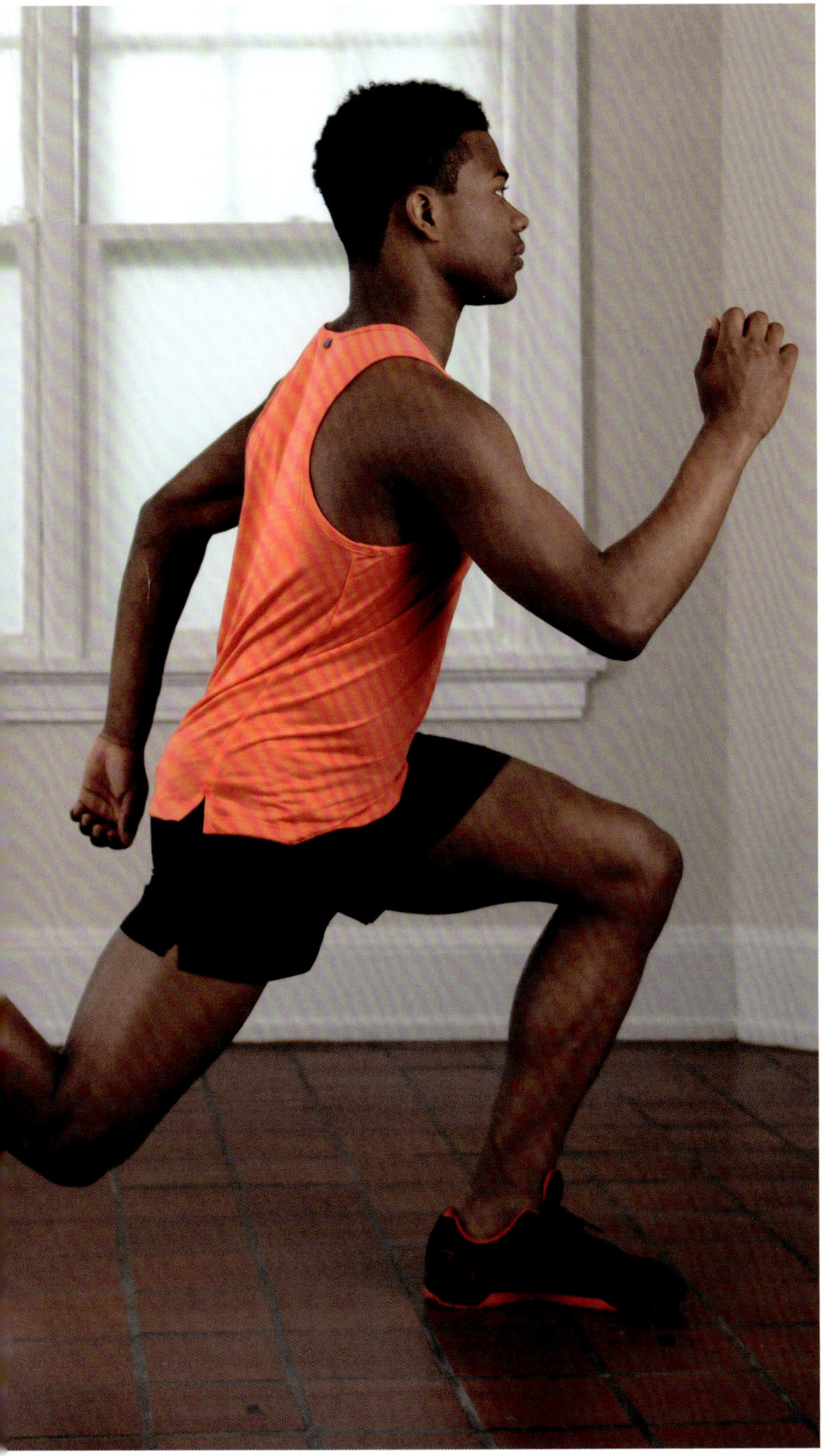

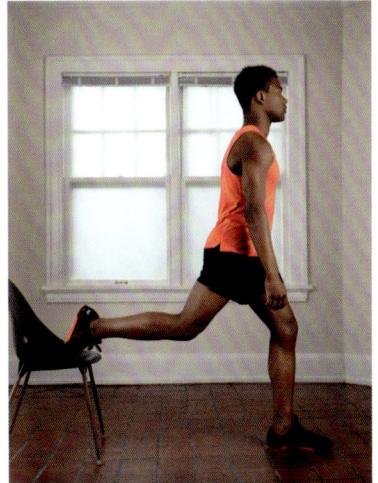

03 Return to a standing position by pressing through the heel of the front foot, standing tall to engage the core.

[Extend your arms out in front for balance, or overhead to increase the challenge.]

REVERSE LUNGE

The reverse lunge is a simple, low-impact way to strengthen the quads, hamstrings, glutes, and calves.

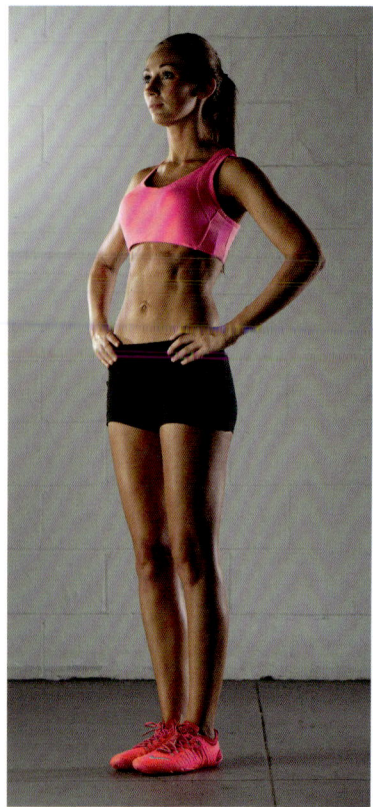

01 Stand tall with hands on your hips.

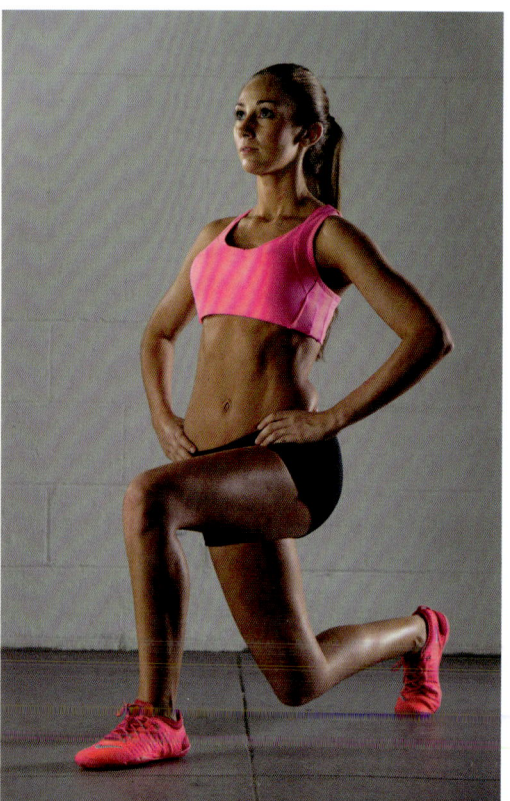

02 Take a large step back with your right foot. Lower your hips so that your left thigh is parallel to the floor and your left knee is directly over your ankle. Your right knee should be bent at 90 degrees, pointing to the floor and directly under your hip.

03 Return to a standing position and repeat, this time leading with the right leg.

SKI JUMP

This exercise is inspired by the movement of downhill skiing. It will condition the calves, quads, and glutes while kicking up your heart rate and challenging your balance, coordination, and core stabilization.

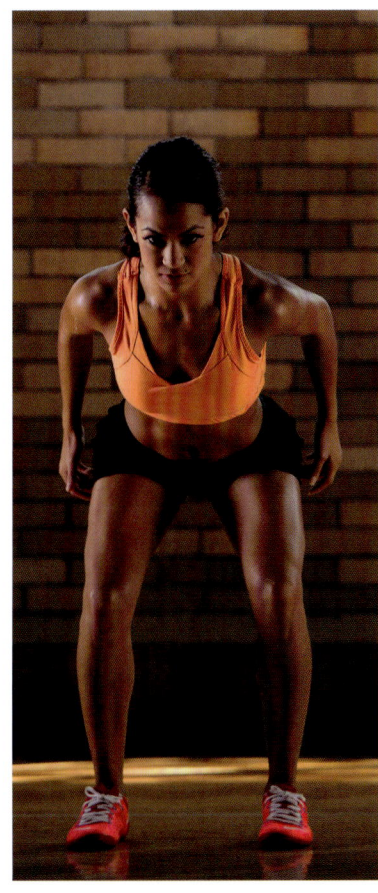 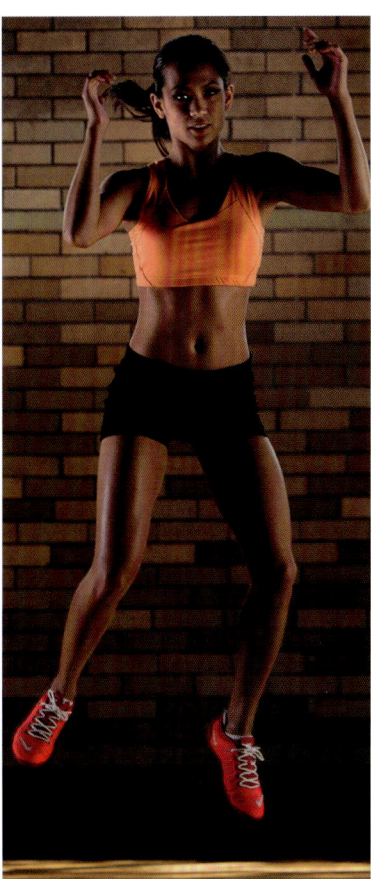 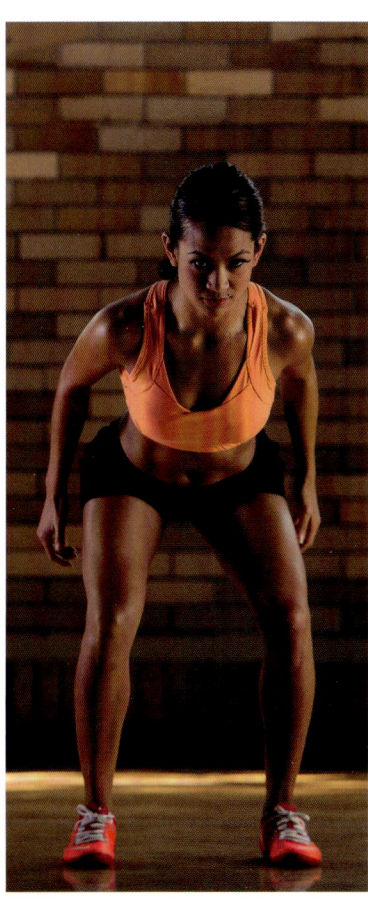

01 Stand tall with your toes pointing forward and your weight in your heels. Inhale as you bend at the knees, lowering into a half squat.

02 Engage your core and exhale as you jump to one side with both feet, maintaining the distance between them. Keep your hips and shoulders facing forward, and bend your arms as though holding ski poles.

03 Land as softly and silently as possible, bending at the ankles, knees, and hips to decelerate the body back to the half-squat position.

FRONT LUNGE

The front lunge is a simple, low-impact way to strengthen the quads, hamstrings, glutes, and calves.

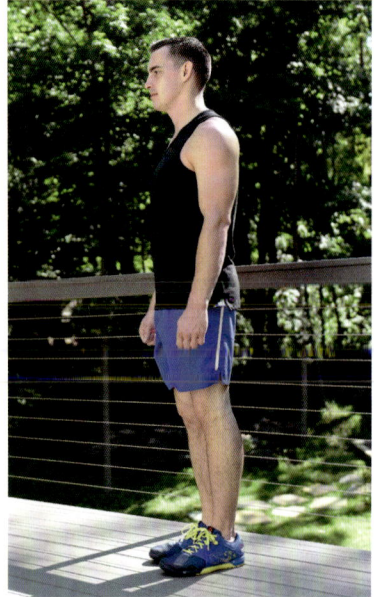

01 Stand straight, with arms at your side and core engaged.

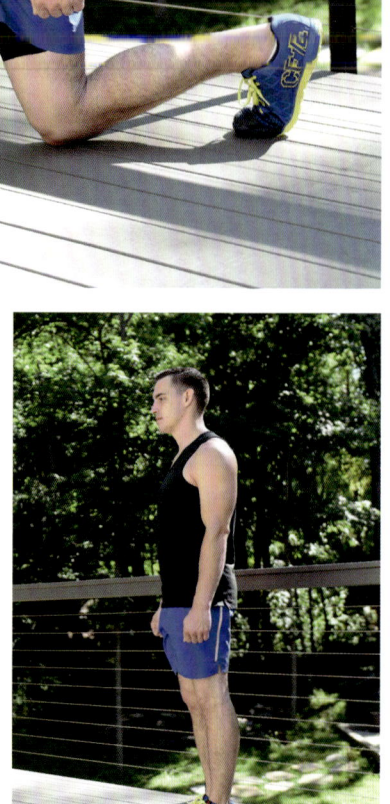

02 Step your left foot forward. Bending your right knee 90 degrees, lower your hips to bring your left thigh parallel to the floor and your left knee directly over your ankle.

03 Return to standing by pressing through the heel of the left foot and bringing the foot backward, standing tall to engage the core.

MORE DIFFICULT ||||||||||||||||||||
Modify stability: For the entire exercise, raise your hands overhead to challenge stability.

LESS DIFFICULT ||||||||||||||||||||
Modify stability: Hold on to any available prop to aid balance.

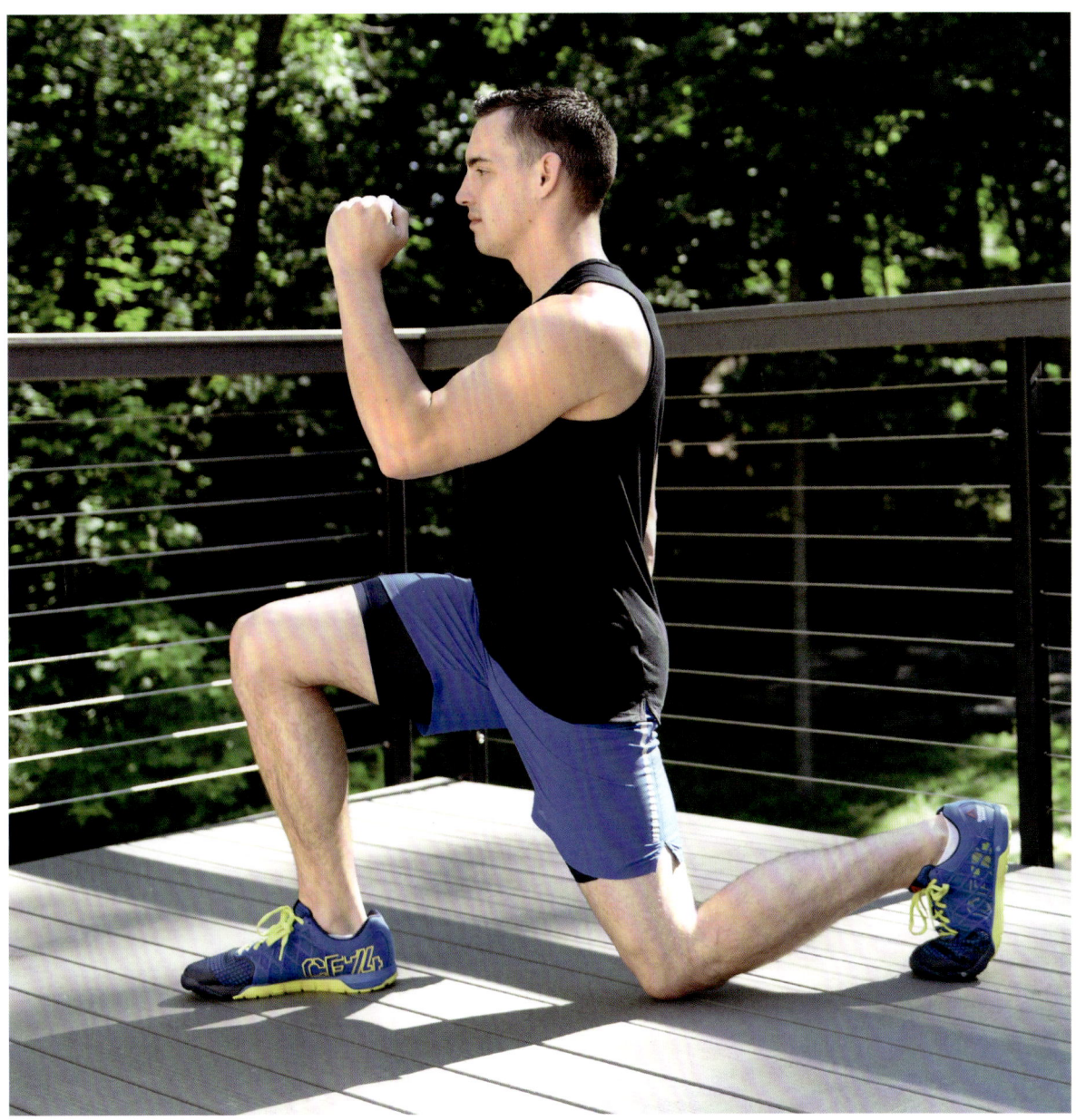

04 Repeat steps 2 and 3, this time leading with the right leg.

According to the American Council on Exercise, lunges are one of the most effective lower-body exercises. Studies prove strengthening the lower body can speed up metabolism and aid fat loss.

UPPER-BODY EXERCISES

SINGLE-LEG BURPEE

Raising a leg throughout the plank and push-up phase of the burpee adds an increased load for the core, challenging the abdominals, lower back, and stabilizing leg.

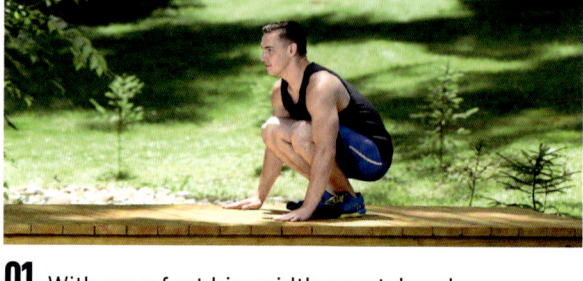

01 With your feet hip-width apart, bend your knees and bring your hands to the ground just in front of your feet.

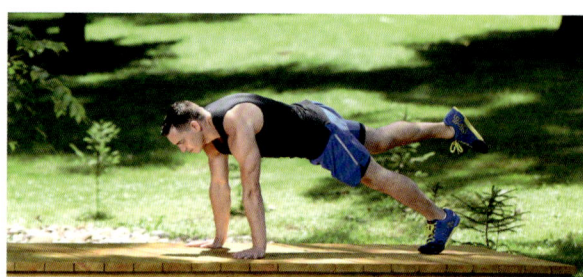

02 Hop your feet back into a plank position with one leg elevated to hip height.

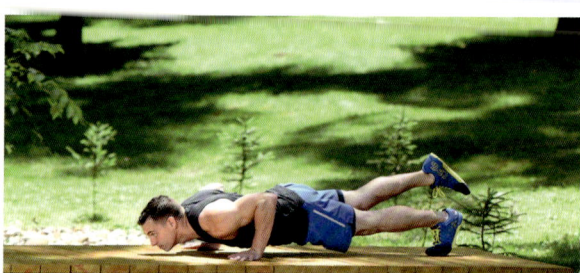

03 Perform one push-up with your core engaged and leg elevated.

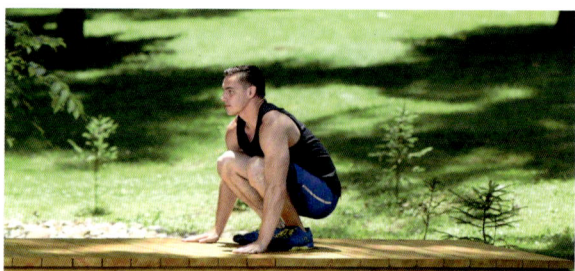

04 Lower the raised leg and jump your feet back to your hands, shifting your weight into the heels and lifting your chest.

MORE DIFFICULT |||||||||||||||||||||||
Modify range of motion and stability:
Extend your arms in all steps. This lengthens your body, making your core work harder.

LESS DIFFICULT |||||||||||||||||||||||
Modify points of contact: In steps 2 and 3, cross the elevated leg on top of the stabilizing one, adding support and increasing balance.

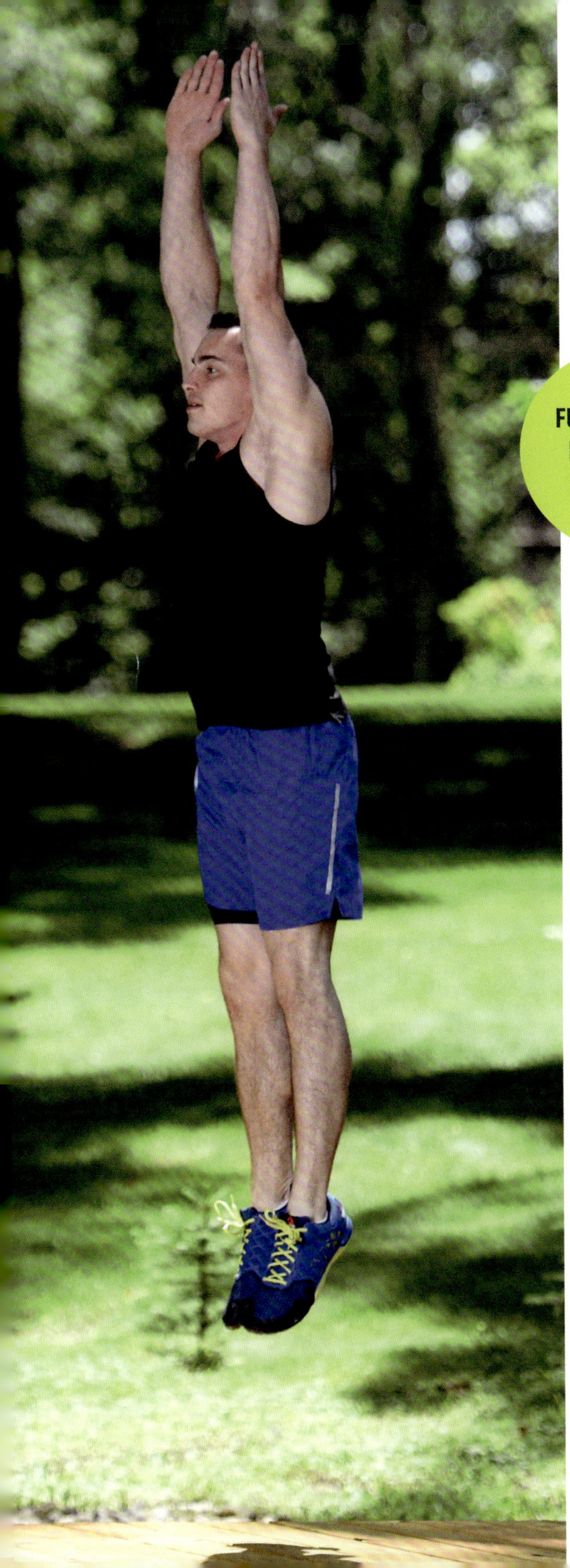

05 Jump up from the crouching position and reach overhead with your hands.

FULLY EXTEND LEGS, HIPS, AND ARMS.

The burpee was created in the 1930s by American physiologist Royal Huddleston Burpee for his doctoral thesis. Burpees are a total-body strength and cardiovascular exercise.

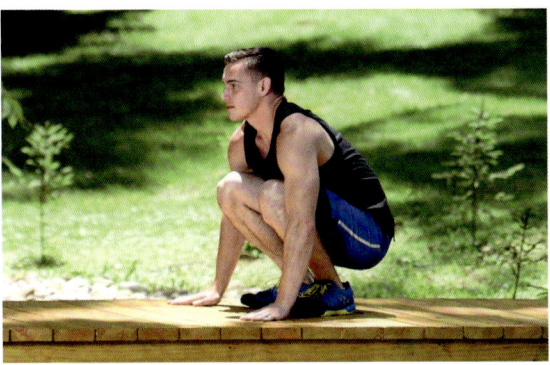

06 Land softly with a slight bend at your knees, hips, and ankles.

BURPEE

The burpee is indisputably the ultimate total body exercise. Each one will work your chest, arms, shoulders, thighs, hamstrings, and core. Burpees can be intimidating, but the benefits are worth the challenge.

MORE DIFFICULT ||||||||||||||||||||
For added challenge, substitute the regular push-up with a triceps push-up, keeping your elbows tight to your rib cage.

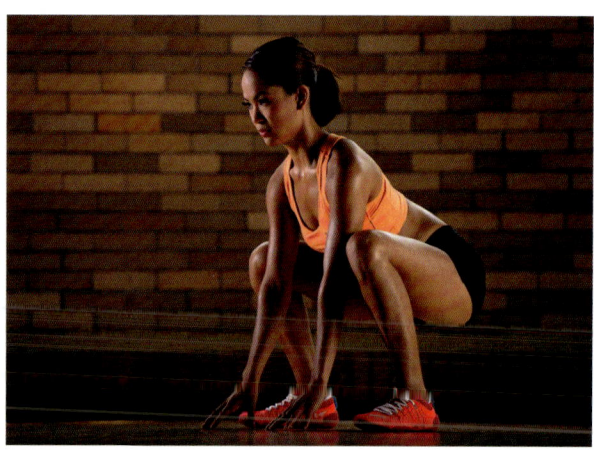

01 With your feet hip-width apart, bend your knees and bring hands to the floor just in front of your feet. Spread your fingers wide and grip the floor.

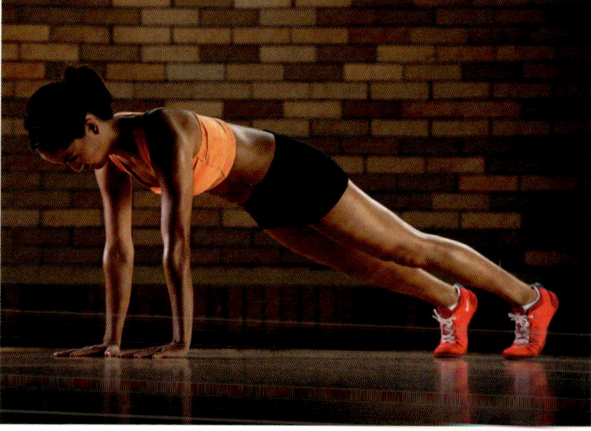

02 Hop your feet back into a plank position. Don't allow your lower back to collapse.

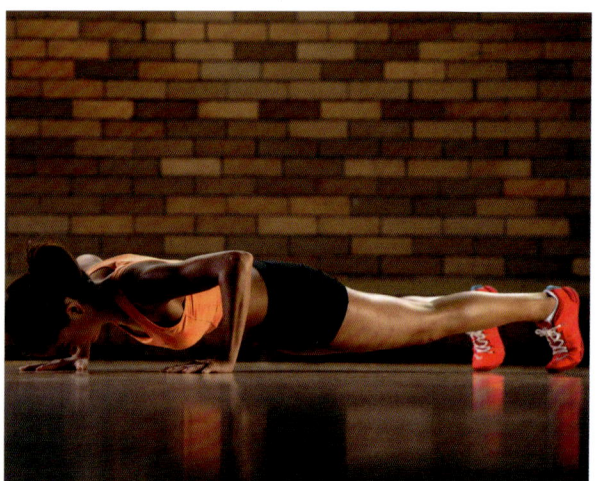

03 Perform one push-up with your core engaged.

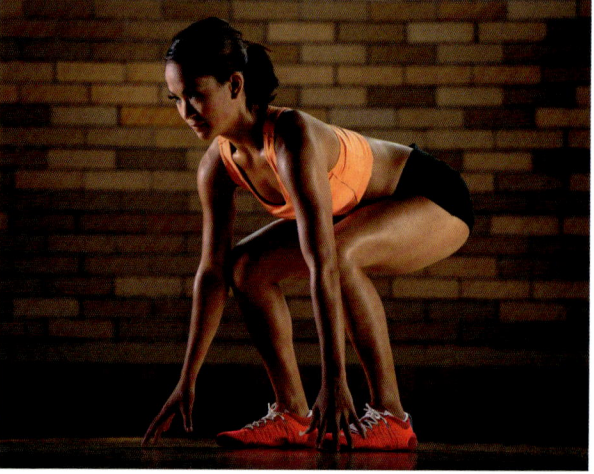

04 Jump your feet back to your hands, shifting your weight to the heels and lifting your chest.

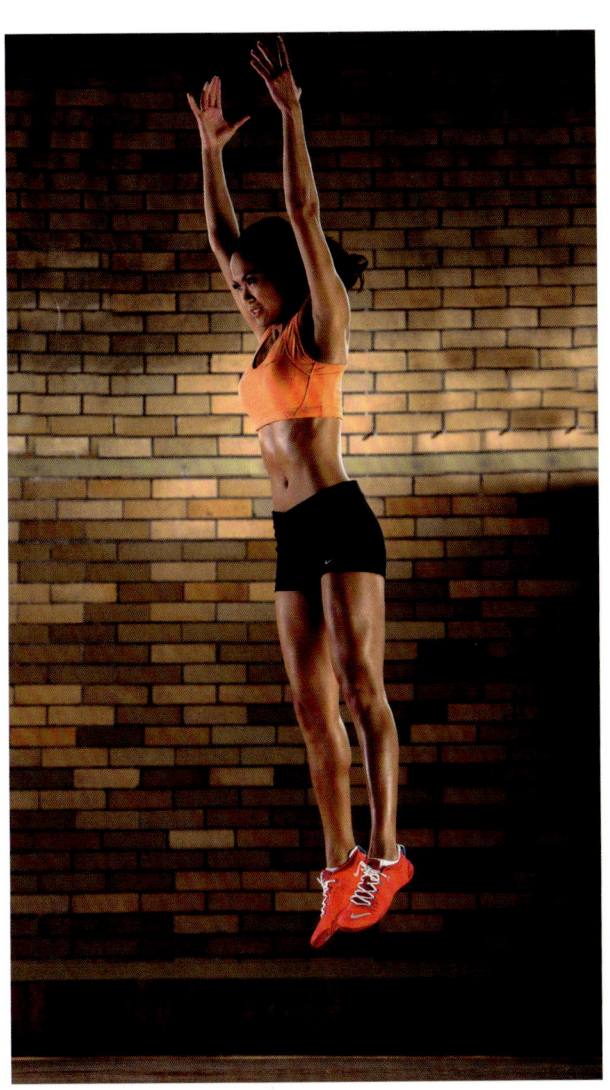

05 Jump up from the crouched position and reach overhead with your hands.

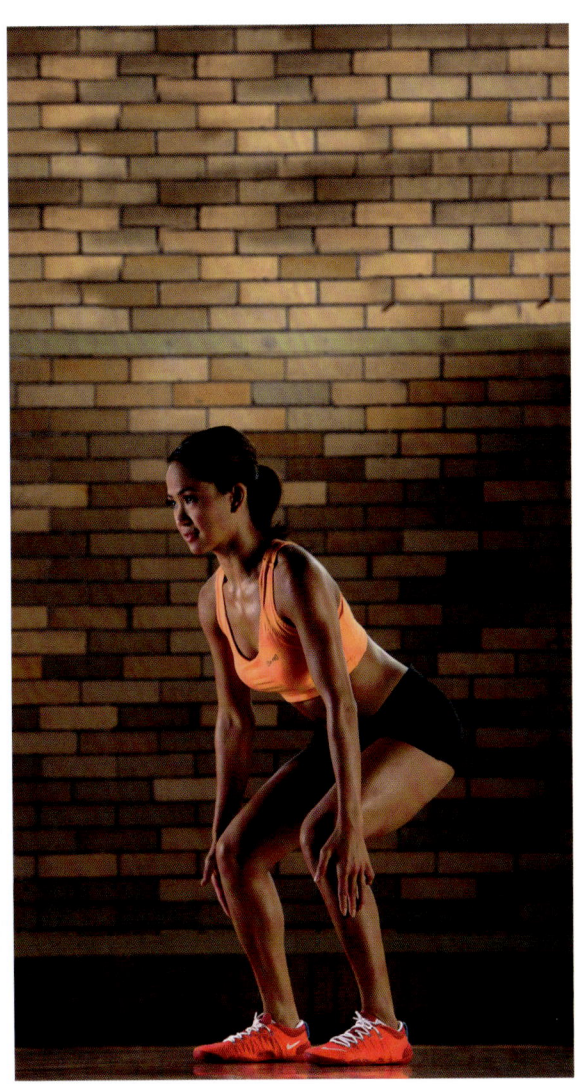

06 Land softly with a slight bend at your knees, hips, and ankles.

SHOULDER PRESS JACK

This twist on the classic jumping jack focuses on the latissimus dorsi, or lats, the largest muscles in your back. Concentrate on keeping the lats engaged and use explosive movements to boost your heart rate.

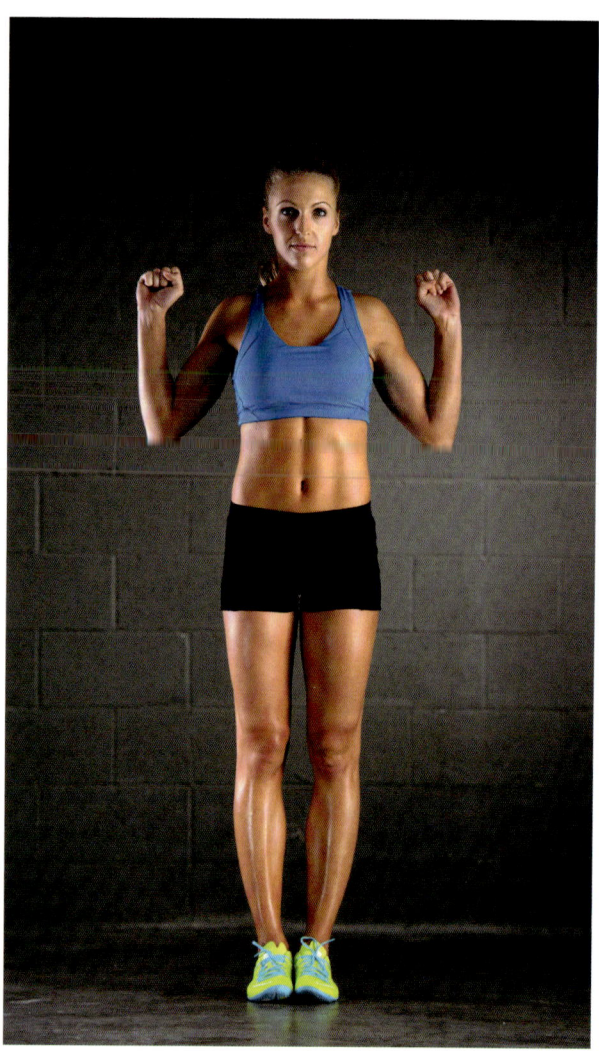

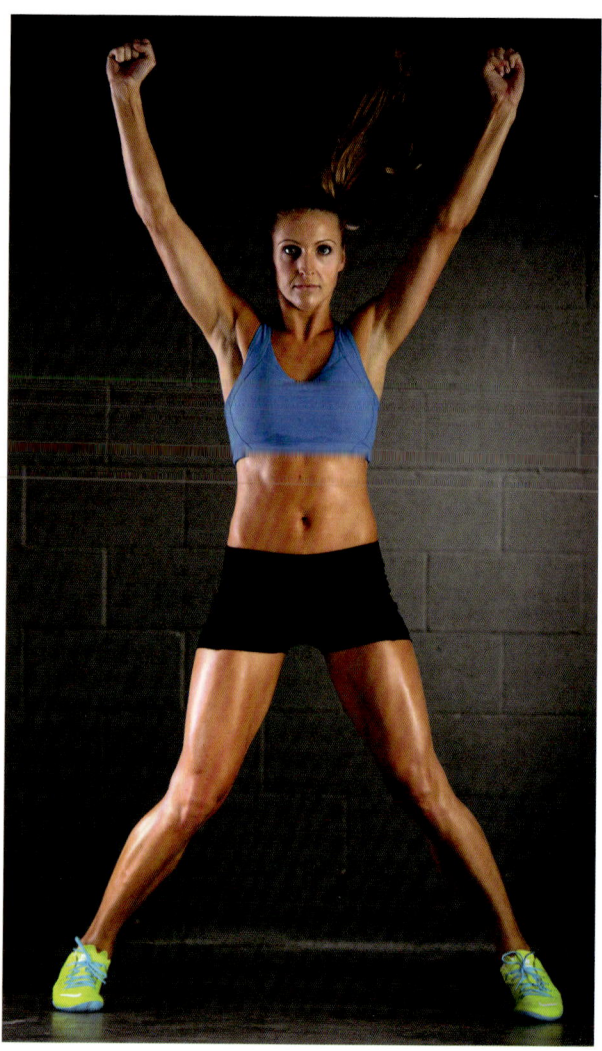

01 Stand with your feet together and your arms bent, elbows by your sides. Make your hands into fists and concentrate on engaging your lats. Engage the core and soften the knees.

02 Jump up, opening your feet wider than your shoulders and simultaneously punching your arms toward the roof. Jump again, bringing the feet together as you tuck your elbows back into your sides and concentrate on squeezing and engaging the lats. Repeat.

TRICEPS DIP

This targeted exercise is specifically designed to strengthen and define your triceps, the muscles on the underside of your arm between the elbow and the shoulder. If you want to banish wobbly underarms, this is the move for you.

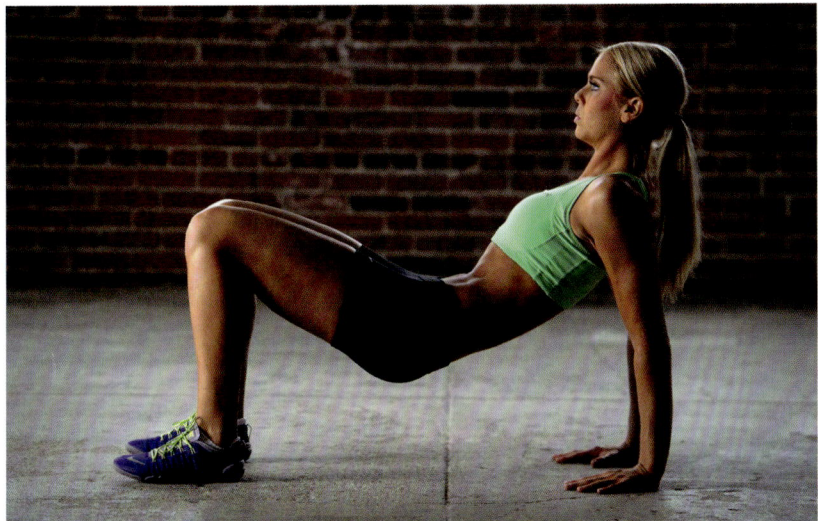

01 Sit with your feet flat on the floor in front of you and knees bent. Lean back slightly and place your hands on the floor behind your hips, fingers pointing toward your toes. Elevate the hips by engaging the core, hamstrings, and glutes.

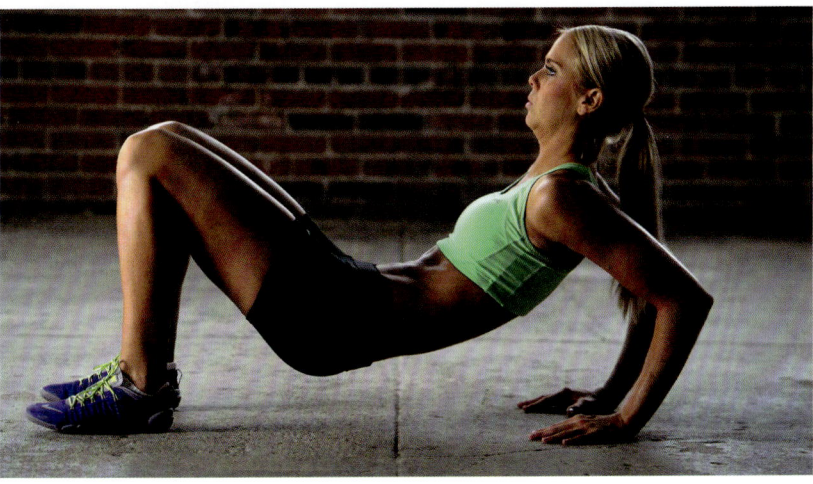

02 Bend your elbows, lowering your hips until they're just above the floor. Don't let your elbows flare out. Imagine squeezing your elbows together as you lower your hips. Extend your arms, bringing your hips back up to the starting position.

MORE DIFFICULT ||||||||||||||||
For a deeper movement, you can do triceps dips with your hands on a stable, elevated surface, such as a bench.

DOWN DOG PUSH-UP

Down dog push-ups are without question one of the best bodyweight exercises for your shoulders, allowing you to build the strength to perform gravity-defying wall walks and even handstand push-ups.

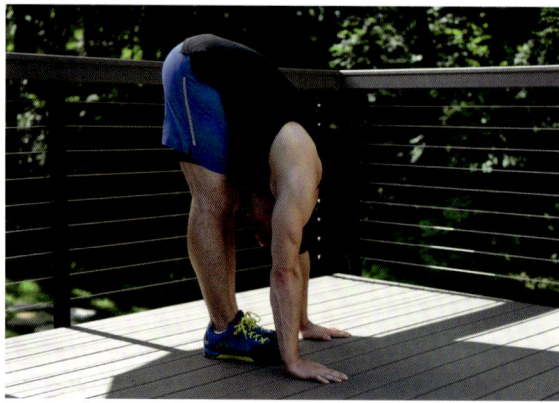

01 Begin by standing tall, then fold forward from the hips until your hands are on the floor.

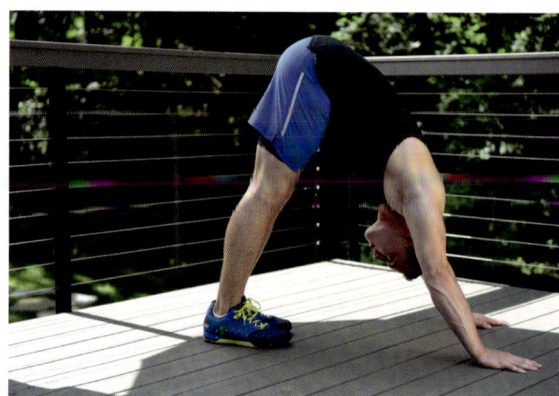

02 Walk your hands away from your body until you form a triangle with the ground. The farther your hands are from your feet, the easier the exercise becomes, because the muscles of the chest and back assist the shoulders. You're now in the down dog position; stay there for the remainder of the exercise.

MORE DIFFICULT ||||||||||||||||||||||
Modify body angle: During the entire exercise, elevate your feet on any available prop to decline the body and transfer a greater proportion of weight into the upper body.

LESS DIFFICULT ||||||||||||||||||||||
Modify body angle: In step 2, move your feet farther from your hands, so weight is more evenly distributed through the core.

> The shoulder is made up of three bones, as well as associated muscles, ligaments, and tendons. It's the most mobile joint in the human body.

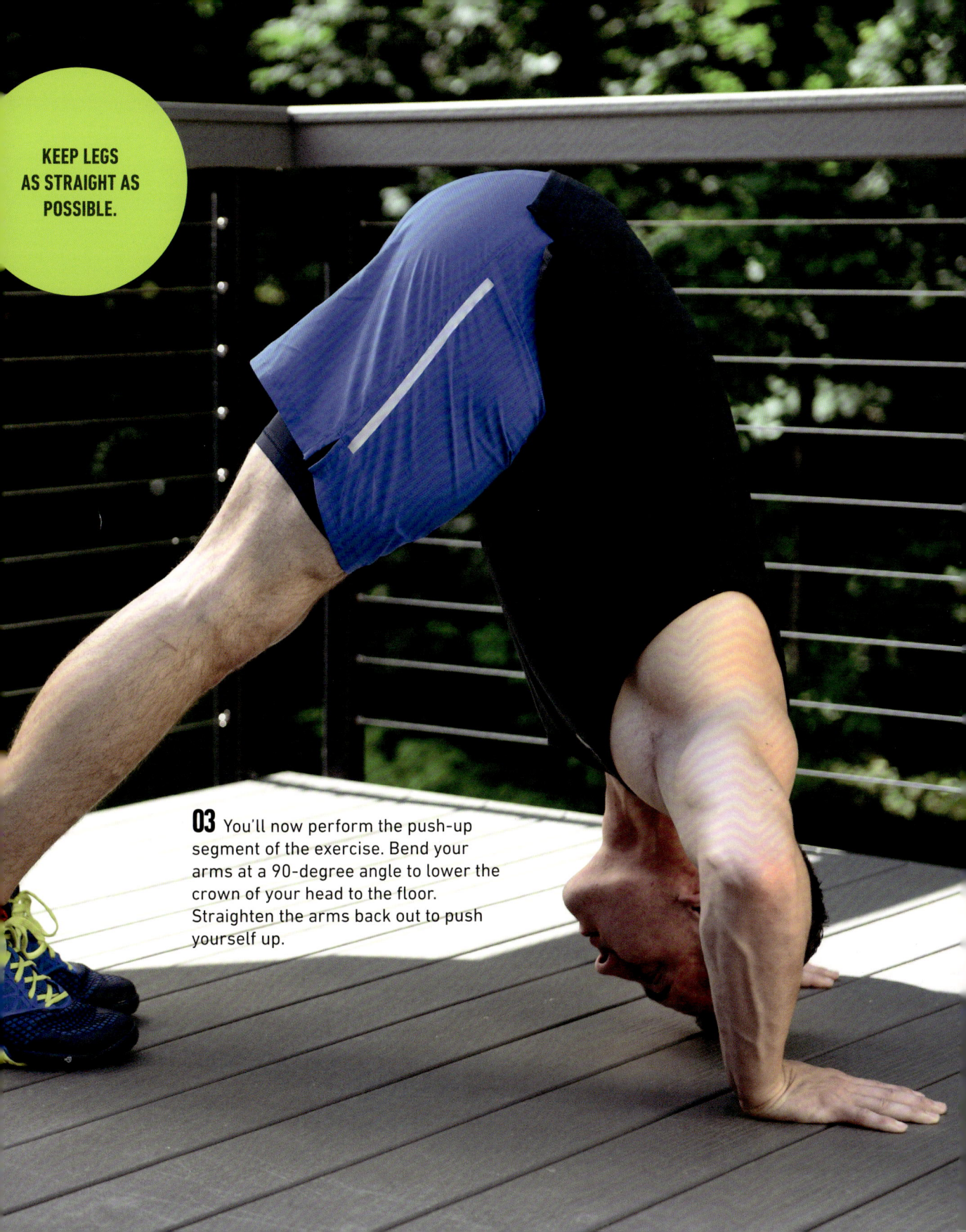

KEEP LEGS
AS STRAIGHT AS
POSSIBLE.

03 You'll now perform the push-up segment of the exercise. Bend your arms at a 90-degree angle to lower the crown of your head to the floor. Straighten the arms back out to push yourself up.

DEAD HANG

This is a great introduction to bodyweight training because it teaches body awareness and helps to develop the fundamental grip strength vital in all hanging exercises.

MORE DIFFICULT ||||||||||||||||||||||
Modify stability: In step 2, gently swing your body from side to side to perform dead swings. This will force you to recruit the muscles in your core for stabilization.

LESS DIFFICULT ||||||||||||||||||||||
Modify stability: Use a resistance band, or place one foot on a chair, to provide support and stability while you build confidence and strength.

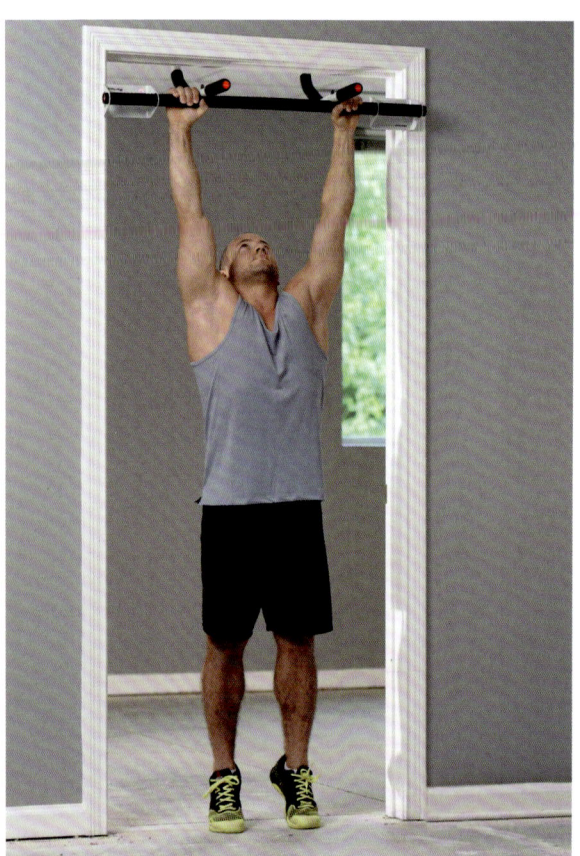

01 Stand directly under your pull-up bar.

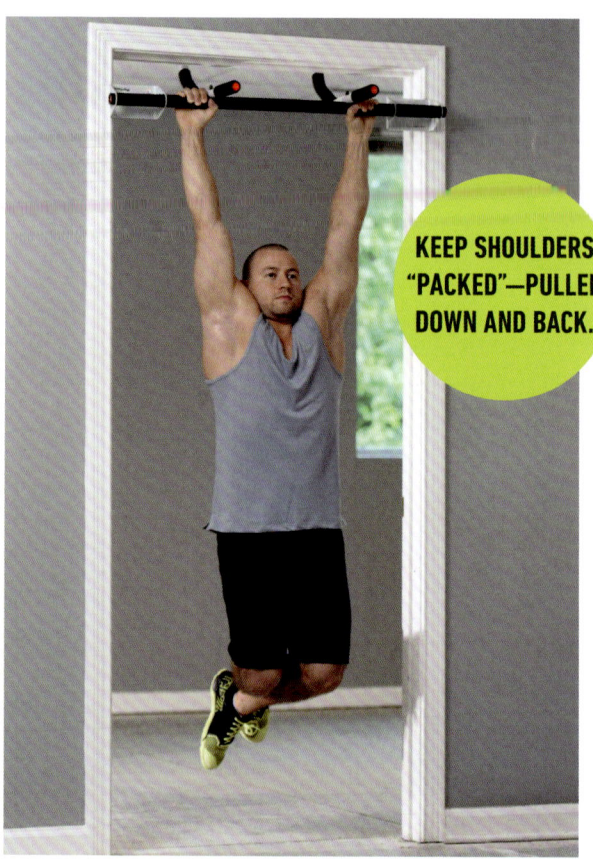

KEEP SHOULDERS "PACKED"—PULLED DOWN AND BACK.

02 Hop up and grab the bar with an overhand grip (palms facing away) wider than your shoulders, and hang from the bar with straight arms. Try to hang with good form for as long as possible.

HANGING SCAPULA RETRACTION

This is a relatively basic exercise, but it's essential for shoulder and back health and will add gains to your bench press.

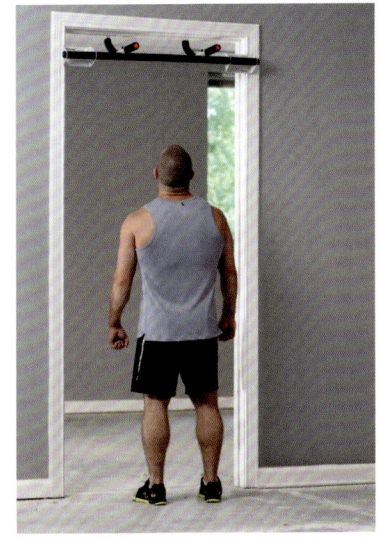

01 Position yourself directly under the pull-up bar.

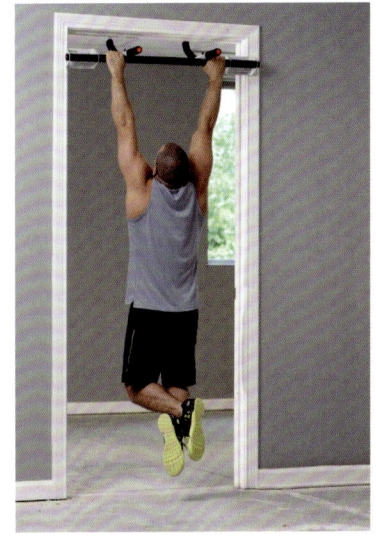

02 Hop up and grab the bar with an overhand grip wider than your shoulders, and settle into a dead hang position with shoulders pulled back and down—known as "packed."

MORE DIFFICULT |||||||||||||||||||||||
Modify speed: Instead of repeating steps 3 and 4, squeeze and hold the shoulder blades for the duration of the exercise. This creates a strength-building isometric hold.

LESS DIFFICULT |||||||||||||||||||||||
Modify speed: After step 2, omit the remaining steps. Instead, hang from the bar without shrugging the shoulders for time. This builds upper-body and grip strength.

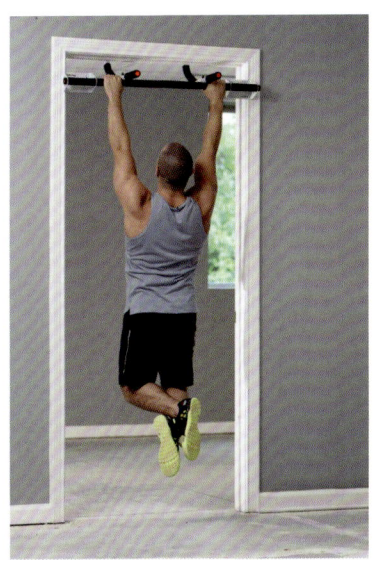

03 Lift your body by squeezing your shoulder blades together, and hold for 3 seconds, with no bend in your arms. As you squeeze, your chest will decline and lower back will arch slightly.

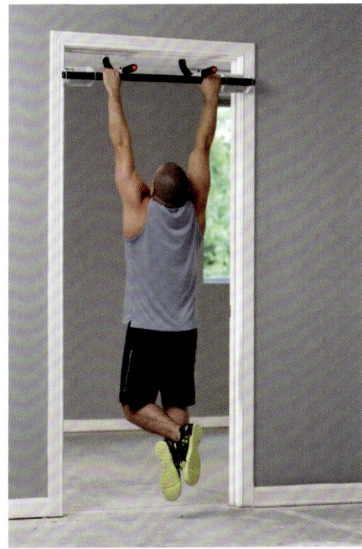

04 Slowly lower back to the dead hang position. Repeat steps 3 and 4 for the duration of the exercise.

TUCK JUMP BURPEE

This is an incredible cardiovascular and strength exercise for those feeling superhuman. Explosive plyometrics combined with the total-body burpee burn fat and improve agility and athletic performance.

MORE DIFFICULT ||||||||||||||||||
Modify range of motion: In step 3, perform two push-ups, and jump twice in step 5. Twice the effort equals twice the gain.

LESS DIFFICULT ||||||||||||||||||
Modify points of contact: Remove the push-up in step 3 and perform a tuck jump squat thrust instead.

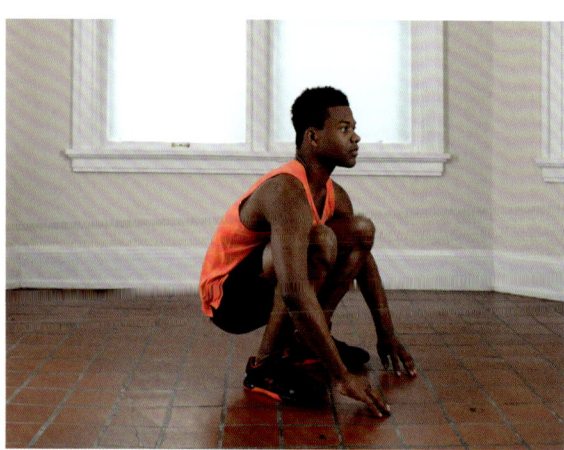

01 With your feet hip-width apart, bend your knees and bring hands to the floor just in front of your feet.

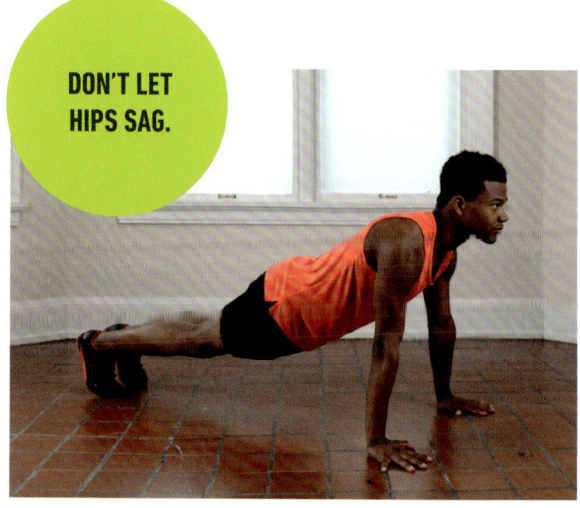

DON'T LET HIPS SAG.

02 Hop your feet back into a plank position with bodyweight evenly distributed between toes and hands, and with the core engaged.

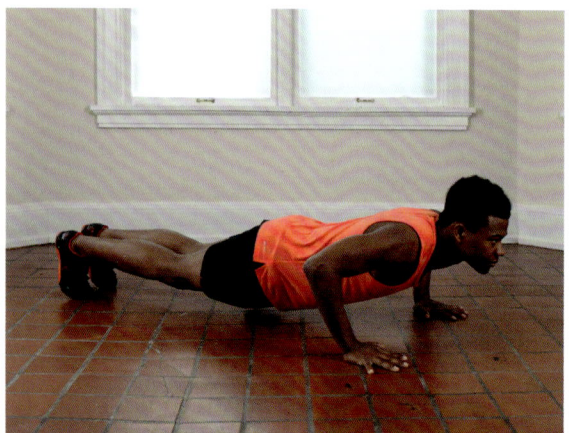

03 Perform one push-up with your core engaged.

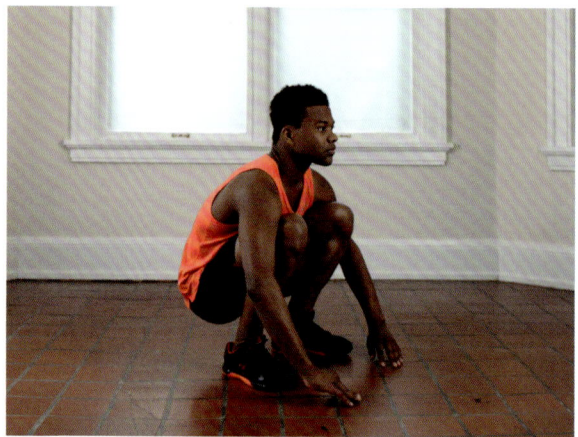

04 Jump your feet back to your hands, shifting your weight into the heels and lifting your chest.

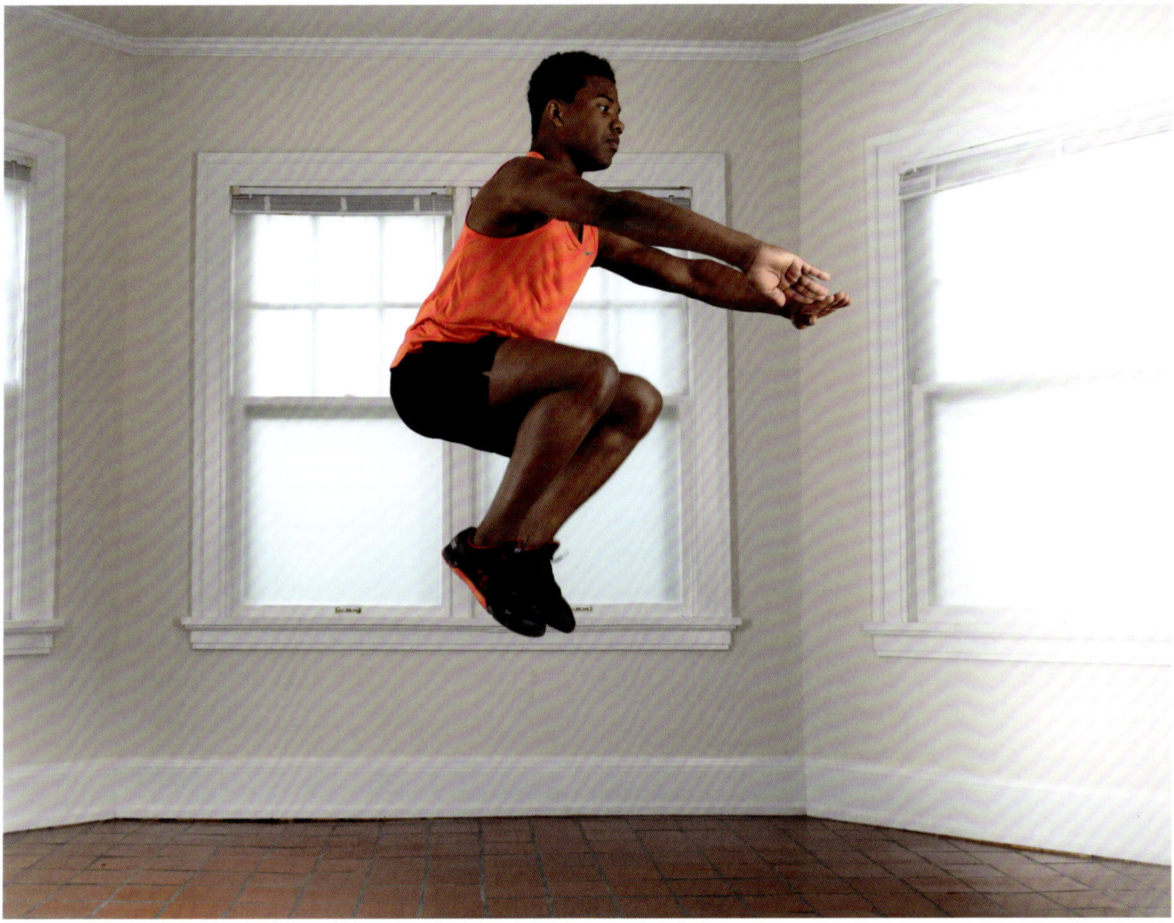

05 Jump up from the crouched position, tucking your knees to your chest.

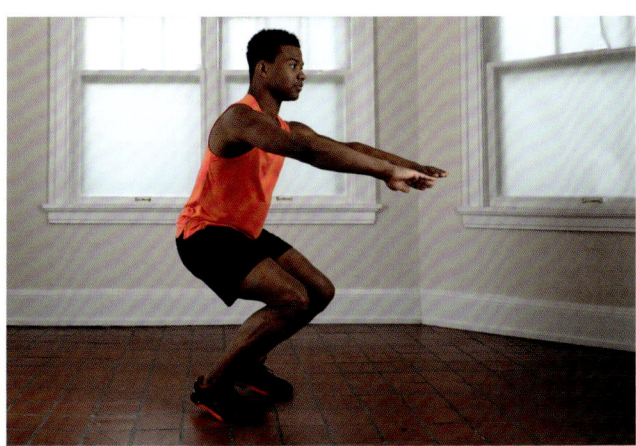

06 Land softly with a slight bend at your knees, hips, and ankles.

A recent study found that performing 10 fast-paced repetitions of a burpee stokes your metabolic furnace as effectively as sprinting for 30 seconds.

PUSH-UP

The push-up may be the perfect compound exercise. If done correctly, it builds upper body and core strength, using the muscles of the chest, back, shoulders, triceps, abs, and even the legs. Keep an eye on your form.

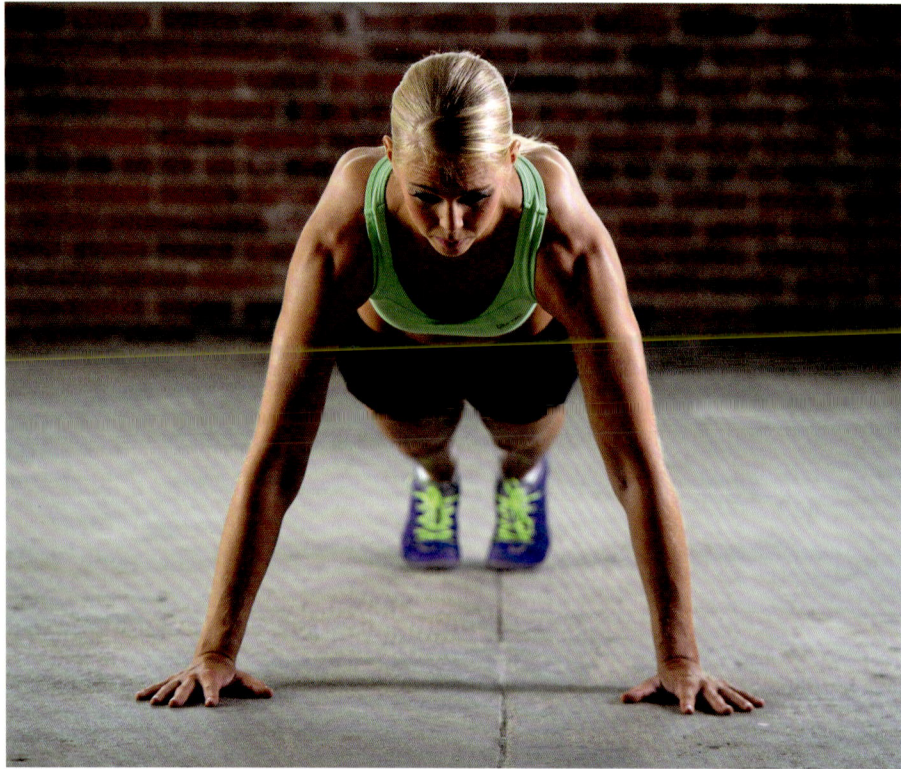

01 Assume a full plank position with your core engaged. Your body should be balanced between your toes and hands, forming a straight line from ankles to head.

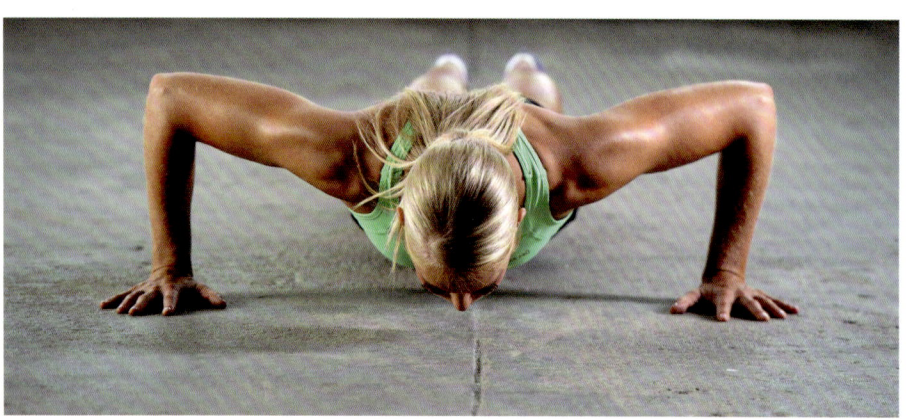

02 Bend your elbows, bringing your chest toward the floor. Once your elbows are slightly beyond 90 degrees, push up through your hands, extending the arms to return to the starting position.

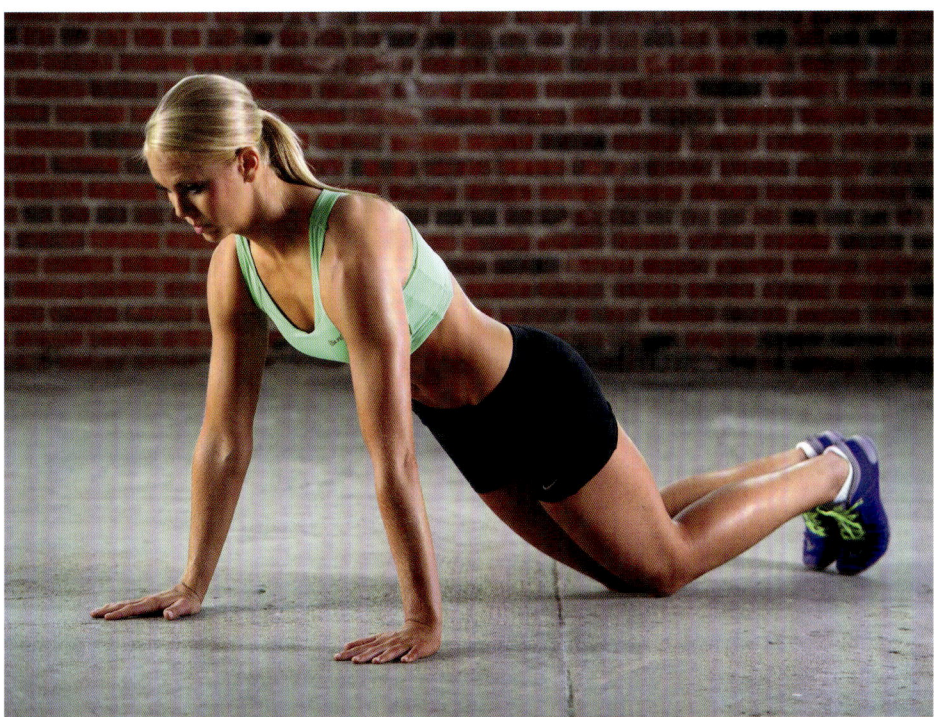

LESS DIFFICULT ||||
If a full push-up is too challenging, place your knees on the floor for stability and support.

CHALLENGE

There are many push-up variations. Try adjusting the position of your hands to work slightly different muscle groups and make the move more challenging.

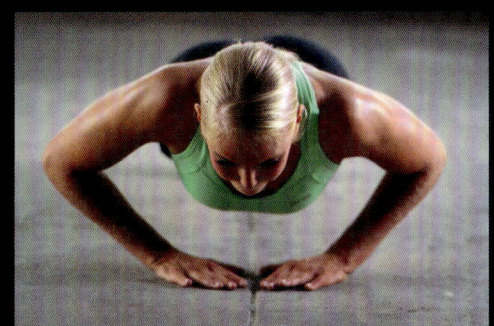

Heart to Hands

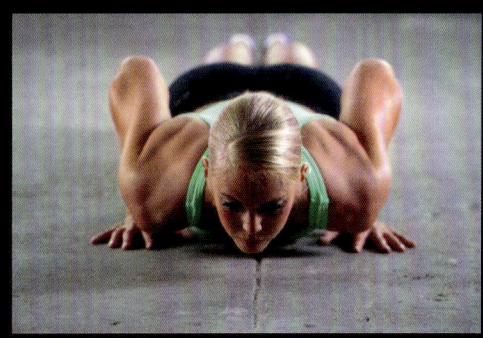

Tricep

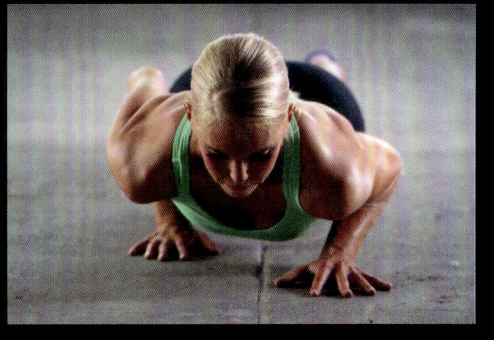

Staggered

PUSH-UP JACK

Push-up jacks fuse cardiovascular jumping jacks with muscle-building push-ups for a killer compound exercise that torches calories.

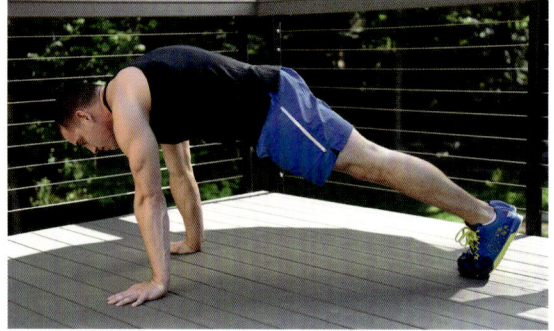

01 Assume a full plank or traditional push-up position with your body balanced between the toes and hands, with hands wider than shoulders and feet side by side.

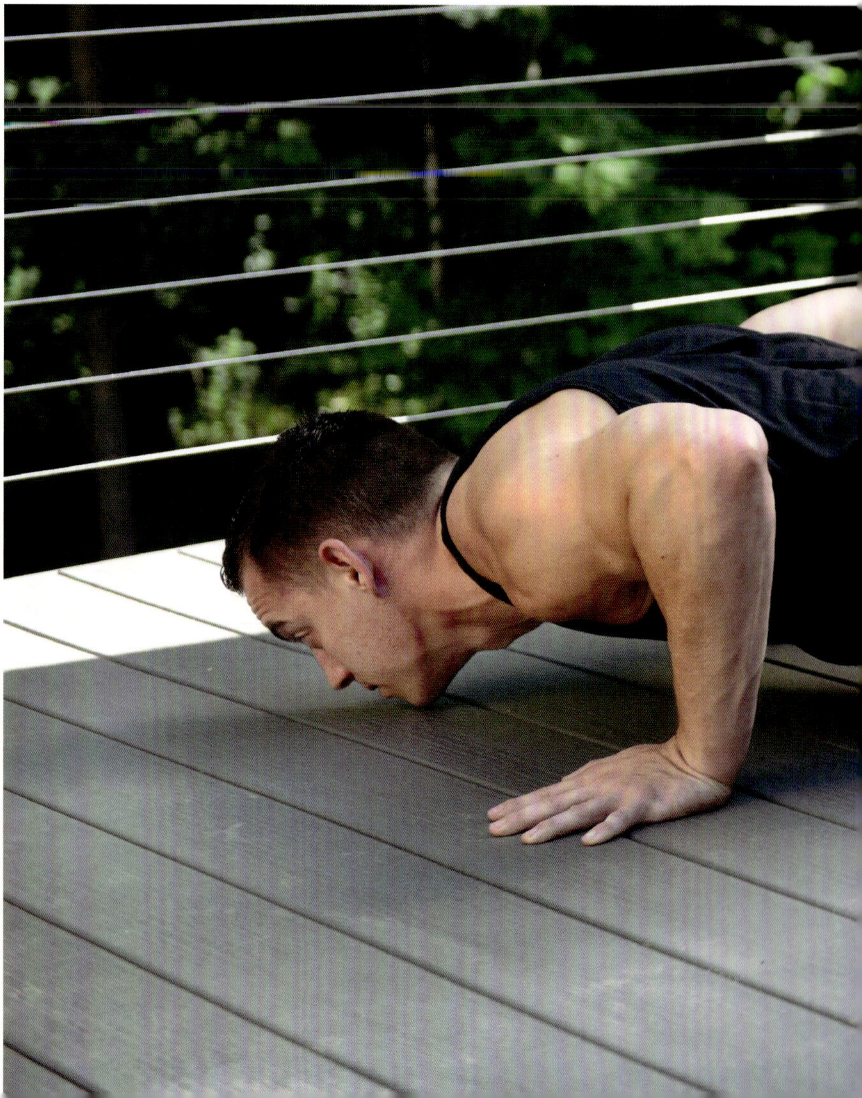

MORE DIFFICULT ||||||||||||||||||||
Modify points of contact: Change hand position to a military, diamond, or staggered push-up position to decrease leverage and stability.

LESS DIFFICULT ||||||||||||||||||||
Modify body angle: During the entire exercise, use any available prop to elevate your upper body into an incline.

X marks the spot. Push-up jacks require incredible trunk stability and core strength and they will help you find some buried treasure—your six-pack abs.

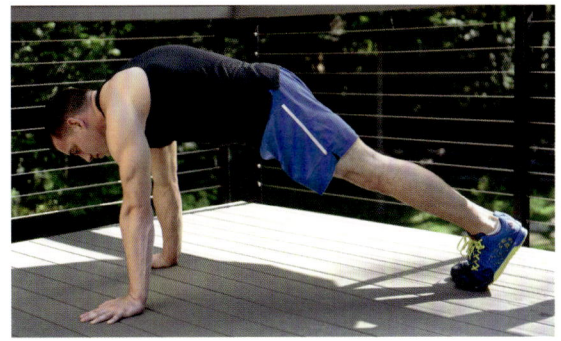

03 Push up through your hands, straightening the arms and hopping the feet closed to return to the starting position. Repeat steps 2 and 3 with controlled speed for the prescribed number of reps.

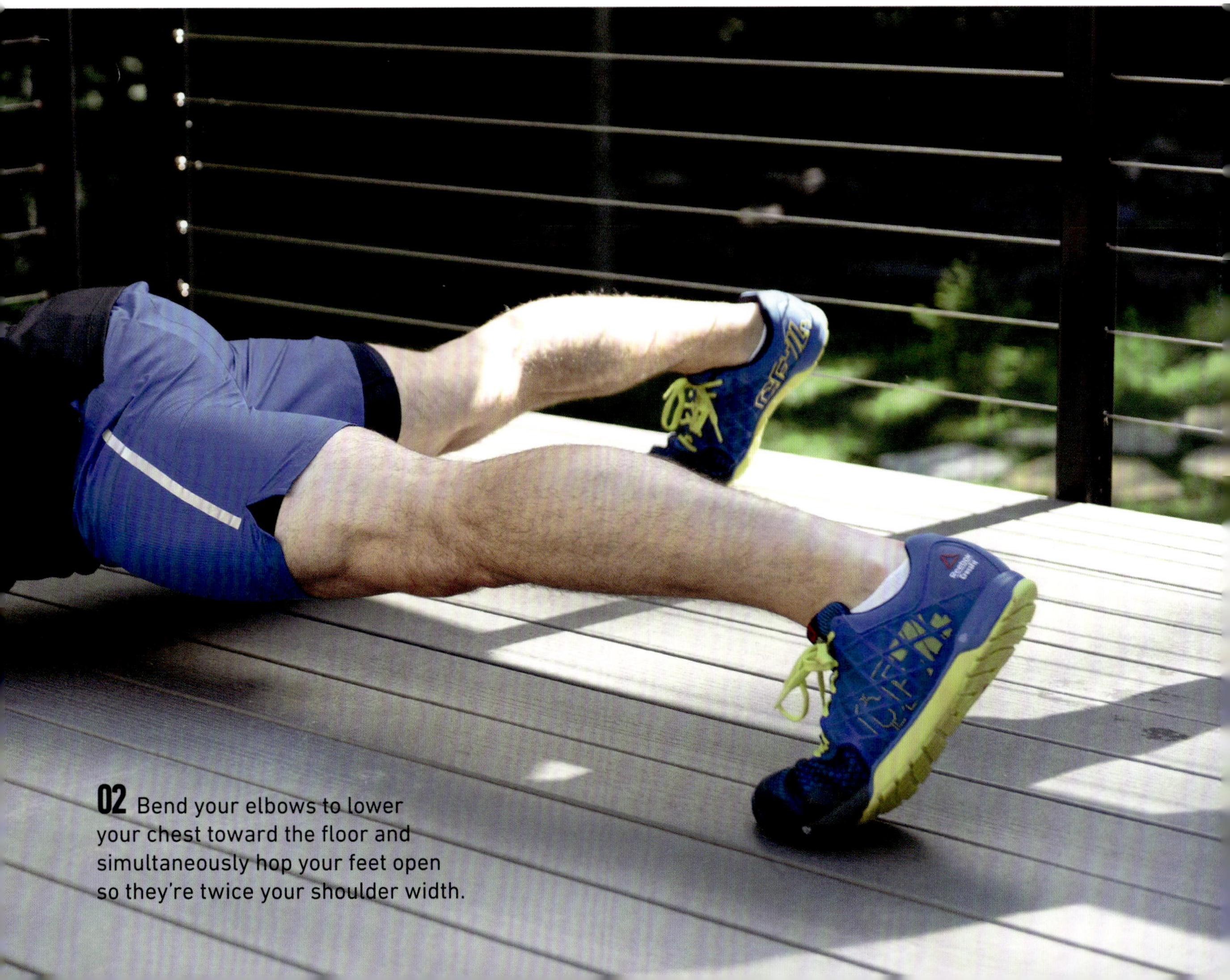

02 Bend your elbows to lower your chest toward the floor and simultaneously hop your feet open so they're twice your shoulder width.

CROSS PUSH

Increased core stability makes the cross push a must-do exercise! As your body weight shifts during the crossing phase of the exercise, the muscles used to stabilize your spine (obliques, transverse abdominals, and erector spinae) all engage, helping to build a stronger, tighter tummy.

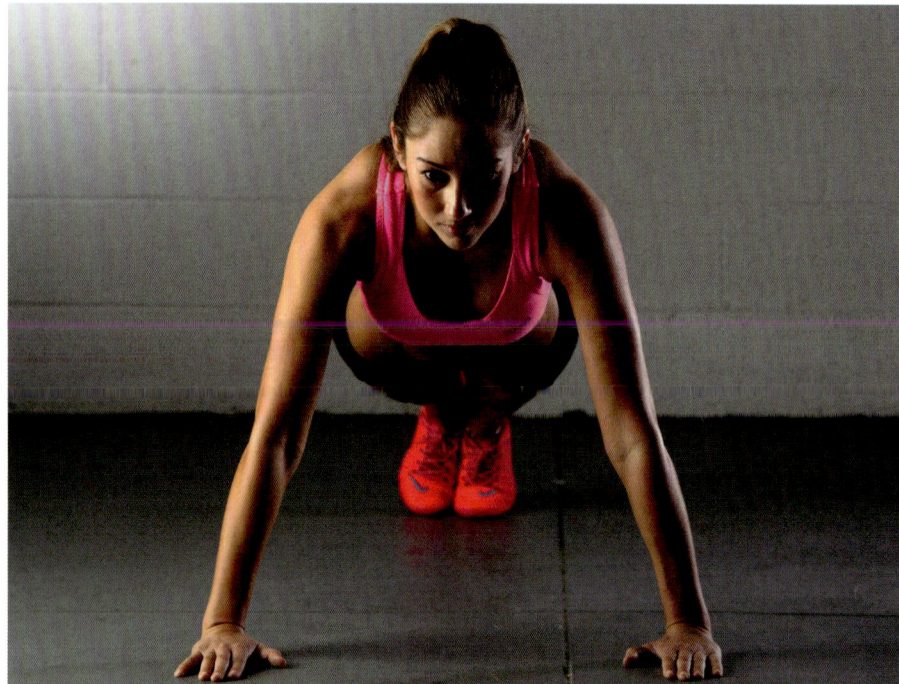

01 Assume a full plank position, with your hands slightly wider than shoulder-width apart and your body forming a straight line from ankles to head. Engage the core.

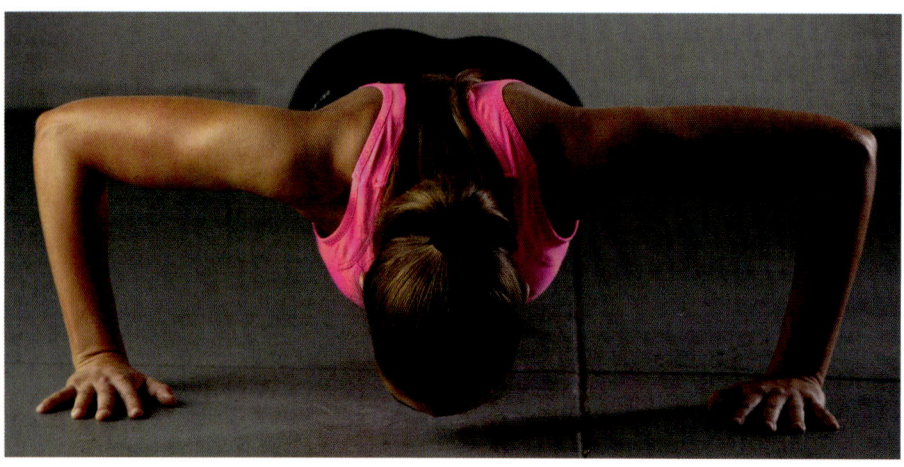

02 Bend your elbows, lowering your chest toward the floor. Once your elbows are slightly beyond 90 degrees, push up through your palms, extending the arms.

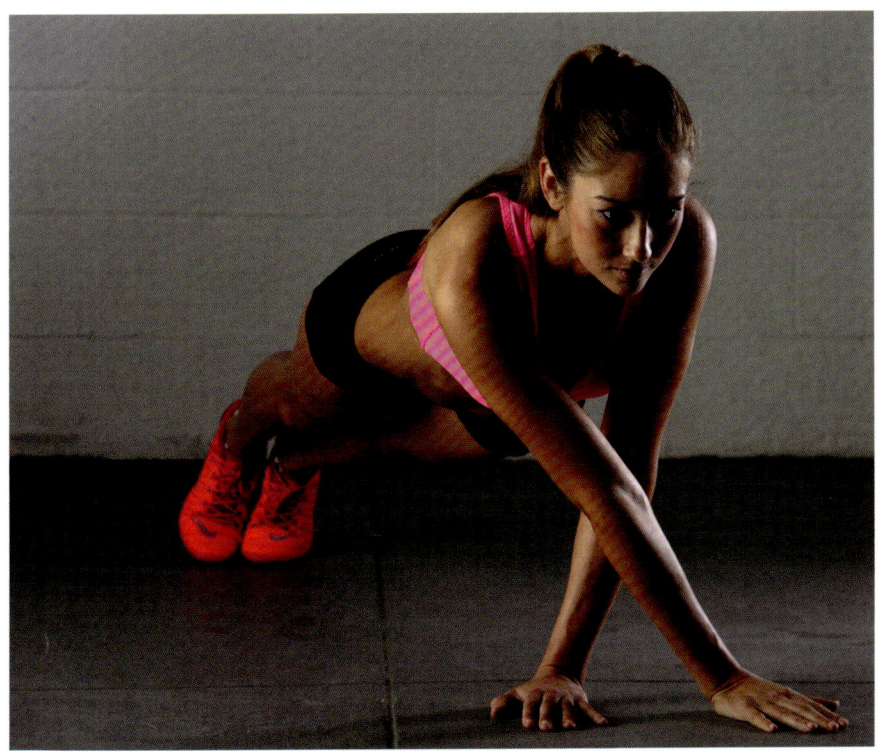

03 Bring your right hand across the body and briefly place the palm of your right hand on the floor just outside of the left hand. Return the right hand to the starting position. Repeat, alternating the crossing arm.

LESS DIFFICULT ||||||||||
Drop your knees: place your knees on the floor for stability and support.

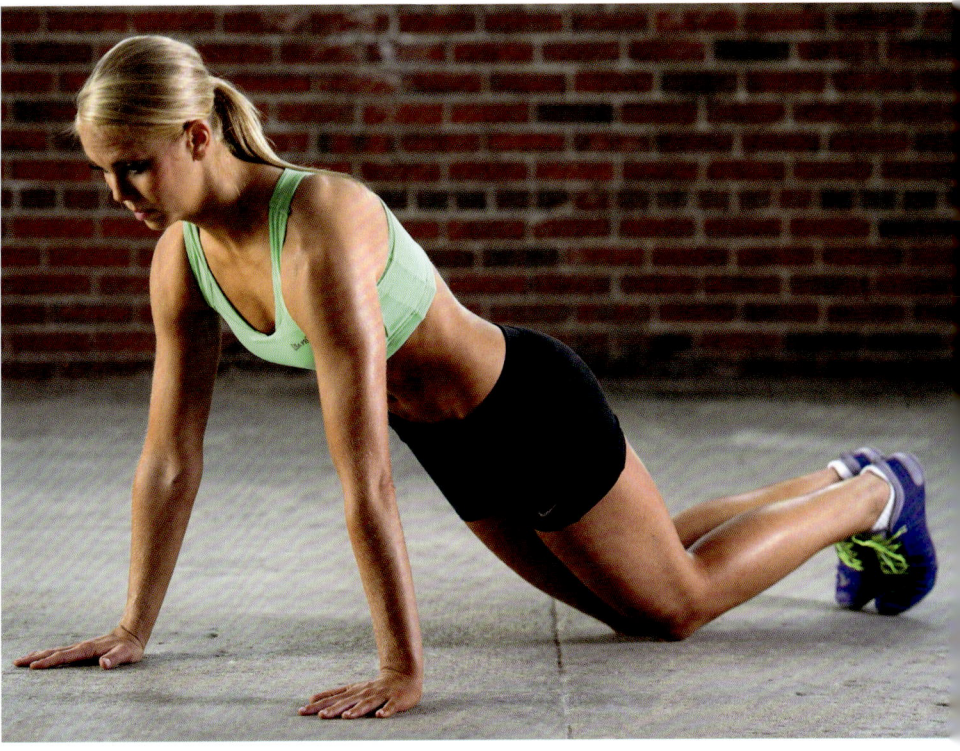

MILITARY PUSH-UP

Military push-ups change the hand position, exerting greater pressure on the triceps than a standard push-up. Narrowing the hand width decreases the base of support, challenging the core.

MORE DIFFICULT ||||||||||||||||||||
Modify body angle: In all steps, elevate your feet on a chair or box to decline the body and transfer weight into the upper body and core.

LESS DIFFICULT ||||||||||||||||||||
Modify body angle: In all steps, elevate your upper body (or kneel) to decrease the weight being moved by arms and shoulders.

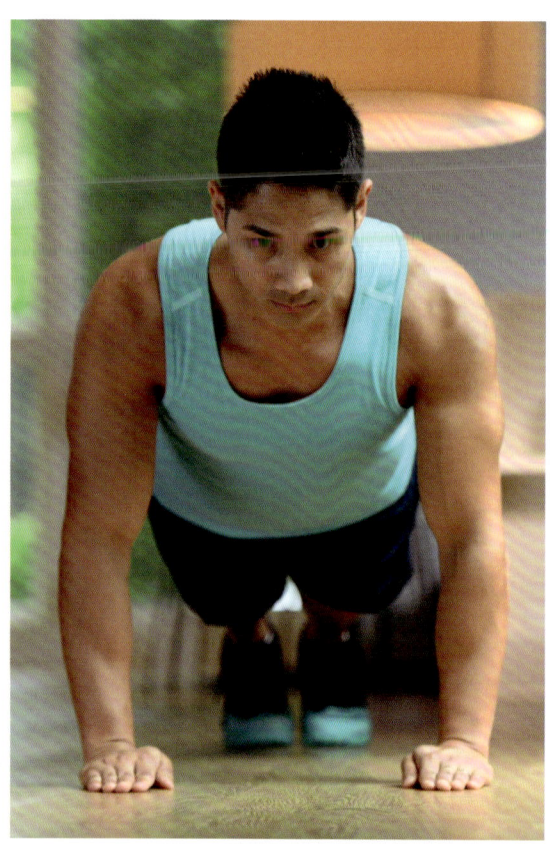

01 Assume a full plank or traditional push-up position, with the body balanced between the toes and hands. Position the hands directly under the shoulders, but not wider than the shoulders.

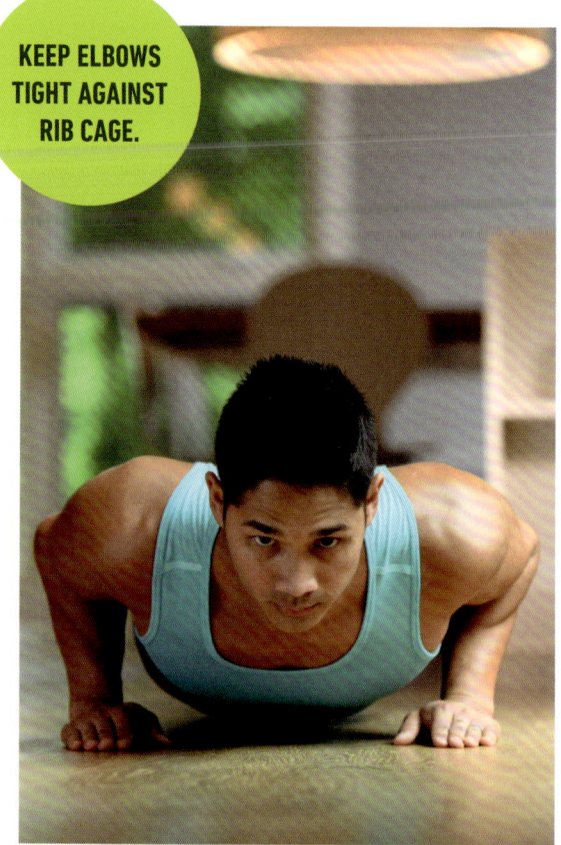

KEEP ELBOWS TIGHT AGAINST RIB CAGE.

02 Keeping the elbows and arms tight against your sides, bend your elbows and lower your body to the floor.

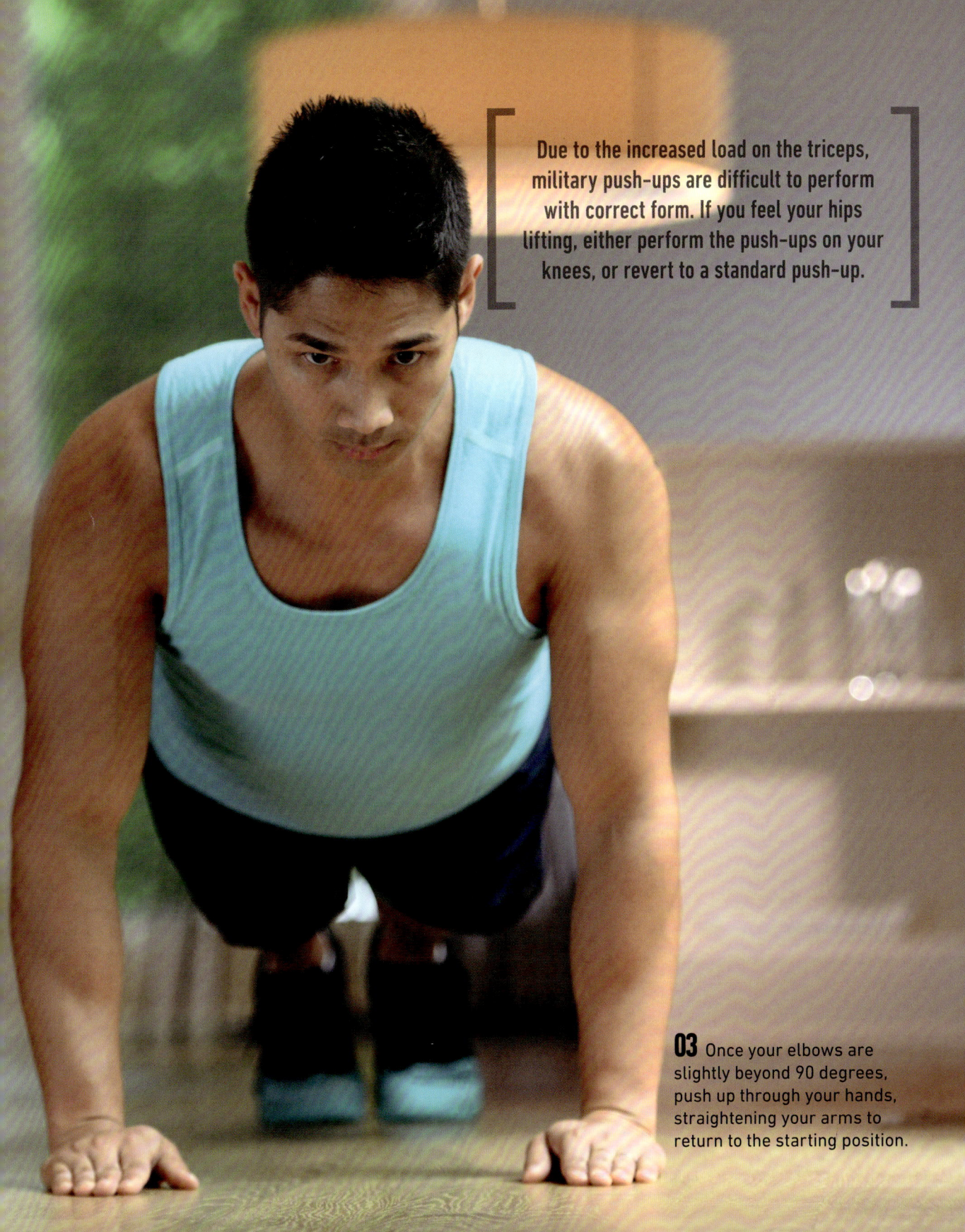

Due to the increased load on the triceps, military push-ups are difficult to perform with correct form. If you feel your hips lifting, either perform the push-ups on your knees, or revert to a standard push-up.

03 Once your elbows are slightly beyond 90 degrees, push up through your hands, straightening your arms to return to the starting position.

ARCHER PULL-UP

Archer pull-ups are the bridge between regular pull-ups and single-arm ones. The motion replicates drawing a bow to shoot an arrow, generating single-arm strength and power.

MORE DIFFICULT ||||||||||||||||||||
Modify speed: In step 3, slowly lower back down to the hanging position over a count of four to accentuate the eccentric muscle contraction and build power.

LESS DIFFICULT ||||||||||||||||||||
Modify stability: Use a resistance band, or place one foot on a chair to increase stability and decrease the amount of weight being moved, and to provide assistance.

> Avoid momentum, don't swing, and pay particular attention to the deceleration—the slow lowering or eccentric contraction—by controlling your descent.

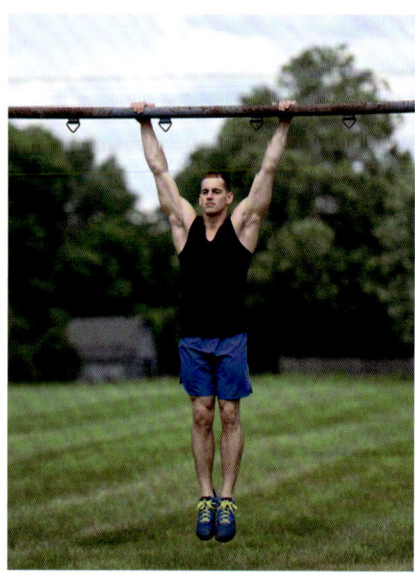

01 Position yourself directly under the pull-up bar. Hop up and grab the bar with an overhand grip (palms facing away) wider than your shoulders. Hang from the bar with arms straight.

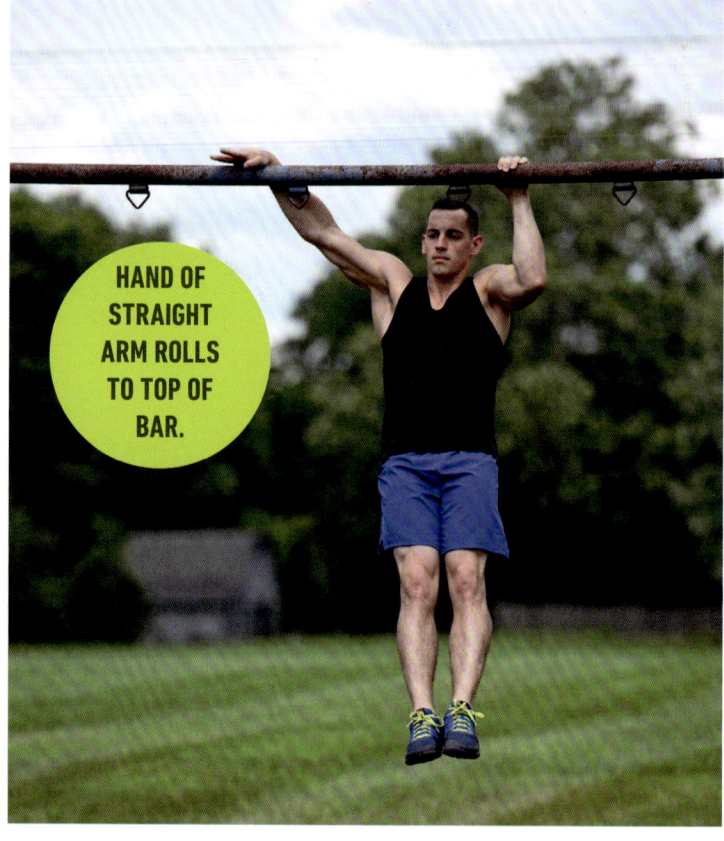

HAND OF STRAIGHT ARM ROLLS TO TOP OF BAR.

02 Pull yourself up to the left, tucking your left elbow tight to the chest so your right arm is extended across the width of the bar, parallel to the ground, at the top of the pull-up.

BALL PRESS

The ball press combines an isolation hold with a press to make your quads, thighs, calves, and butt burn while sculpting your shoulders, back, and arms. Keep your movements quick and explosive while maintaining proper form.

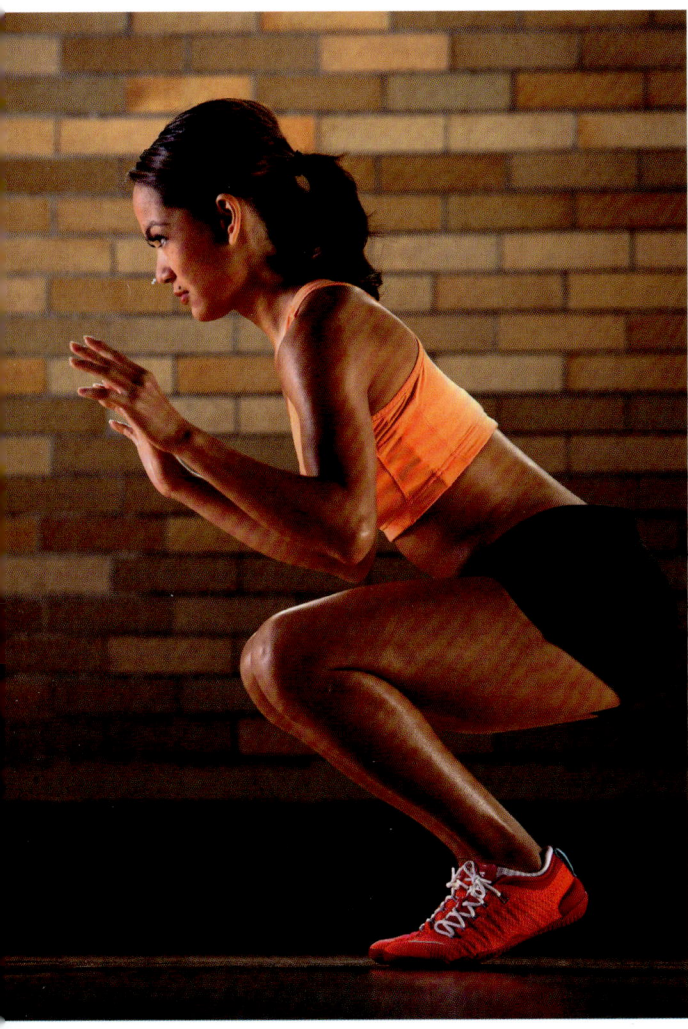

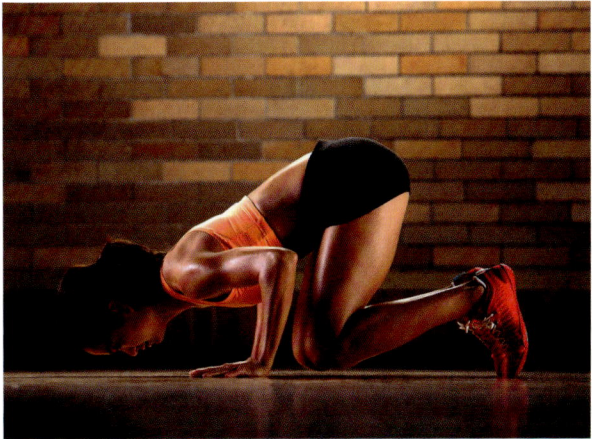

02 Allow your body to fall forward, catching yourself with your hands and lowering into a mini push-up.

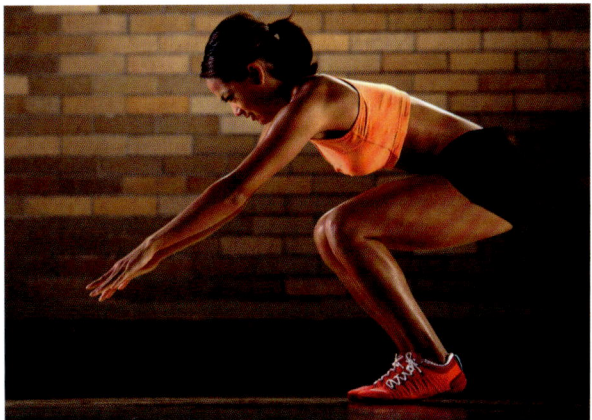

01 Stand with feet hip-width apart. Rise onto the balls of your feet and lower into a squat position by bending at the hips and knees. Hold your hands in front of your chest with arms bent. This is the "ball" position.

03 Drive aggressively through the hands to extend the arms and project yourself back onto the balls of your feet, never leaving the "ball" position.

CHIN-UP

Chin-ups are a bodyweight training essential because they work the biceps, back, and core while supercharging your metabolism.

ISOLATE BACK, SQUEEZE BICEPS. DON'T SWING!

MORE DIFFICULT |||||||||||||||||||||||
Modify speed: In step 3, lower slowly, straightening arms over a count of four to produce an eccentric muscle contraction that builds strength.

LESS DIFFICULT |||||||||||||||||||||||
Modify points of contact and stability: For all steps, use a resistance band or place your foot on a chair to assist the chin-up by adding leverage.

01 Position yourself directly under your pull-up bar. Hop up and grab the bar with an underhand (palms facing you/supine) shoulder-width grip and hang from the bar with straight arms.

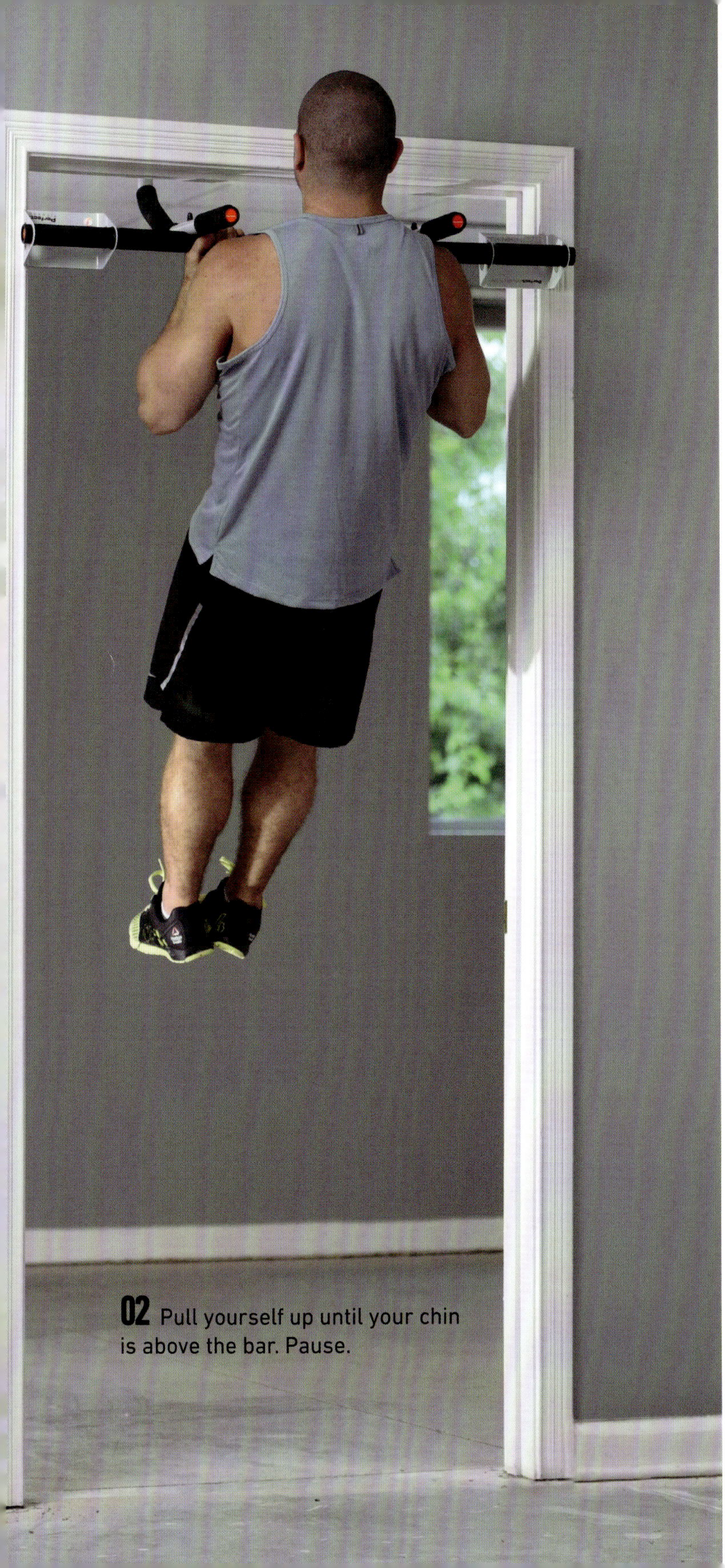

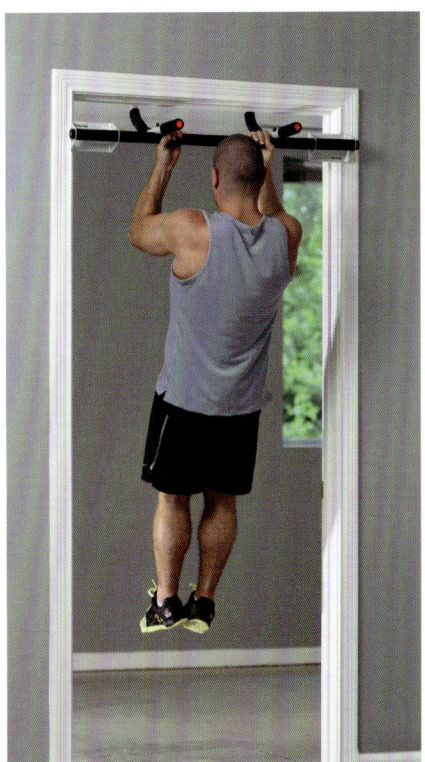

03 Lower yourself down with control. Repeat steps 2 and 3 as prescribed.

Chin-ups are slightly easier than pull-ups because the supine position of the hands allows for greater activation of the biceps.

02 Pull yourself up until your chin is above the bar. Pause.

SPHINX

Named after the Egyptian statue, this exercise combines a forearm plank and push-up to work the chest, triceps, back, core, and hips. It is essential to engage your core throughout this exercise for stability and to protect your lower back.

If you find it difficult to extend both arms at the same time, build strength by extending one at a time. Follow a pattern of up, up, down, down, switching the lead arm with every rep.

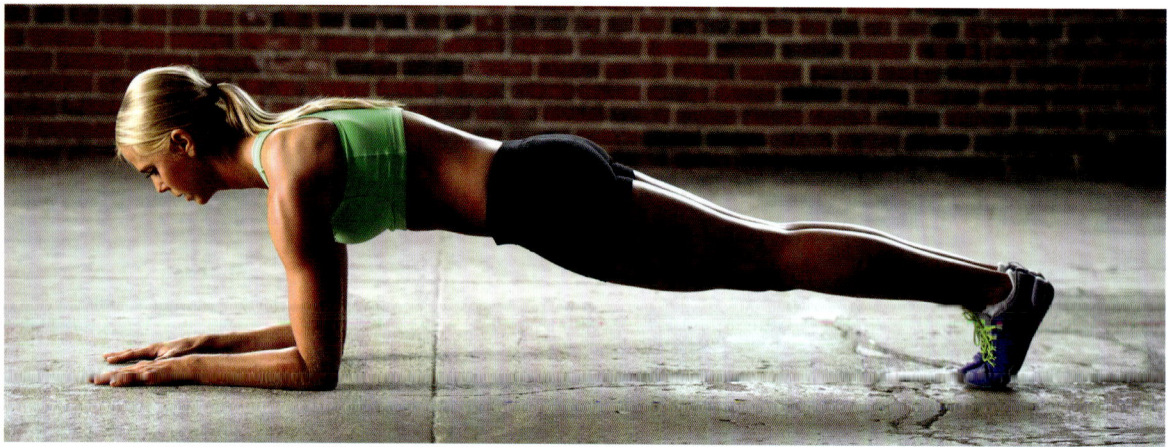

01 Start in a basic forearm plank position. Your body weight should be evenly balanced between your forearms and toes. Open your hands so that your palms are flat on the floor. Keep your core engaged and body straight.

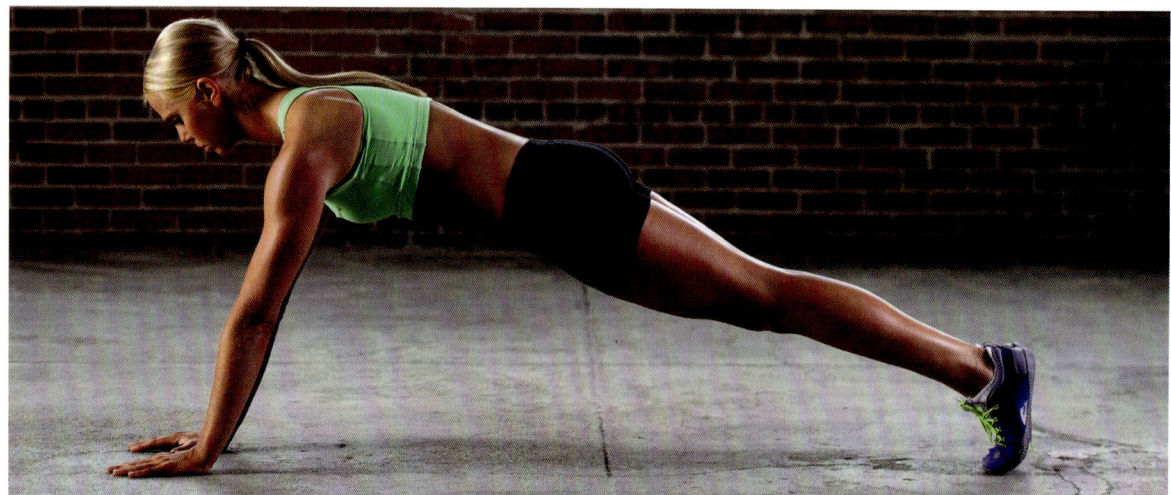

02 Push down through the palms of your hands, elevating your body until arms are straight. Slowly lower back down into a forearm plank and repeat.

SPIDERMAN

This variation on the push-up is inspired by the agile superhero of the same name. It will increase hip mobility and flexibility, and build core strength.

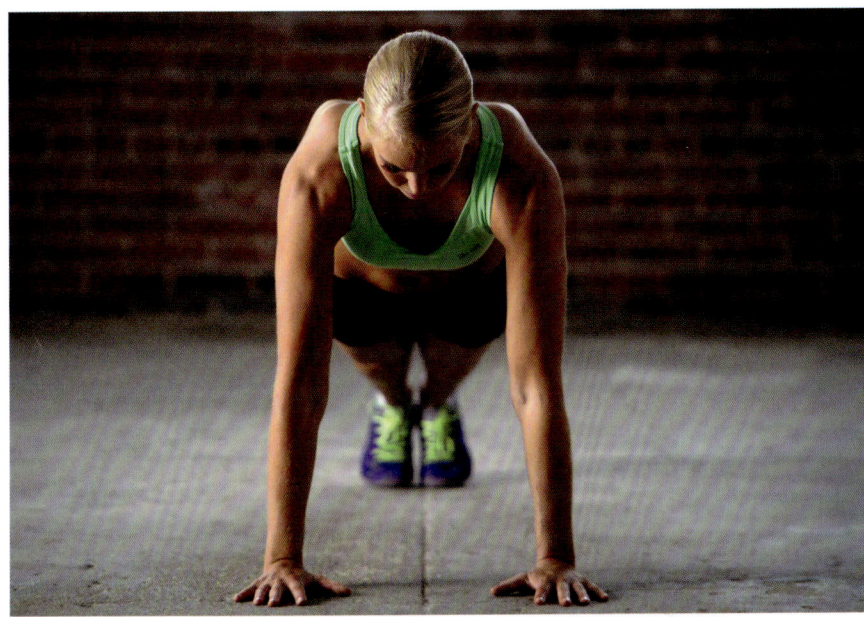

01 Assume a standard push-up position, with palms just wider than shoulders, arms straight, and body in a straight line balanced between arms and toes.

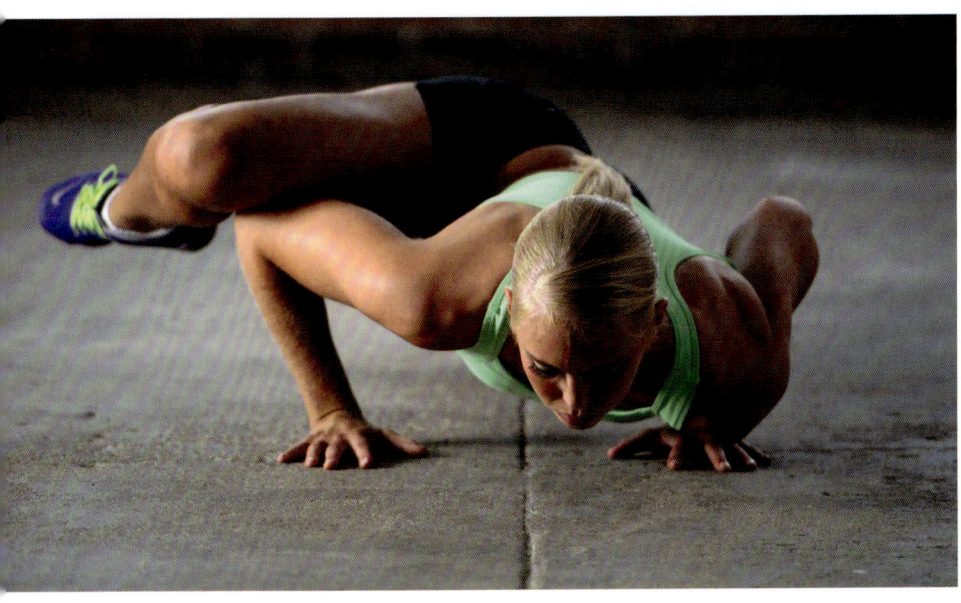

02 Bend your arms, bringing the chest down as you lift your right foot off the floor. Swing the right leg out sideways, bring your right knee up toward your right shoulder.

Bring your right foot back to the floor and push your body back to the starting position. Repeat, alternating legs.

INVERTED BODYWEIGHT ROW

This exercise balances the muscles used in push-ups and bench presses, helping with back strength and shoulder stability.

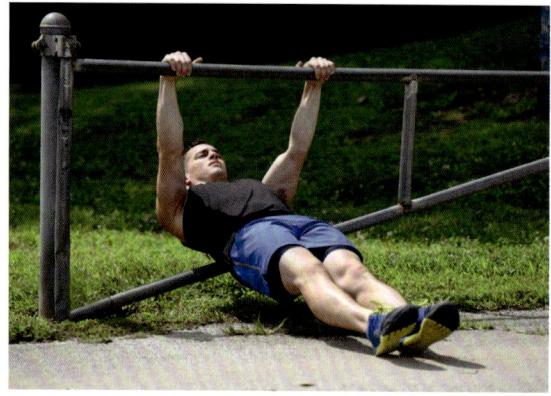

01 Lie on your back directly under the bar. Grab the bar with an overhand grip (palms facing away), and your hands wider than your shoulders.

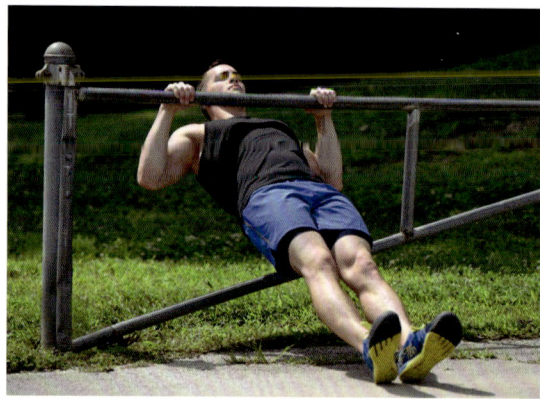

02 Pull yourself up until your chest touches the bar. Pause.

MORE DIFFICULT ||||||||||||||||||||||
Modify stability and range of motion:
Raise a foot to decrease stability and challenge trunk stabilization. Switch feet halfway through the reps.

LESS DIFFICULT ||||||||||||||||||||||
Modify stability and points of contact:
Perform this exercise standing or seated with a resistance band to build confidence.

Keep your scapular retraction going during both the concentric and eccentric motions of the row. More specifically, try to pinch your shoulder blades together for the entire duration of the exercise.

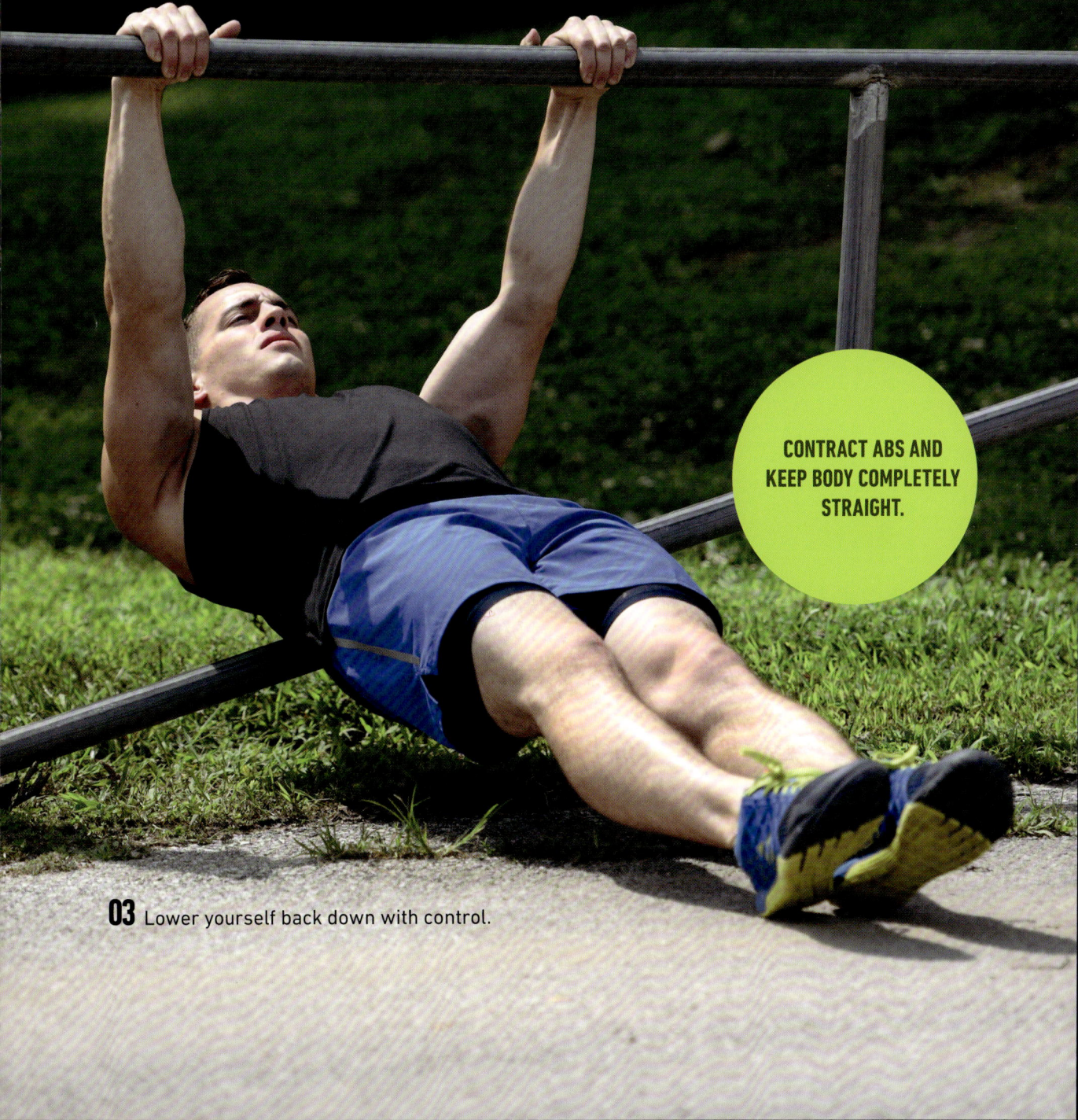

CONTRACT ABS AND KEEP BODY COMPLETELY STRAIGHT.

03 Lower yourself back down with control.

1-2 PUSH

The 1-2 push is an intense, full-body move that will elevate your heart rate while working your core, arms, and legs. Complete the move as quickly as you can, but remember that correct form takes priority.

MORE DIFFICULT |||||||||||||||||||||
Modify range of motion: In step 3, add a plyometric (clap) push-up to generate explosive upper-body power.

LESS DIFFICULT |||||||||||||||||||||
Modify body angle: For all steps, place your hands on a tall prop, shifting most of the weight into the lower body.

01 Begin in the plank position with hands on the floor slightly wider than shoulders, legs extended, and on your toes. Engage the core and form a straight line from ankles to head.

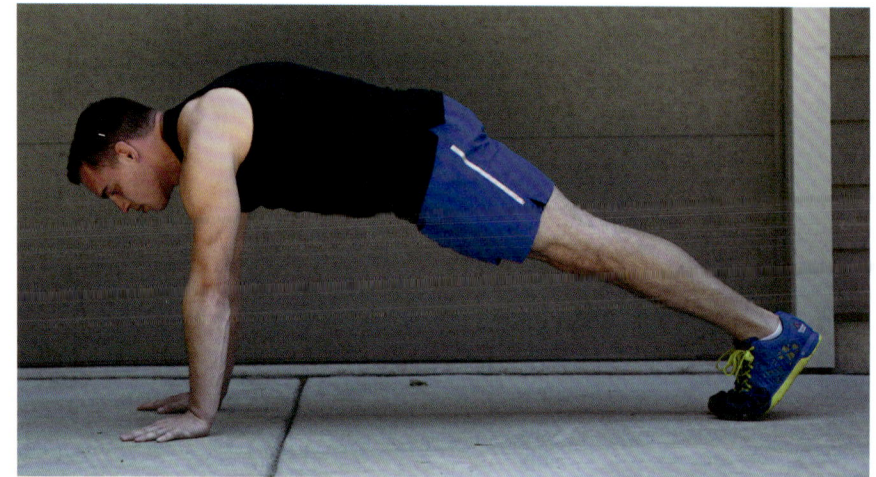

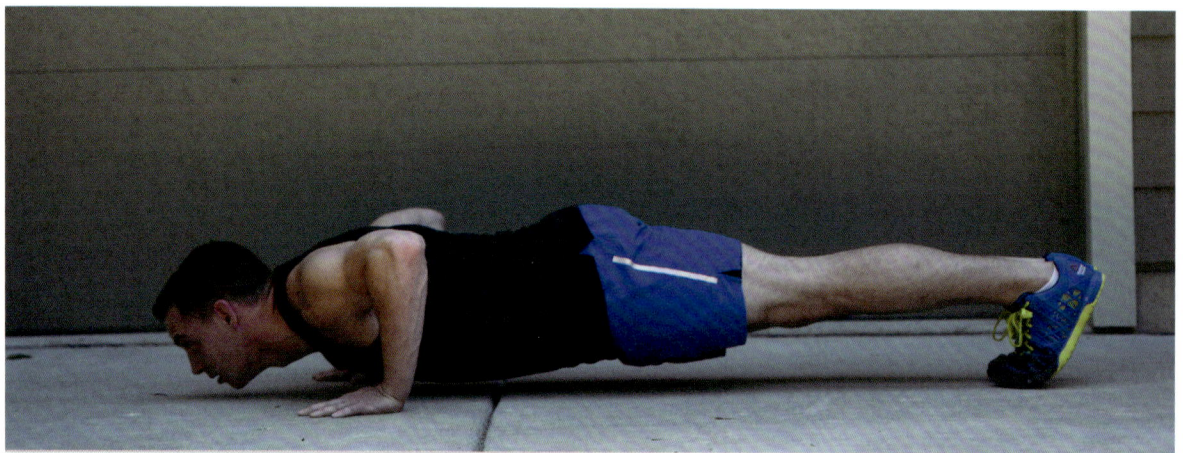

02 Bend your elbows, bringing the chest toward the floor until your elbows are bent slightly beyond 90 degrees.

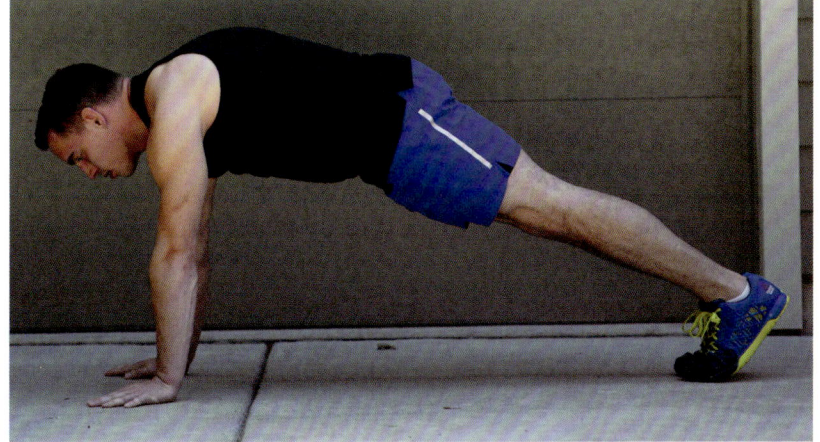

[
Remember: Form comes first, speed second.
]

BRING KNEES COMPLETELY THROUGH ELBOWS.

03 Push up off the floor and straighten the arms.

04 As arms reach full extension, bring your right knee to your chest and quickly switch legs, bringing the left knee to the chest. Then return to the starting position. Repeat steps 2 through 4, alternating legs.

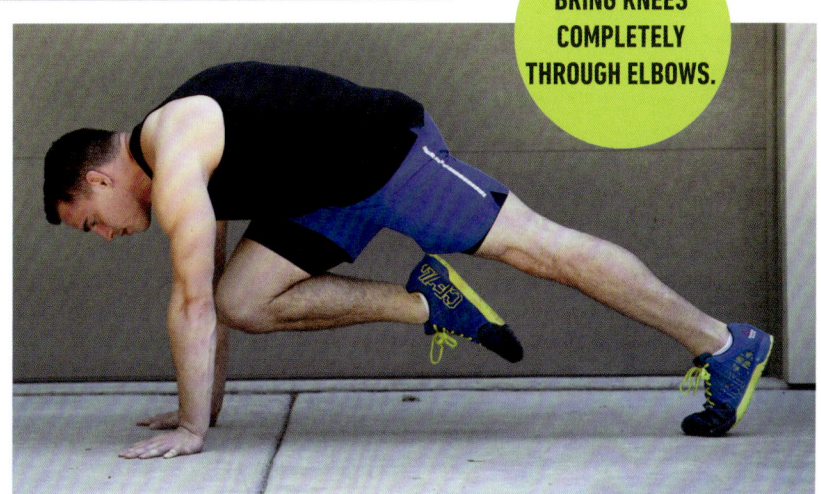

CHALLENGE

By changing the angle of the legs when you bring the knee to the chest, you can create greater activation of the obliques.

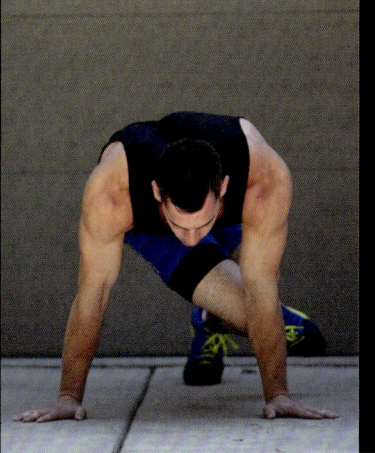

DIAGONAL MOUNTAIN CLIMBER

In the last step, take the knee across the body to the opposite elbow.

PULL-UP

Pull-ups are hands-down the best exercise for your upper back, and arguably one of the best exercises for the human body.

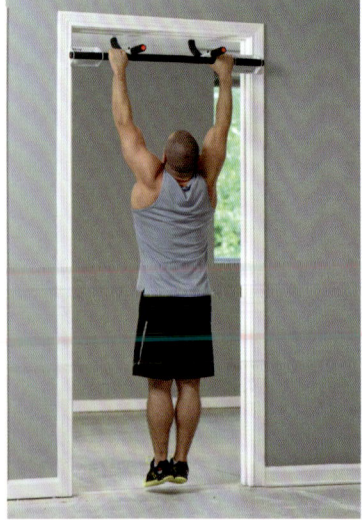

01 Hop up and grab the pull-up bar with an overhand grip (palms facing away) wider than your shoulders, and hang from the bar with straight arms.

MORE DIFFICULT |||||||||||||||||||||||
Modify speed: In step 3, slowly straighten your arms as you lower over a count of four to perform an eccentric muscle contraction that builds strength.

LESS DIFFICULT |||||||||||||||||||||||
Modify points of contact and stability: For the entire exercise, use a band or place a foot on a chair to assist the pull-up by adding leverage.

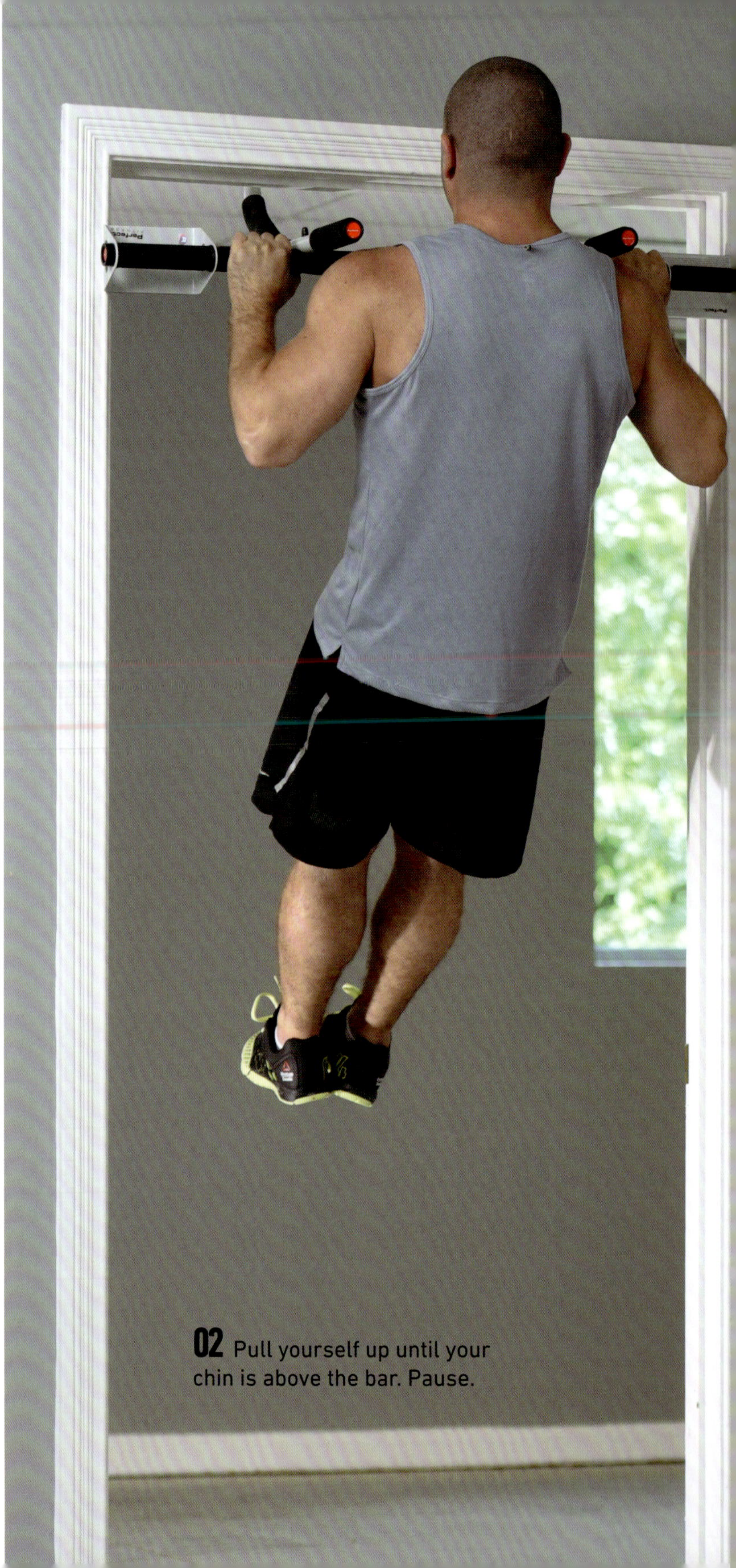

02 Pull yourself up until your chin is above the bar. Pause.

ISOLATE BACK
AND BICEPS.
DON'T SWING!

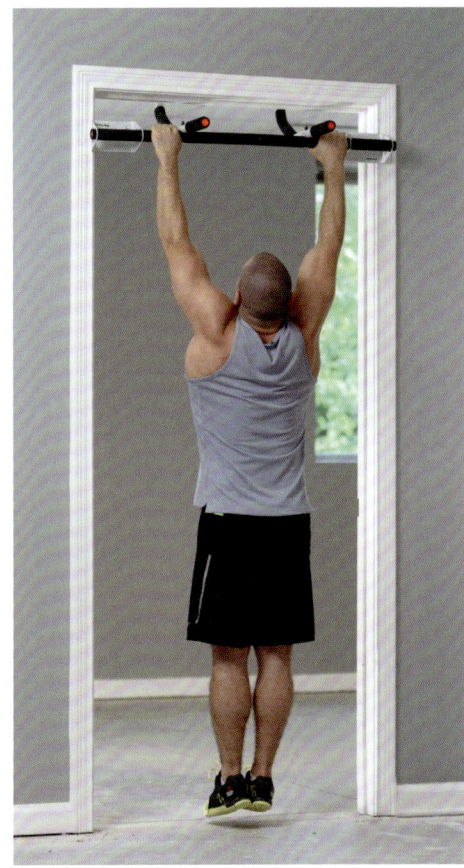

03 Lower yourself down with control. Repeat only steps 2 and 3 when performing reps.

The Guinness World Record for most pull-ups in one minute is 77 repetitions, performed by Adam Sandel on April 20, 2024.

CORE
EXERCISES

HIGH KNEES

This is an excellent exercise for runners and athletes who want to improve running form and foot speed. The dynamic running motion will challenge your cardiovascular endurance and help to strengthen your hip flexors.

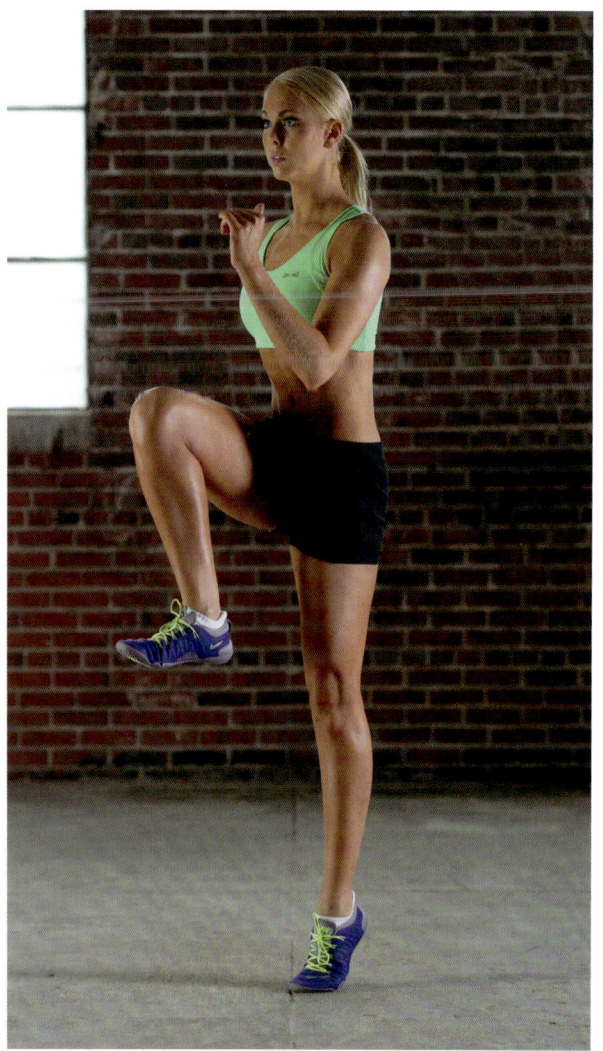

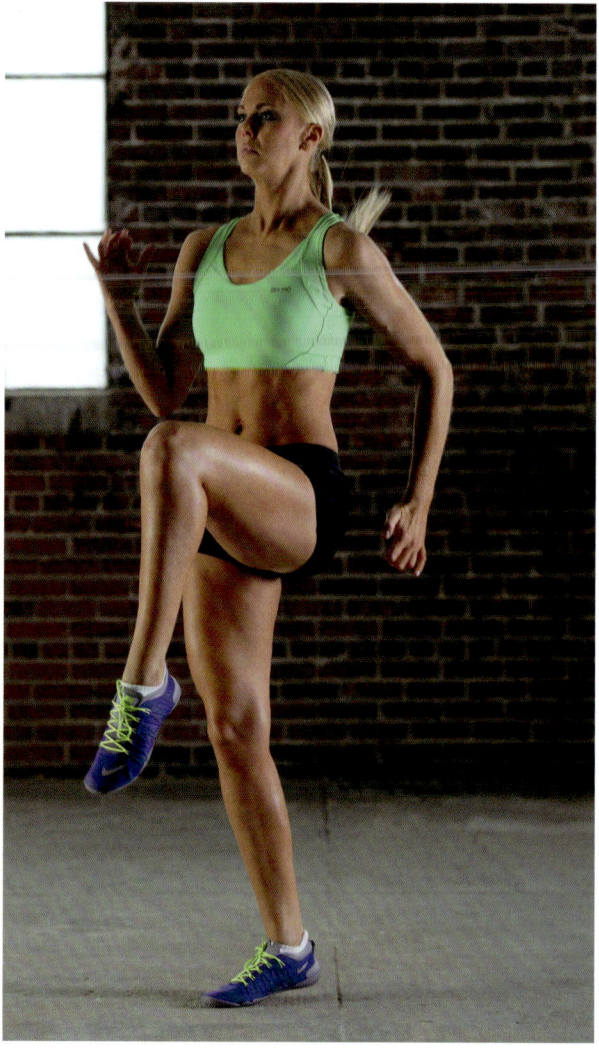

01 Stand with feet hip-width apart. Drive your right knee toward your chest and quickly place it back on the ground.

02 Immediately follow by driving the left knee to the chest. Alternate knees as quickly as you can. Bring your knees to your belly button or higher.

HANGING LEG RAISE

This is the Holy Grail of abdominal exercises! It will build a bulletproof core, increase grip strength and flexibility, and decompress your spine.

MORE DIFFICULT ||||||||||||||||||||
Modify range of motion: In step 2, bring your toes to touch the bar between your hands. This almost doubles the working range of the exercise and increases the work for abs, back, and hips.

LESS DIFFICULT ||||||||||||||||||||
Modify points of contact: In preparation for eventually performing a hanging exercise, start by practicing leg raises on the floor to increase stability and focus on controlling the raising and lowering of the legs.

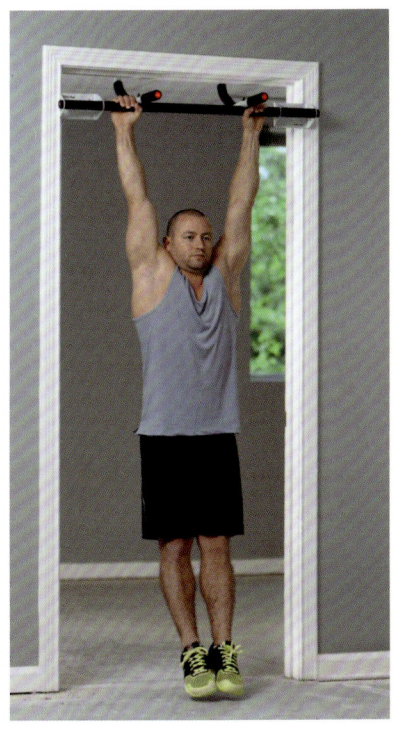

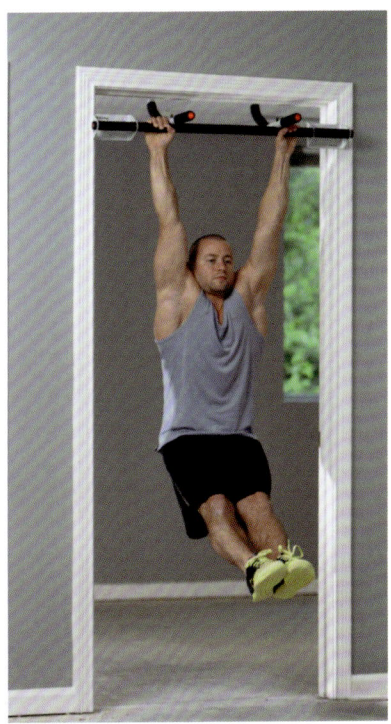

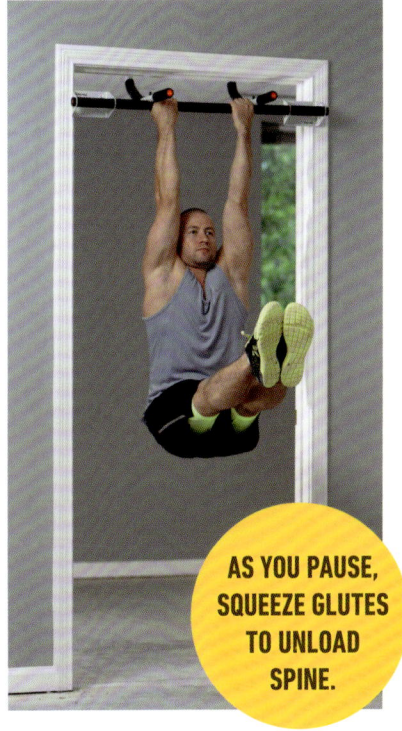

AS YOU PAUSE, SQUEEZE GLUTES TO UNLOAD SPINE.

01 Stand directly under the pull-up bar. Hop up and grab the bar with an overhand grip (palms facing away), hands wider than shoulders, and hang with arms straight.

02 With shoulders open and packed and legs kept straight, raise your legs with control until they're just beyond parallel to the floor. Pause for 2 seconds.

03 Lower your legs under control, and repeat.

SQUAT TO L-SIT

This total-body exercise utilizes the lower body and core, and it also engages the hip flexors and triceps isometrically.

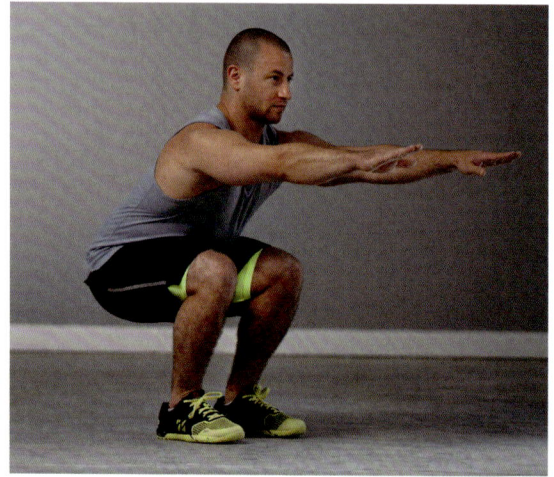

02 Inhale and lower into a deep squat (glutes below knees) as if trying to make glutes touch the back of the calves, arms extended for balance.

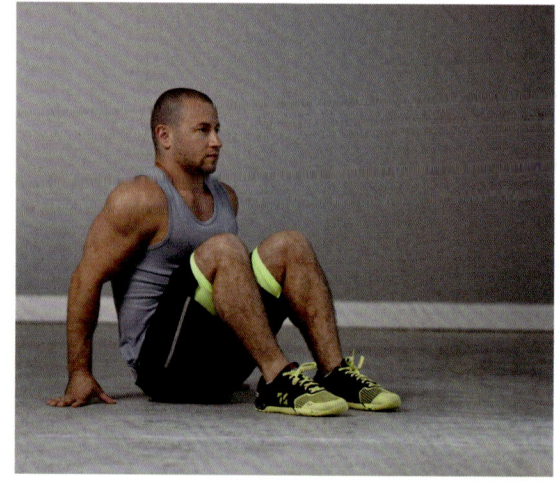

03 Place your hands on the floor slightly behind your hips, and sit, weight shifted back, palms directly under shoulders, fingertips facing out.

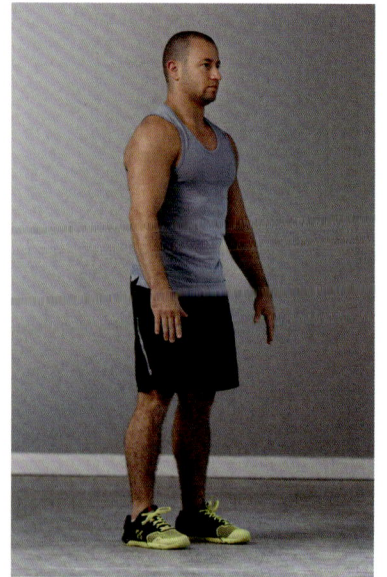

01 Stand tall, with your feet hip-width apart and toes pointing forward.

MORE DIFFICULT ||||||||||||||||||||||
Modify speed: Hold both steps 2 and 5 for a count of four to build strength in the toughest two phases of the exercise.

LESS DIFFICULT ||||||||||||||||||||||
Modify range of motion: In step 5, either extend the legs partially or simply hold them off the floor in a tucked position.

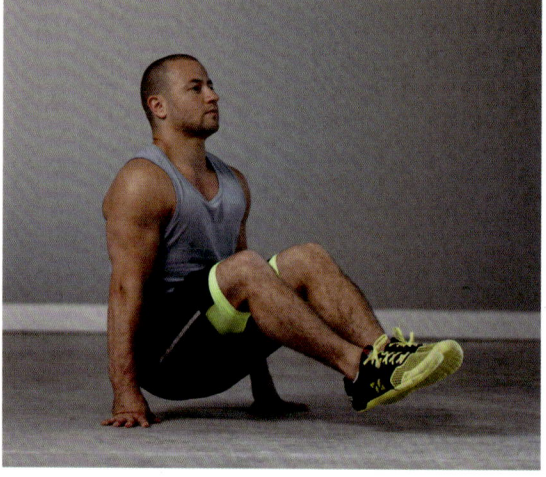

04 Push into the floor with your hands, straighten your arms, and bring your shoulders down in order to lift your butt off the floor.

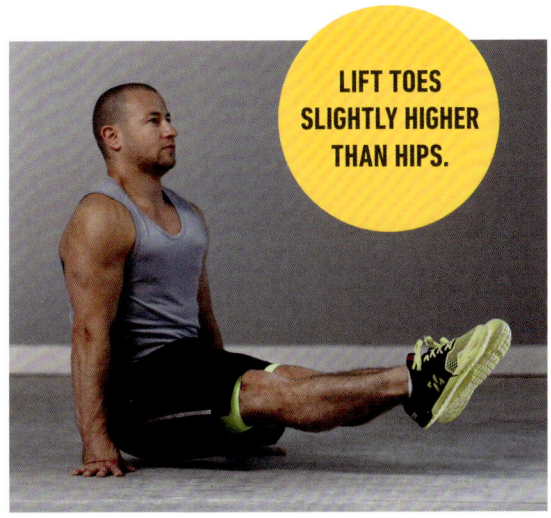

LIFT TOES SLIGHTLY HIGHER THAN HIPS.

05 Straighten and elevate the legs, squeezing the inner thighs and pointing the toes. Hold this position briefly.

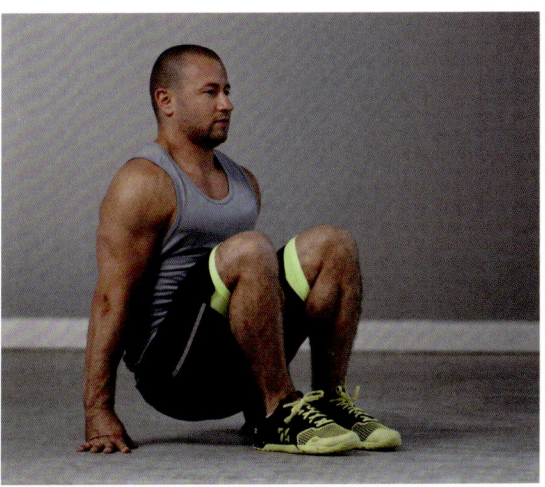

06 Bend and then lower the legs, placing the soles of your feet on the floor.

The deeper you can sit into your squat, the easier the transition to L-sit will become.

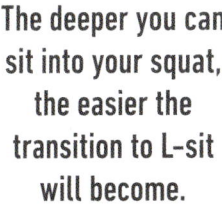

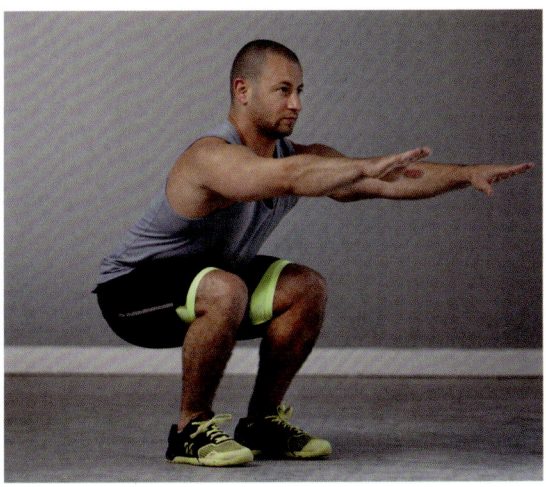

07 Extend your arms in front of you for balance and lift your hips from the floor, rocking yourself slightly forward into a deep squat.

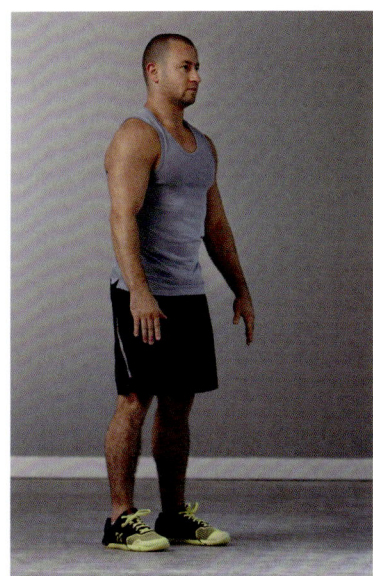

08 Straighten your legs and stand tall, engaging the core, squeezing the glutes, and tucking the hips under.

HOLLOW BODY ROCKER

While the motion is only small, adding a "rock" to the hollow body position will challenge your core like never before!

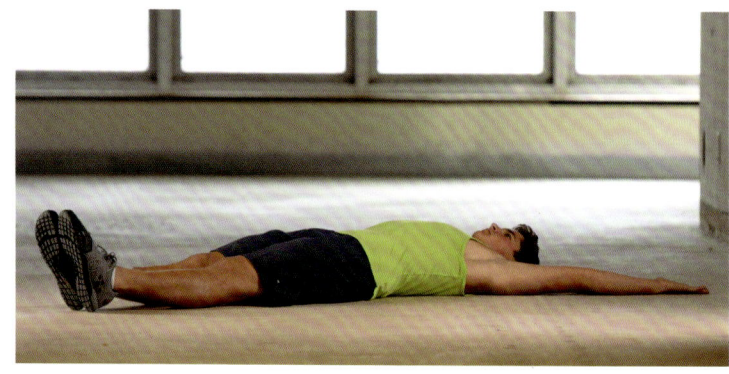

01 Lie on your back with arms and legs extended, pull your belly button in toward the floor, and tuck your pelvis to connect your lower back to the floor.

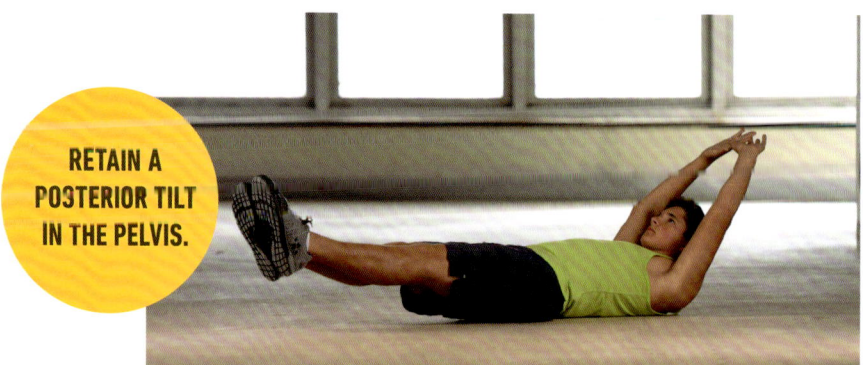

RETAIN A POSTERIOR TILT IN THE PELVIS.

02 Slowly raise your legs, shoulders, and head off the floor. Hold this "hollow" curved position as you proceed to the next step.

MORE DIFFICULT ||||||||||||||||||||
Modify range of motion: In step 3, rock until your hips lift off the floor to increase the range of motion and generate greater force for your core to control.

LESS DIFFICULT ||||||||||||||||||||
Modify speed: Omit step 3. Instead, hold the position in step 2, building strength and preparing to add motion later.

03 Gently rock back and forth on the curve of your lower back. Don't swing your arms or legs. Rock for the duration of the exercise.

PLANK

This deceptively simple exercise is the secret to rock-hard abs. The plank position engages the transverse abdominals, which aid in stabilization of the spine and pull in the tummy. It helps develop strength in the core, shoulders, and glutes.

MORE DIFFICULT |||||||||||||||||||||
Supercharge your plank with these modifications.

Lift one leg: Lift one leg and extend it upward. Keep your hips square with the ground and resist the urge to rotate.

Lift one arm: Extend one arm straight out in front of you.

Use a stability ball: Rest your forearms on the ball while keeping your toes on the floor.

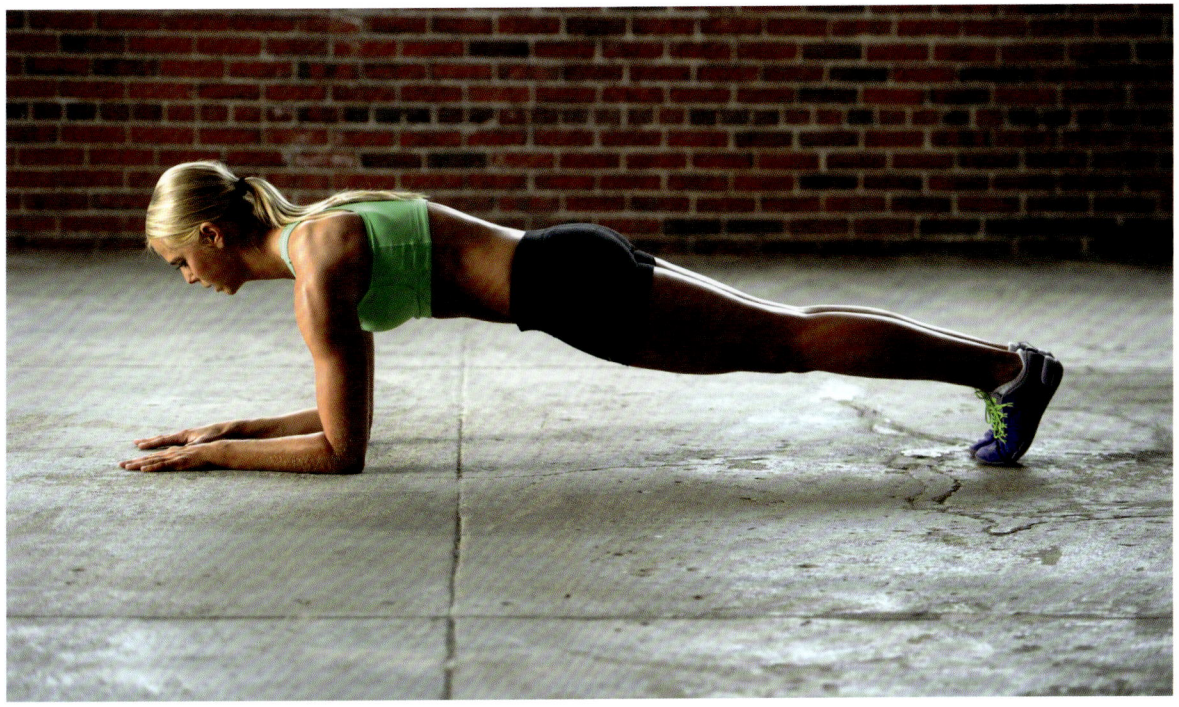

Place your forearms on the floor and extend your legs until your body is balanced between your toes and forearms. Your elbows should be directly beneath your shoulders, and your body should form a straight line from head to heels. Keep your eyes directly over your hands.

BACK BRIDGE

Stretch the front of your body, strengthen the muscles supporting your spine, and work almost every muscle on the back of the body in this familiar and fun exercise.

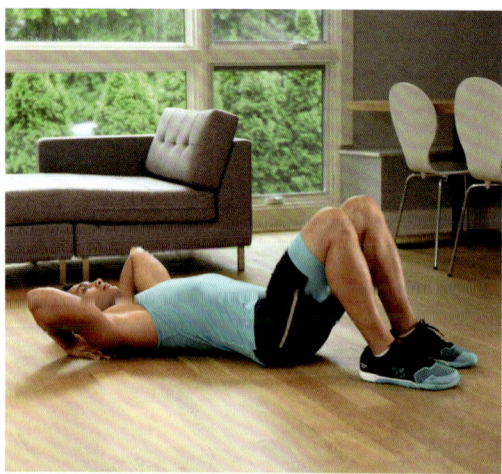

01 Lie on your back on the floor with knees and elbows bent, palms on the floor by the side of your head, and fingers pointing at your toes.

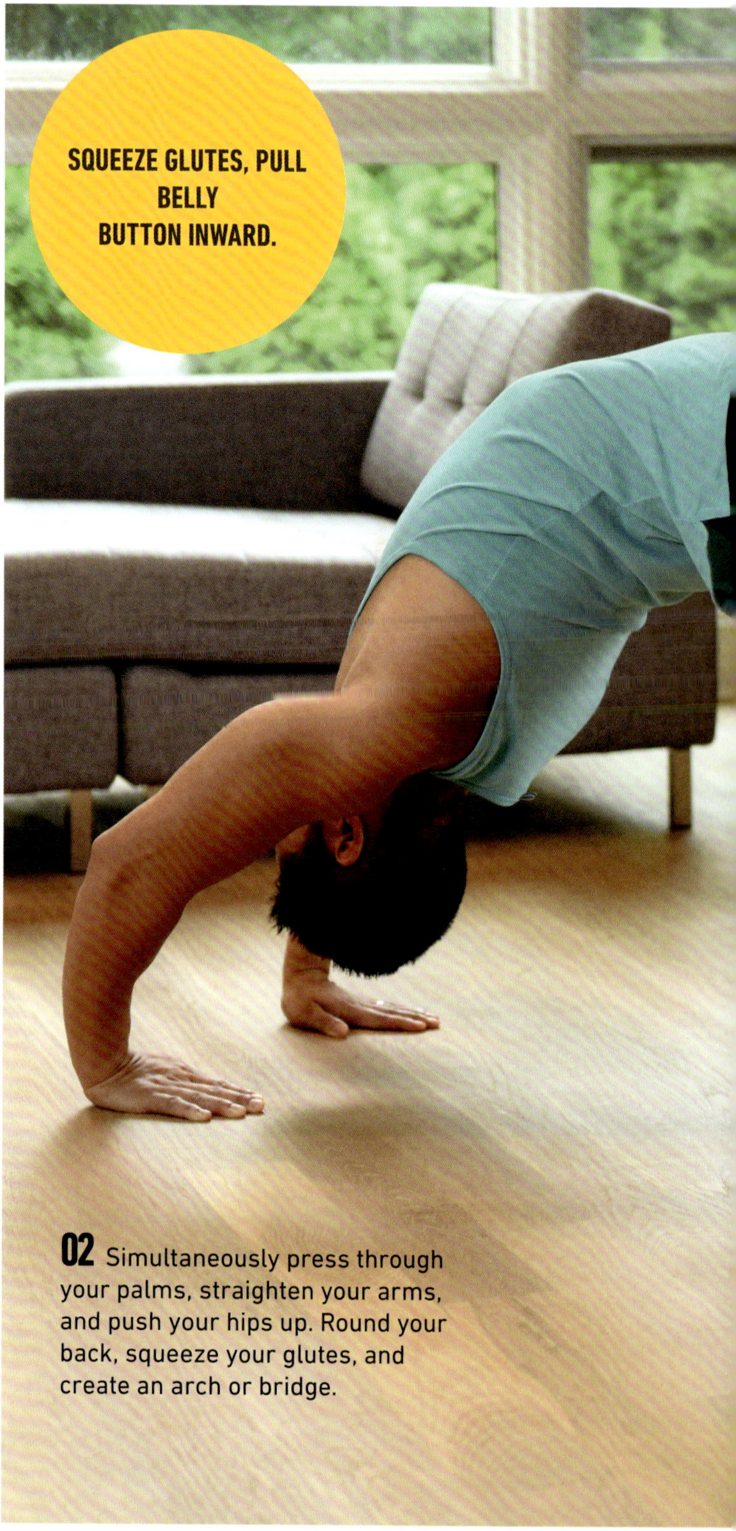

MORE DIFFICULT ||||||||||||||||||||
Modify range of motion: After reaching full extension in step 2, lower halfway, press back to full extension, and then lower completely.

LESS DIFFICULT ||||||||||||||||||||
Modify speed: Instead of doing repetitions, hold the highest point of the exercise in step 2 for the duration..

SQUEEZE GLUTES, PULL BELLY BUTTON INWARD.

02 Simultaneously press through your palms, straighten your arms, and push your hips up. Round your back, squeeze your glutes, and create an arch or bridge.

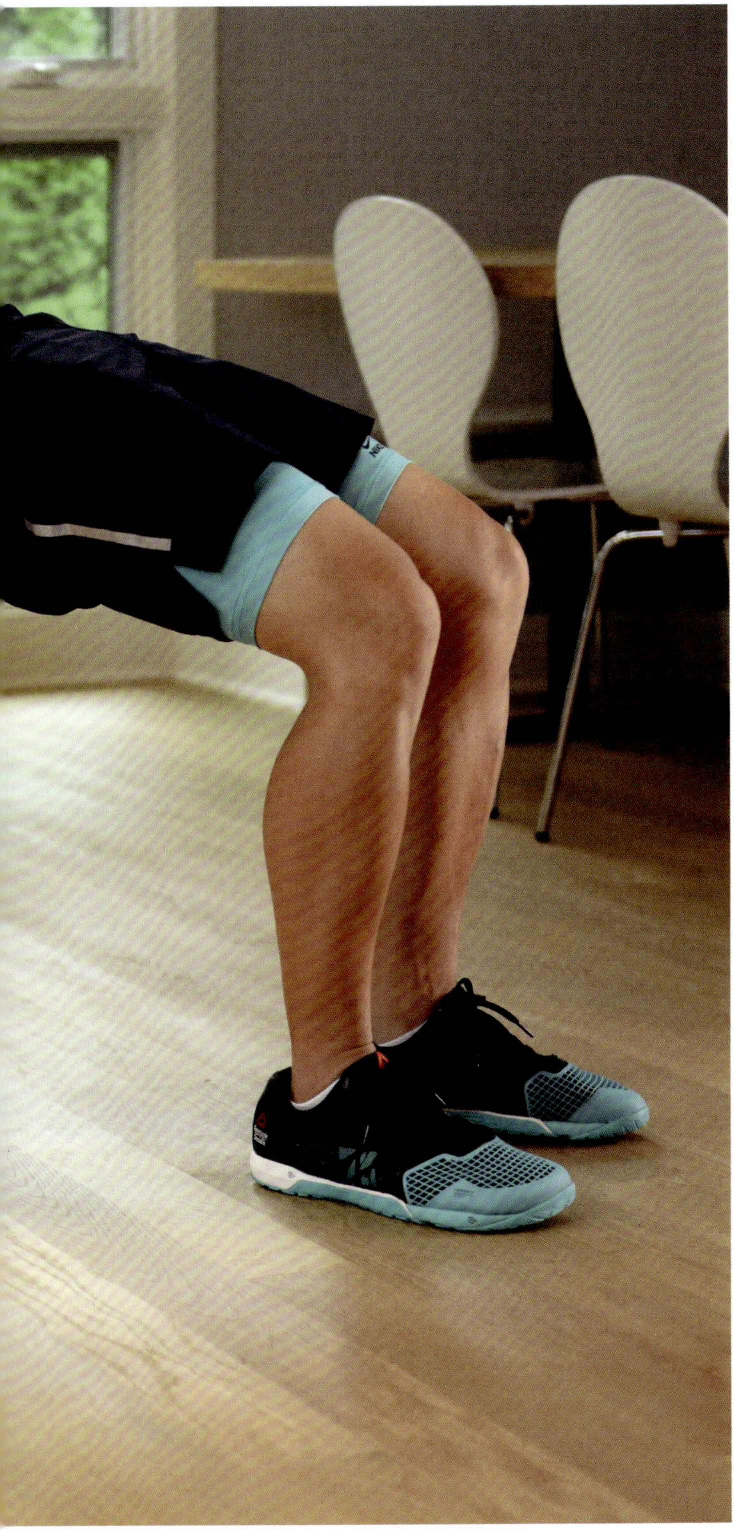

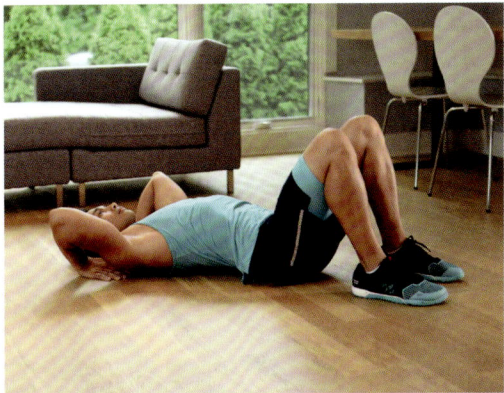

03 Hold for the prescribed duration, then lower with control.

Quality, not quantity!
If you can't hold for 30 seconds, break these into smaller, more manageable chunks—perform 3 for 10 seconds or 2 for 15 seconds.

FLUTTER UP

This advanced core exercise engages the abdominals, erector spinae, and hip flexors as you fight to elevate the upper and lower body in unison.

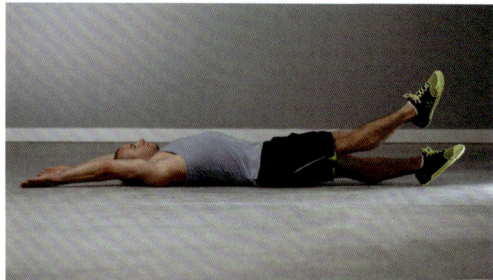

01 Lie on your back with arms and legs extended, and with one leg approximately 1 foot (30cm) higher than the other.

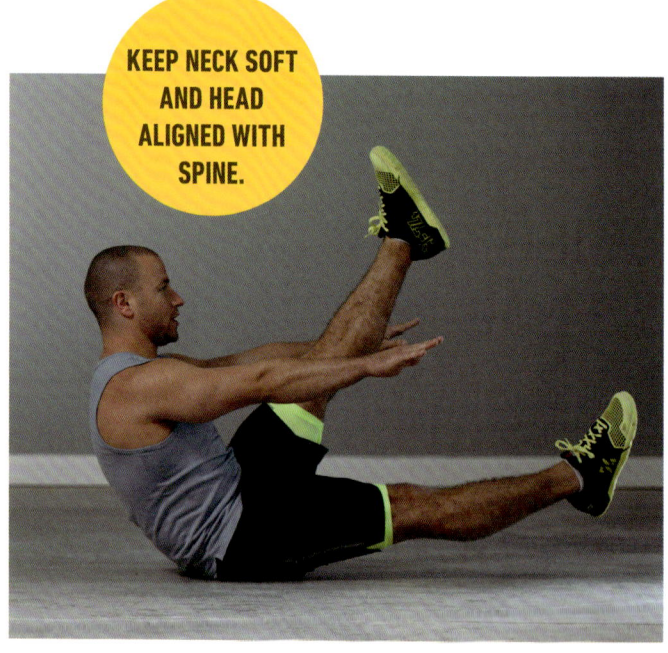

KEEP NECK SOFT AND HEAD ALIGNED WITH SPINE.

02 Switch the feet in 1-foot (30cm) increments as you simultaneously lift the torso and legs to form a V, with the arms reaching toward the fluttering toes.

MORE DIFFICULT ||||||||||||||||||||||||||
Modify range of motion: In steps 2 and 3, add a half rep after each full rep by lowering halfway and raising back up, performing 50 percent more work and punishing your core.

LESS DIFFICULT |||||||||||||||||||||||||
Modify range of motion: Keep your upper body still and only flutter your legs. Focus on proper form in your posterior pelvic tilt.

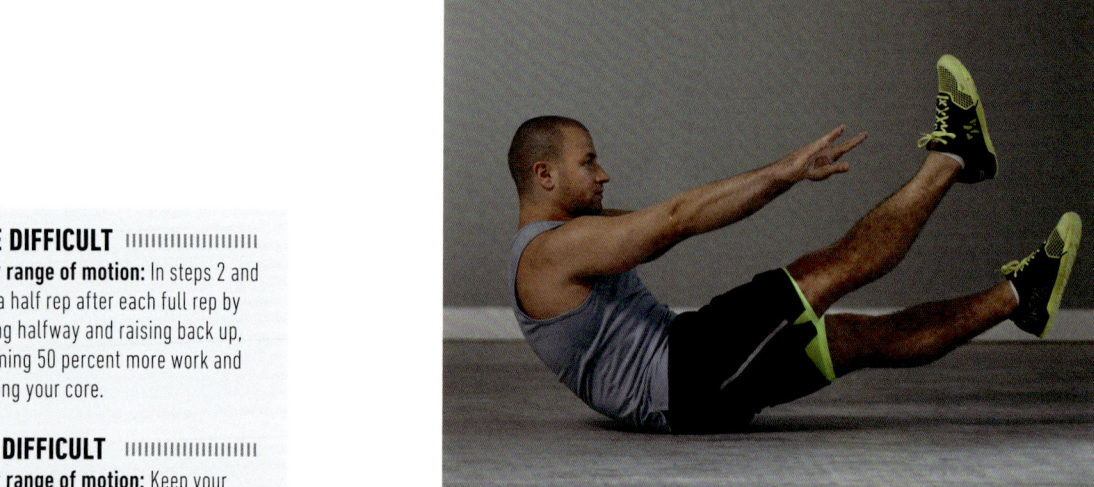

03 Continue to flutter the legs as you slowly lower your torso back to the floor. Repeat steps 2 and 3 for the duration of the exercise.

PLANK ROTATION

Plank rotations are a fun alternative to the traditional side plank. Rotating the body through multiple planes of motion challenges your balance and coordination and will tone the obliques, back, hips, thighs, and shoulders.

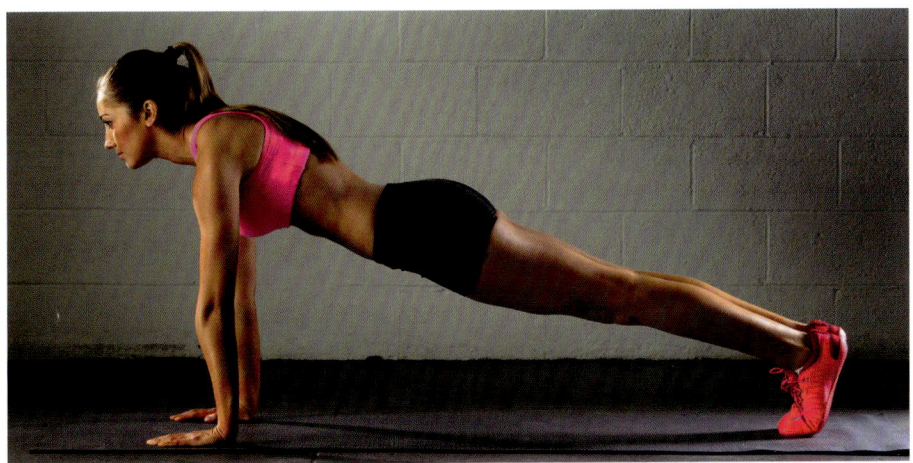

01 Begin in a full push-up position, with wrists under shoulders, core engaged, and legs extended.

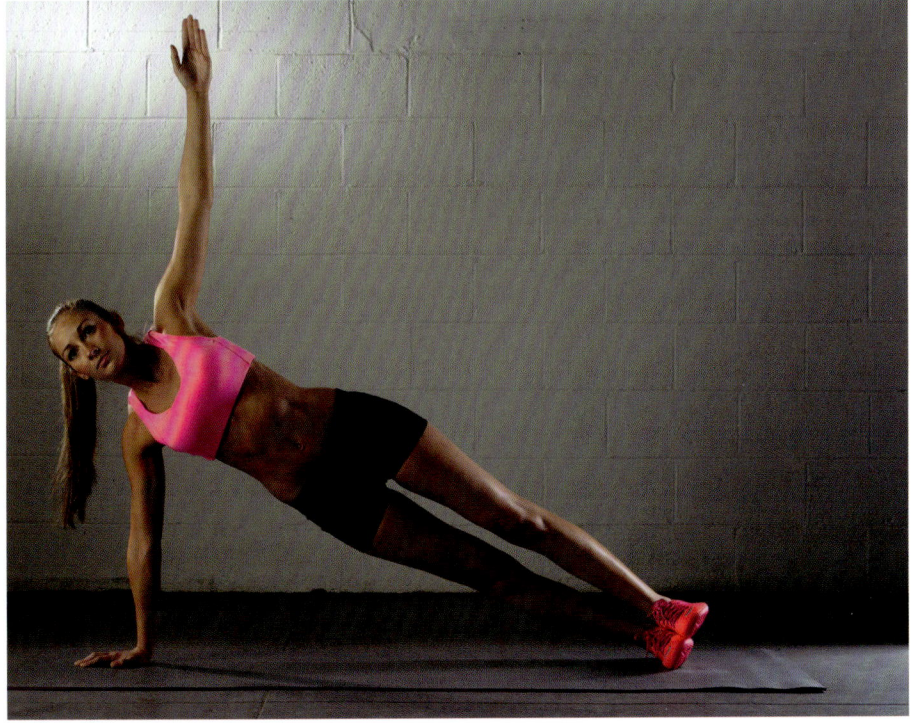

02 Raise your left arm toward the ceiling as you slowly rotate your body to the left. Lift from the bottom of the rib cage, opening the chest. Return to the starting position and repeat on the opposite side.

SPRINTER SIT-UP

This is no ordinary sit-up. The alternating movements of the arms and legs force your stabilizing core muscles to work, while aggressively driving the knees works the hip flexors.

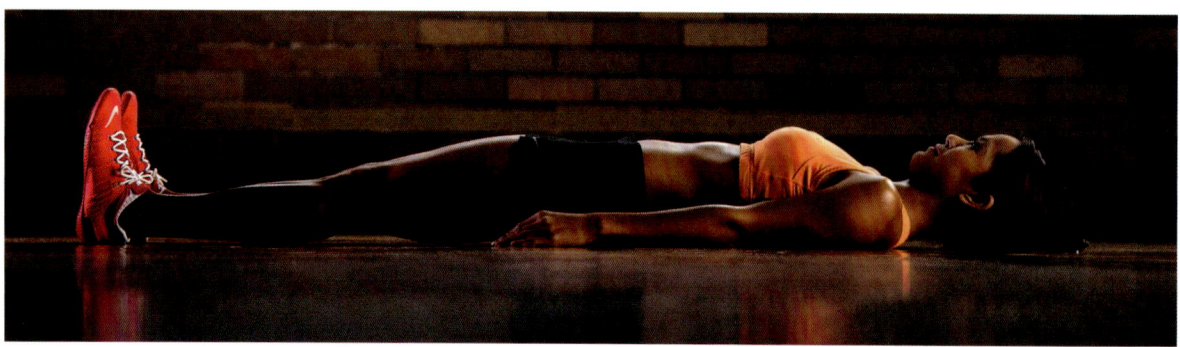

01 Lie on your back with your arms at your sides and legs extended.

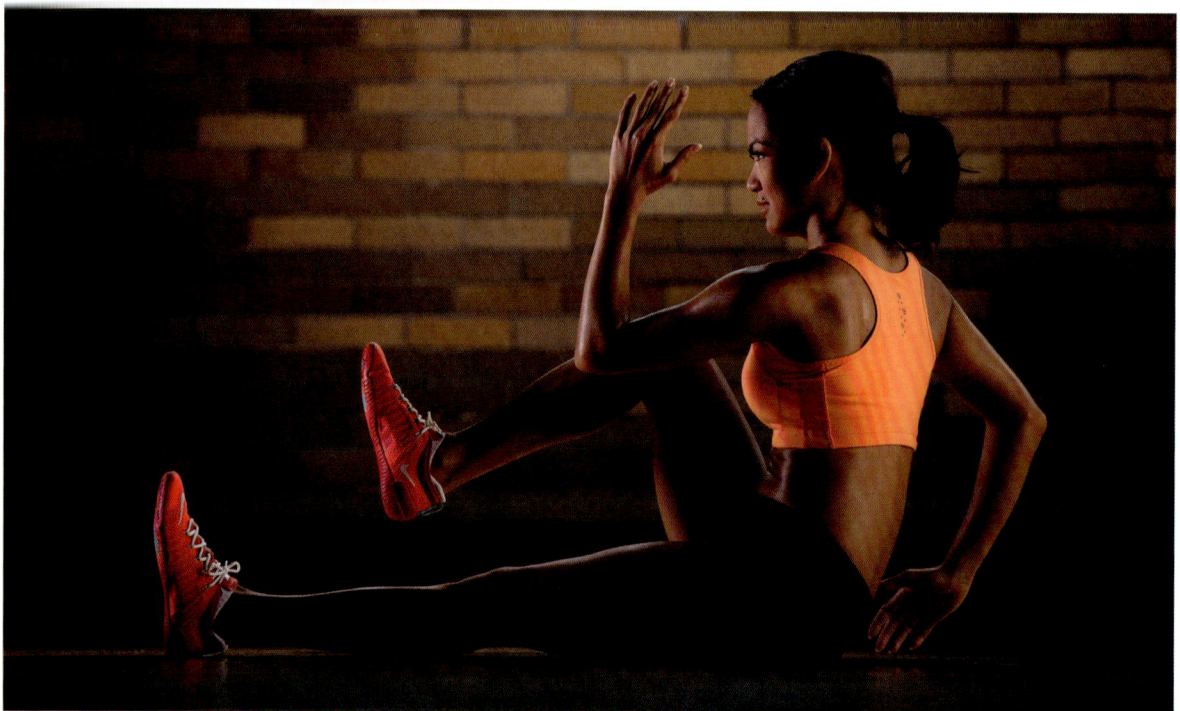

02 Sit up with an explosive movement, simultaneously bringing the right knee to your chest and swinging the left arm forward as if running.

> Do not rotate your torso while swinging your arms. Keep your hips and shoulders facing forward.

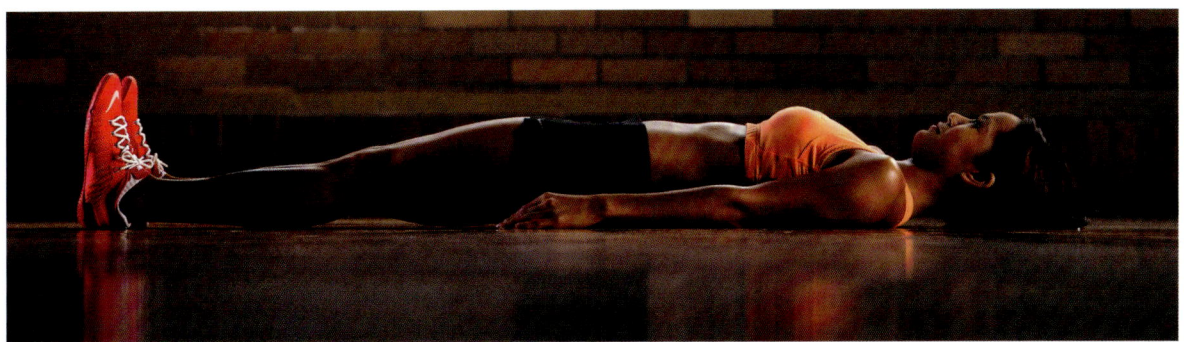

03 Fully extend the right leg and return the left arm to the starting position.

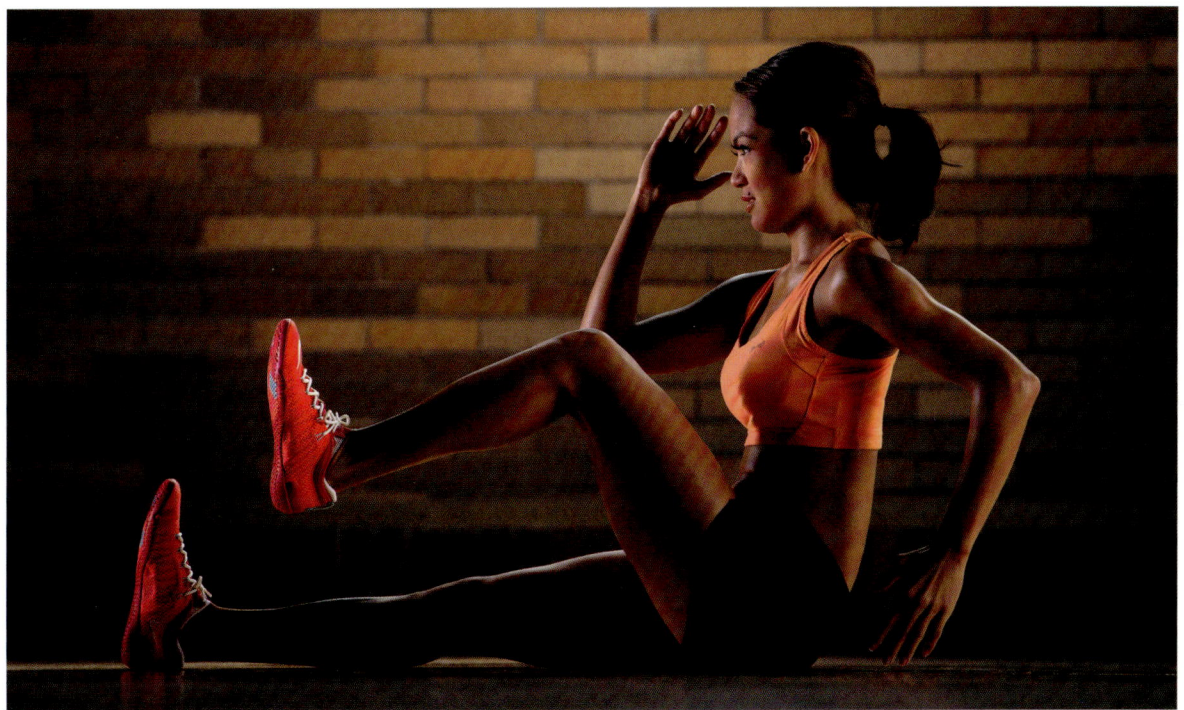

04 Sit up again, this time bringing the left knee in to the chest as you swing the right arm forward. Repeat, alternating arm and leg movements as though sprinting.

MOGUL JUMP

The inspiration for this fat-blasting move comes from downhill skiing. Mogul jumps specifically target the lower abdominals and obliques, but also engage the shoulders, chest, hips, and thighs. Working all those muscles in unison makes your heart rate skyrocket and body fat percentage plummet.

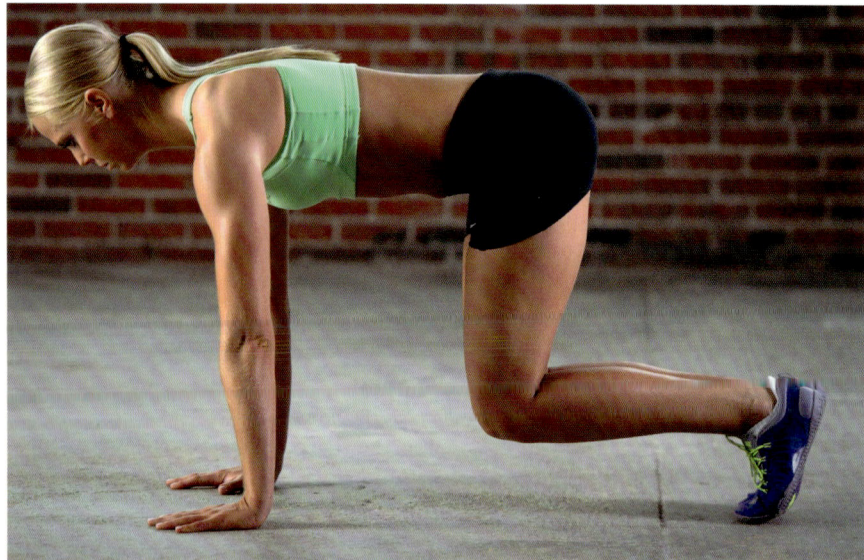

01 Begin on all fours with your arms straight and your legs together. Lift your knees off of the ground so that your legs are bent at a 90-degree angle and your weight is balanced between your hands and the balls of your feet. Your shins should be parallel to the floor.

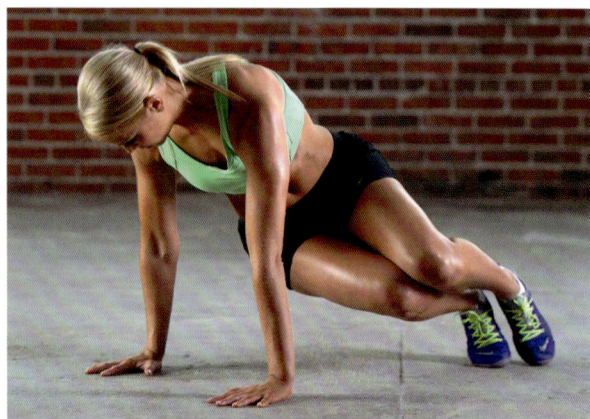

02 Keeping your arms straight and your knees together, hop and rotate your feet and knees to the left, rotating as much as possible. The knees should be perpendicular to the body and the hips in line with the shoulders.

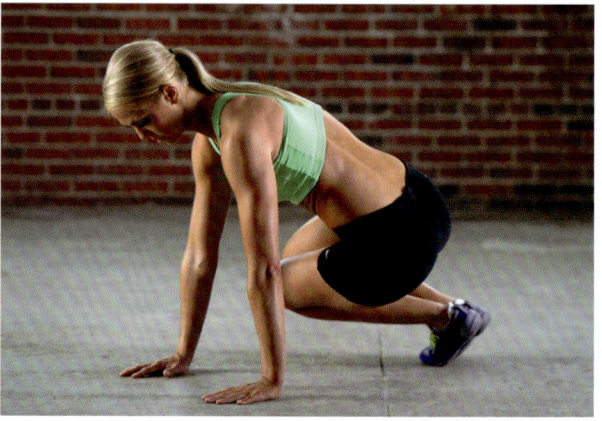

03 Jump and rotate feet and knees to the opposite side, keeping arms straight and knees together. Repeat, moving as quickly as possible while maintaining proper form.

MOUNTAIN CLIMBER

A challenging cardiovascular exercise, mountain climbers mimic finding a foothold while climbing a summit and work your core, hip flexors, and legs.

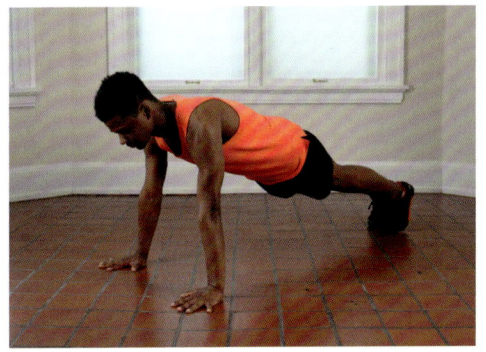

01 Position your hands on the floor slightly wider than your shoulders. Rise up onto your toes, and engage the core to form a straight back and balance your weight between your toes and head. This is the plank position.

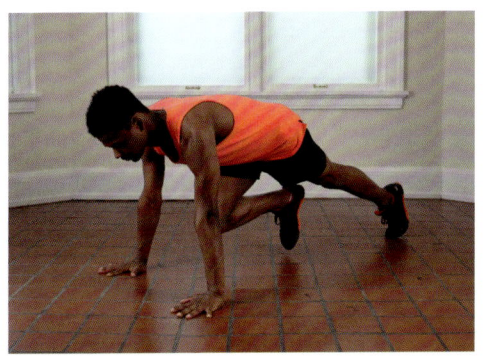

02 Bending your right leg, pull your knee in toward your chest while keeping your core engaged.

ELBOWS STRAIGHT, MAINTAIN A RIGID PLANK POSITION THROUGHOUT.

MORE DIFFICULT ||||||||||||||||||||
Modify range of motion and reps: During step 2, extend partially, then add a second pull of the knee to the chest before switching legs..

LESS DIFFICULT ||||||||||||||||||||
Modify body angle: For all steps, elevate your hands on a prop, shifting weight to the lower body so it's easier to sustain the plank.

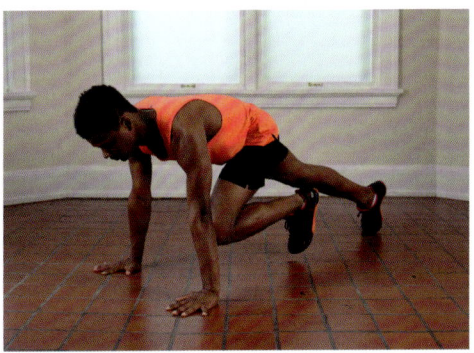

03 Straighten the right leg back into its original position and simultaneously pull the left knee toward the chest. Repeat, alternating leg positions, with controlled speed.

HANGING REVERSE CURL

This targets your lower abdominals and lower back. A strong, flexible core makes you more powerful in all endeavors.

MORE DIFFICULT |||||||||||||||||||||||||
Modify range of motion and repetitions: In step 2, add a smaller second knee tuck/crunch at the top of the motion before fully straightening legs in step 3, increasing the work by 50 percent.

LESS DIFFICULT |||||||||||||||||||||||||
Modify range of motion: In step 2, tuck and raise the knees only until thighs are parallel to the ground to decrease the work for the knees and the time the core needs to be engaged.

KNEECAPS POINT DIRECTLY AT CHEST.

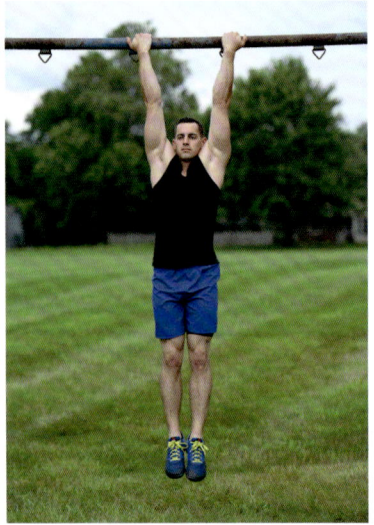

01 Position yourself directly under your pull-up bar. Hop up and grab the bar with a shoulder-width underhand grip (palms facing you).

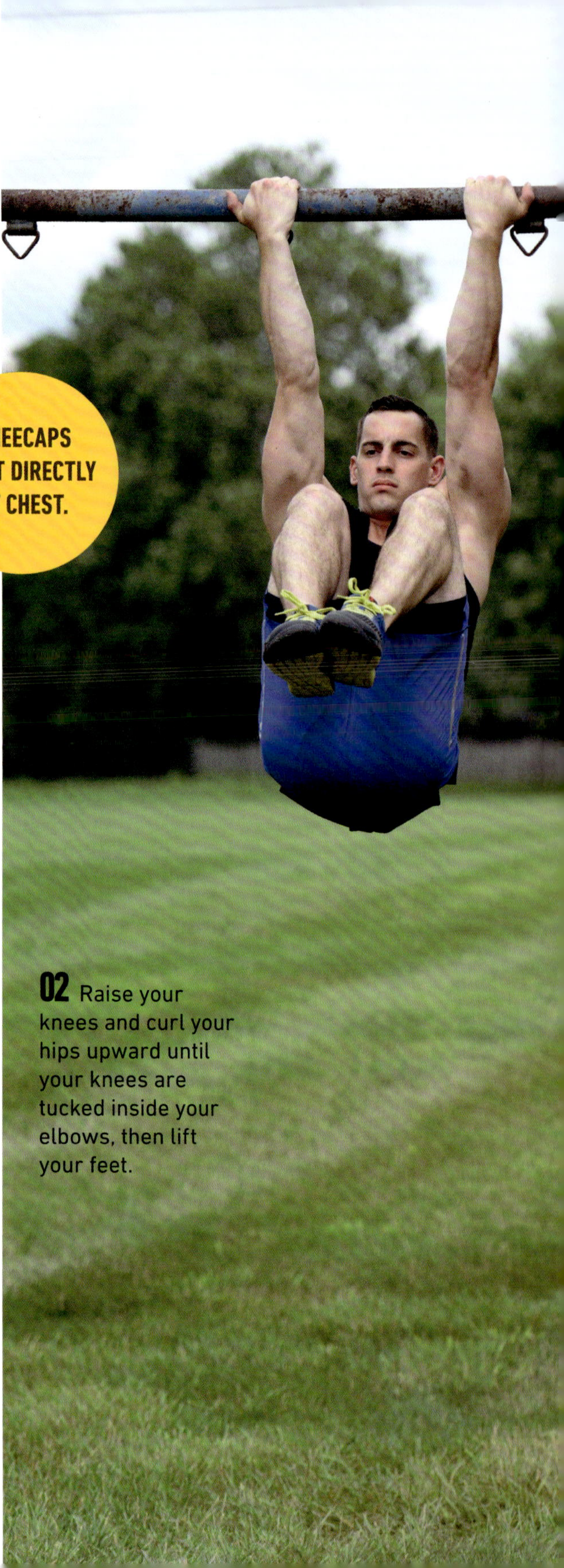

02 Raise your knees and curl your hips upward until your knees are tucked inside your elbows, then lift your feet.

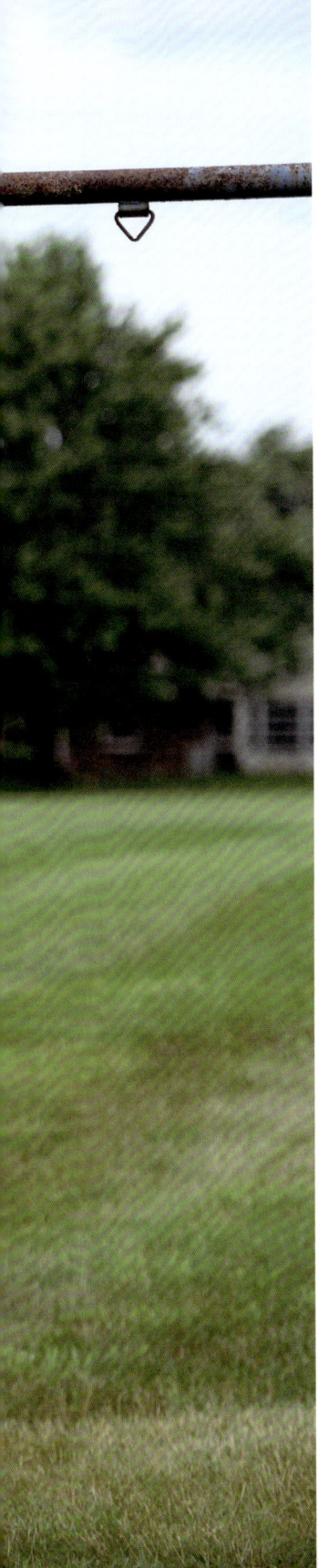

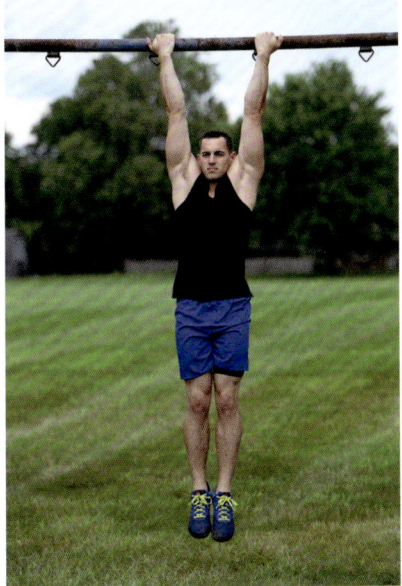

This exercise can be performed from a dead hang—hanging from the bar with arms straight and shoulders packed—but make sure you're not swinging and using momentum.

03 Lower back down slowly until your feet nearly touch the ground.

CHALLENGE

Twist both knees across the body as you curl upward, as if skiing moguls, to engage the obliques.

SKI TUCKS

Bring both knees across the body to one elbow, lower, and repeat to the opposite elbow.

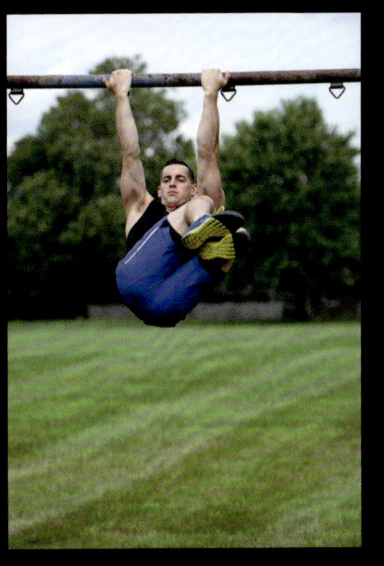

PIKE

The pike, or leg raise, is the one ab exercise we always come back to in the gym. Pikes are a simple yet highly effective way to target your lower abs and hip flexors.

> If your back arches as the legs lower, you are taking your legs too low. The weight and leverage of the legs is too much for your core to control. Adjust the angle of the legs accordingly to keep the work in the abs and hip flexors.

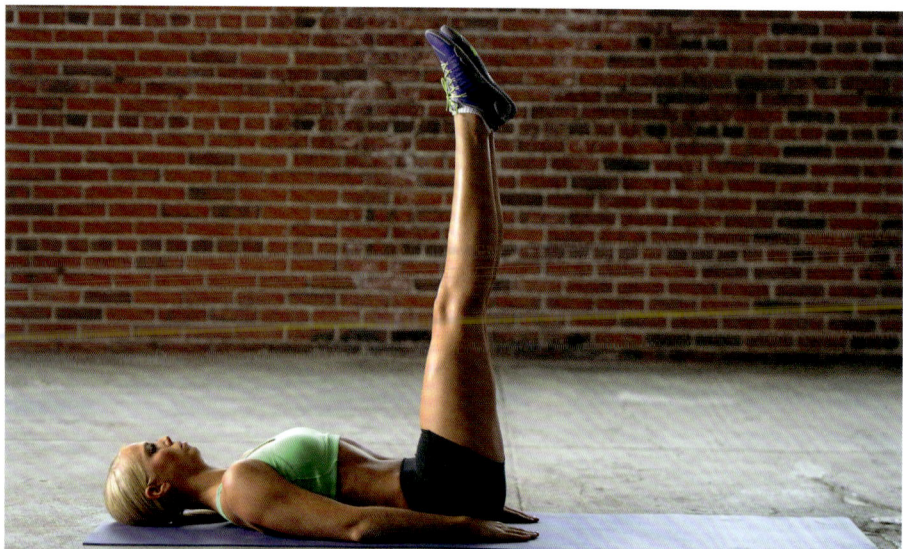

01 Lie on your back and place your hands under your butt with palms facing down. Squeeze your legs together and slowly raise them until they are perpendicular to the floor, keeping them as straight as possible. Hold the contraction for 1 second.

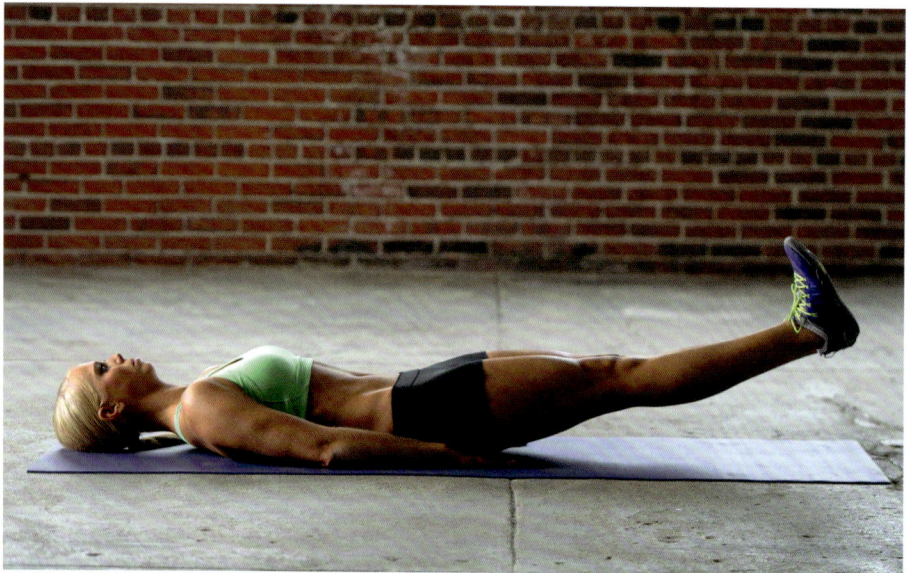

02 Maintaining straight legs, slowly lower your feet to within an inch of the floor.

IN-AND-OUT ABS

In-and-out abs combines the core work of the classic plank with a dynamic tuck that challenges the thighs and hips and engages stabilizing muscles.

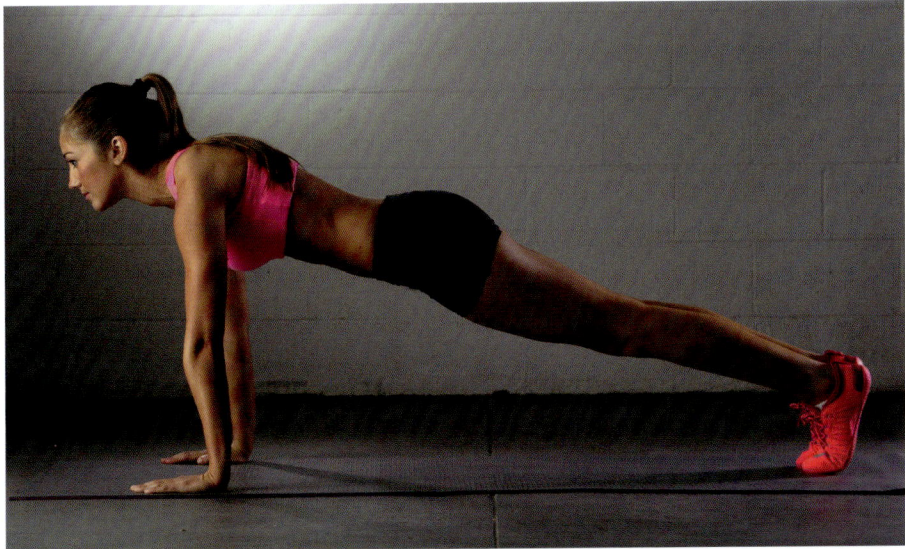

01 Position your hands on the floor, slightly wider than shoulder-width apart. Rise up onto your toes and engage the core to form a straight line from ankles to head. Squeeze the glutes to support your lower back.

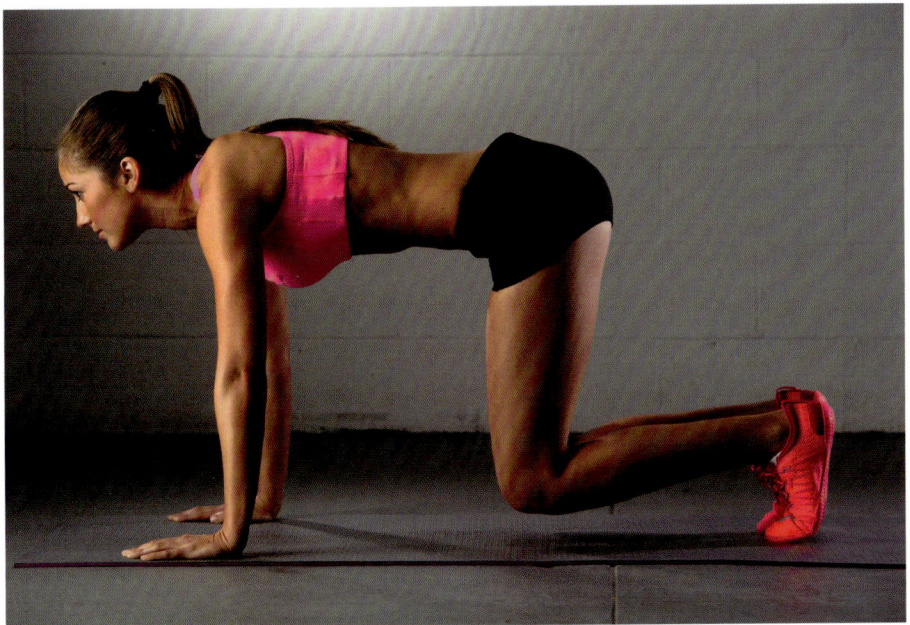

02 Jump in, tucking both knees under your body and landing on the toes with legs bent at 90 degrees. Do not bring your knees past your hips.

Jump back to the starting position, engaging the core for stability.

REVERSE PLANK BRIDGE

Create stability and balance through the back side with this simple bodyweight staple.

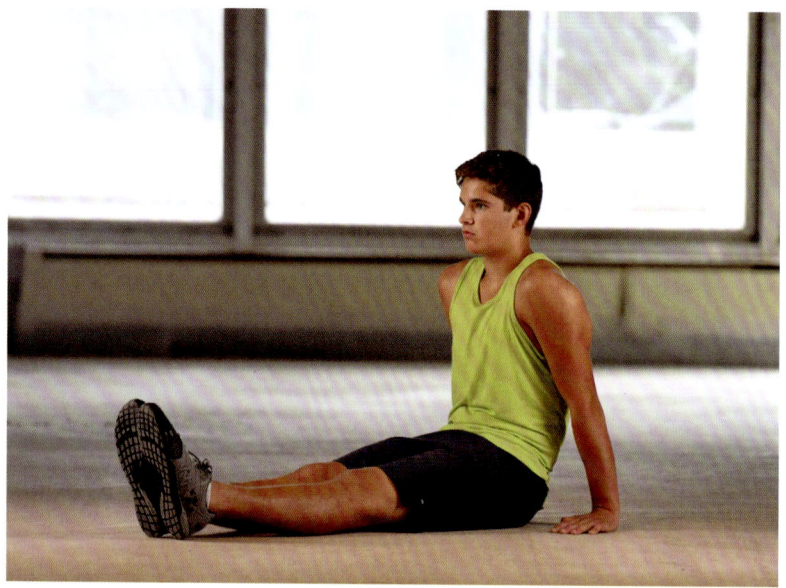

01 Sit on the floor with your legs extended in front of you. Place your palms on the floor with fingers slightly spread and pointing toward your toes.

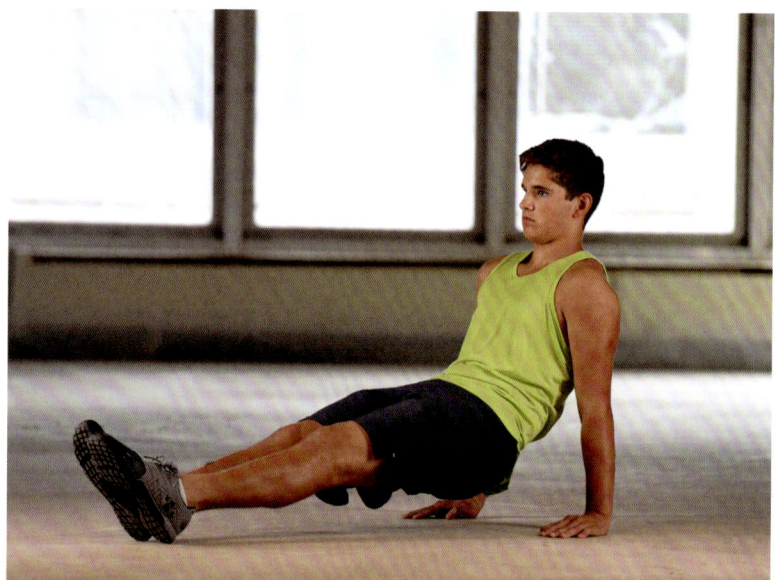

02 Press into your palms and lift your hips and torso toward the ceiling.

MORE DIFFICULT |||||||||||||||||||||
Modify reps: Add a small pulse to step 2 by lowering halfway down and then re-engaging the core and glutes to perform 1.5 reps, then repeat.

LESS DIFFICULT |||||||||||||||||||||
Modify speed and points of contact: In all steps, bend your knees to decrease the length of the body.

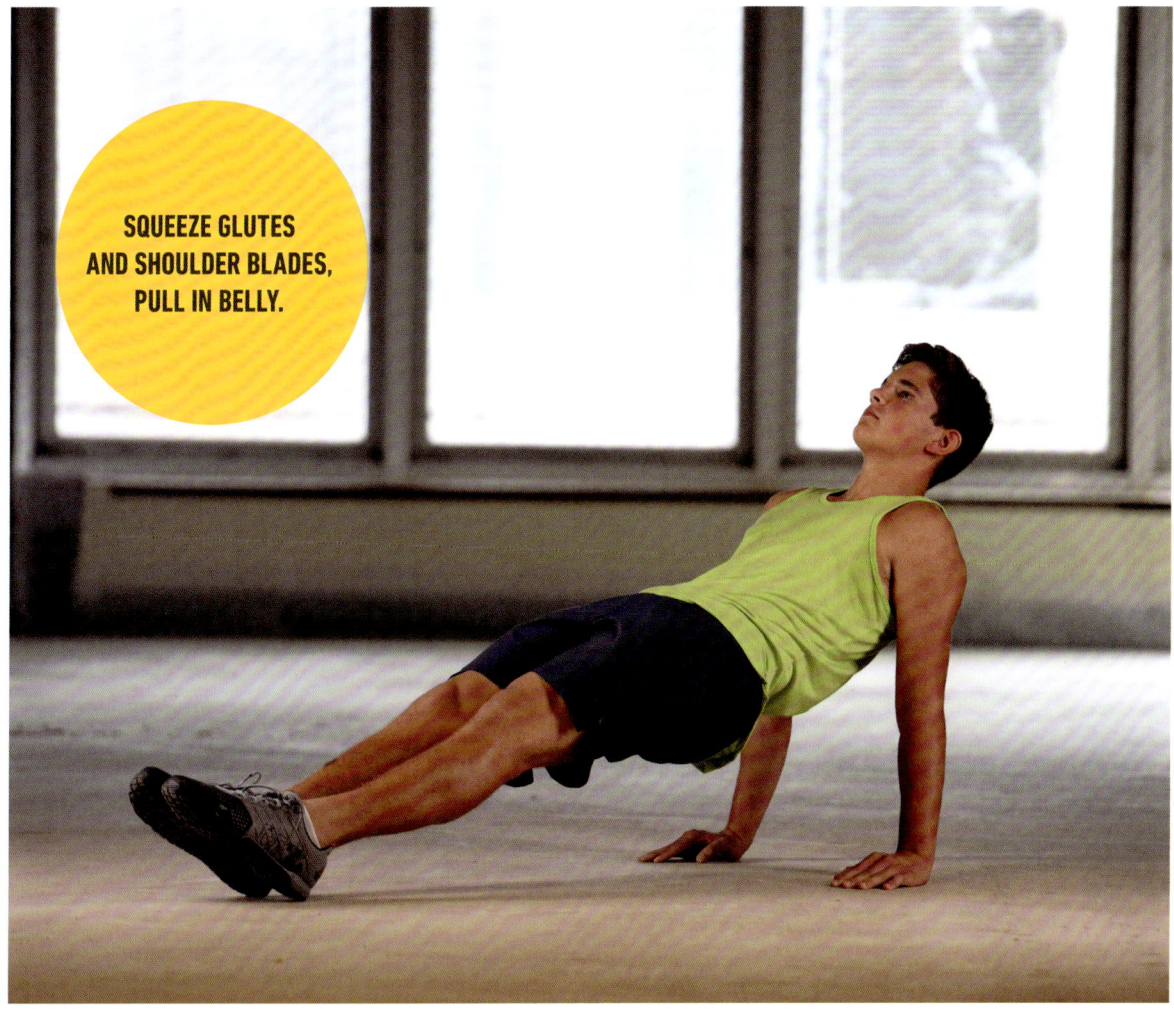

SQUEEZE GLUTES AND SHOULDER BLADES, PULL IN BELLY.

03 Look at the ceiling. Fully straighten but do not lock your arms and legs. Squeeze and engage the glutes, pulling your belly button to your spine, and hold.

The goal is to maintain a straight line and hold for up to 30 seconds. You may need to begin by holding the position for only a few seconds as you build your strength. Quality, not quantity!

BICYCLE CRUNCH

The bicycle crunch is an excellent exercise for building core strength and toning the thighs. The movement of your legs mimics the motion of riding a bike.

MORE DIFFICULT |||||||||||||||||||||

To increase the difficulty of this exercise, elevate the feet. For an even greater challenge, elevate and extend the legs.

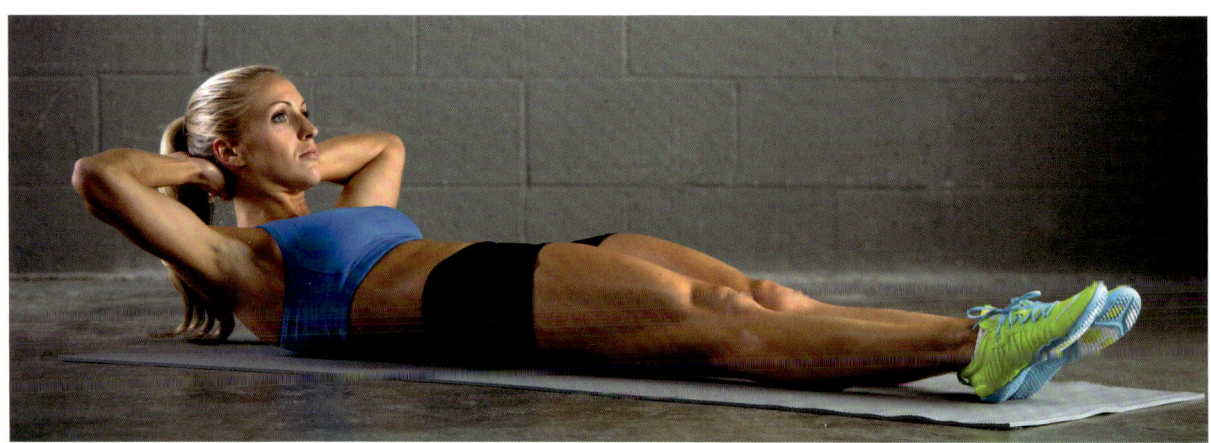

01 Lie flat on the floor with your hands behind your head, elbows out wide, and fingers interlocked. Pull your shoulder blades off of the floor by activating the abs. Don't pull on your neck.

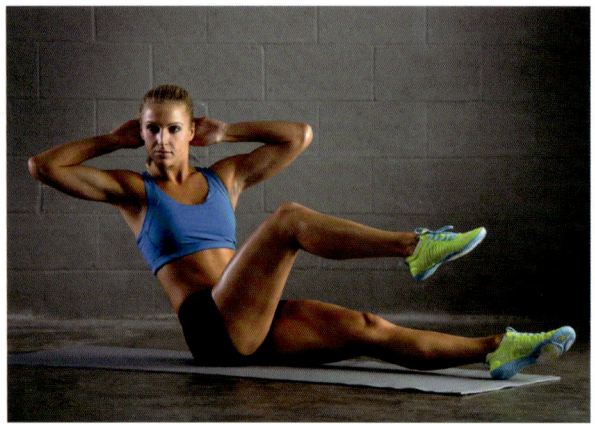

02 Bring your right knee toward your chest until it is bent at 90 degrees. Simultaneously rotate your core to pull your left shoulder toward the right knee.

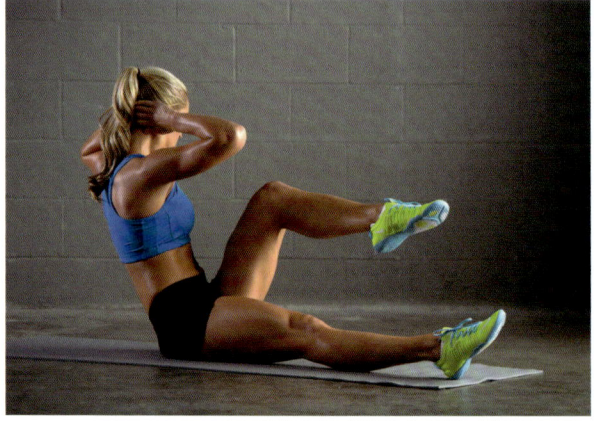

03 Switch sides, extending the right leg and simultaneously pulling the left knee toward your chest. Rotate your core and pull your right shoulder toward the left knee. Repeat, alternating sides.

RUSSIAN TWIST

This classic ab exercise targets the obliques, but your back muscles will also be engaged to stabilize and support your spine.

[Do not do this exercise if you have lower back pain or injury. Substitute the bicycle crunch instead.]

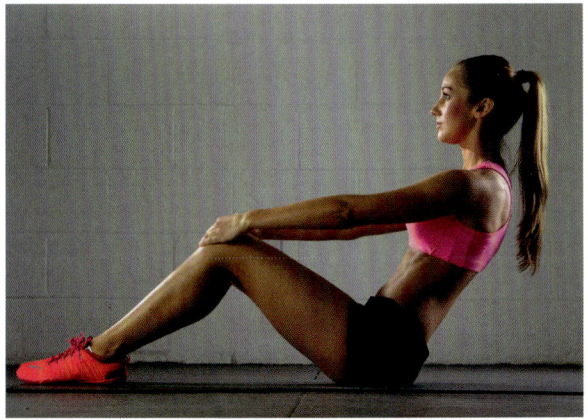

01 Sit with knees bent and heels approximately one foot (30cm) from your glutes. Hold your knees and straighten your arms as you lean back without rounding your spine. This is the perfect position for your spine; don't let it curve during the exercise.

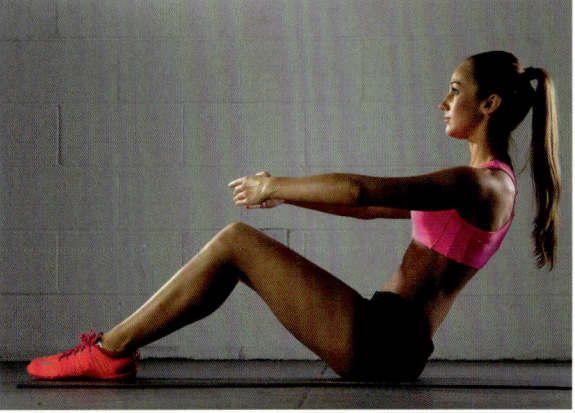

02 Lift arms from knees and extend in front of rib cage. Arms should remain slightly rounded as if holding a beach ball to your chest.

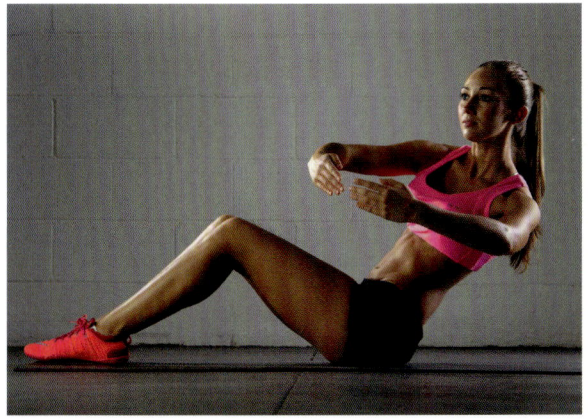

03 Pull the belly button to the spine and rotate to the left. This is a small, controlled motion; do not swing your arms. If you feel pain in your lower back, reduce the amount of twist.

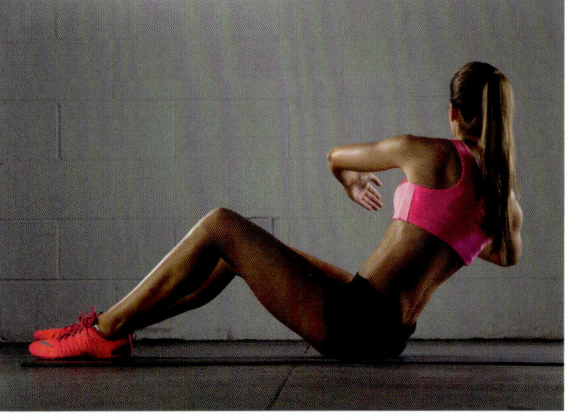

04 Inhale to center and rotate to the right. Repeat, keeping your abs engaged and spine straight.

KNEE TUCK EXTENSION

The knee tuck extension amps up the classic chin-up by adding a challenging isolation hold for hip flexors, quads, and abdominals.

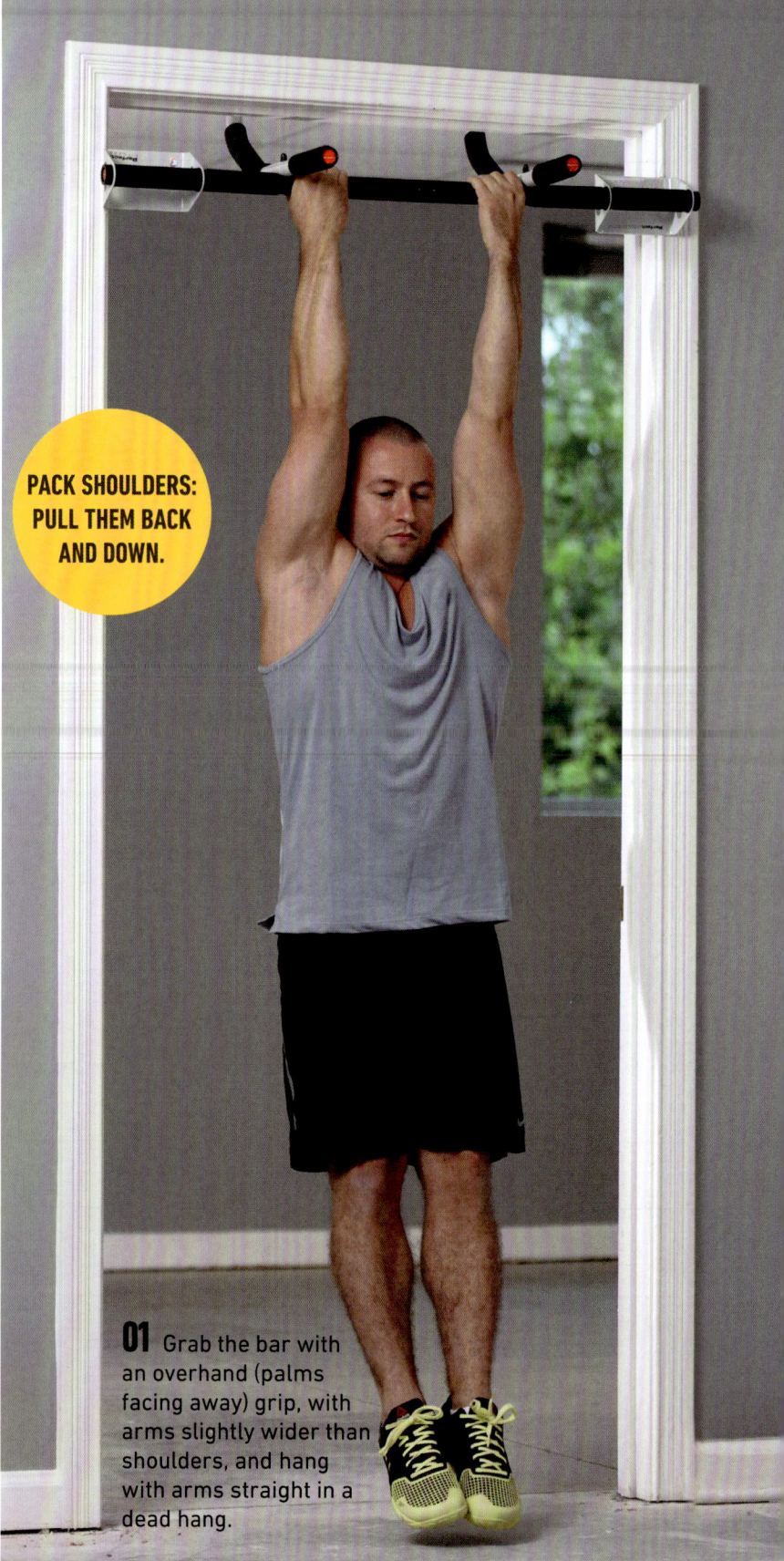

PACK SHOULDERS: PULL THEM BACK AND DOWN.

MORE DIFFICULT |||||||||||||||||||||||
Modify speed: Hold step 3 for a count of four to create a brief isolation hold, which will build strength in the position where you're working against the greatest leverage.

LESS DIFFICULT |||||||||||||||||||||||
Modify stability: Perform the exercise lying on the floor instead of hanging to increase stability and to build confidence and strength before eventually going to the bar.

01 Grab the bar with an overhand (palms facing away) grip, with arms slightly wider than shoulders, and hang with arms straight in a dead hang.

> Knees up, chin down: The rectus abdominis (six-pack abs) are flexors. If you bring the knees up and tuck the chin slightly, it will encourage the abs to contract.

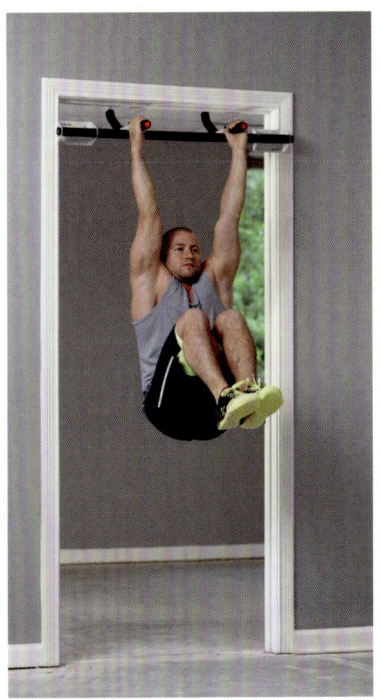

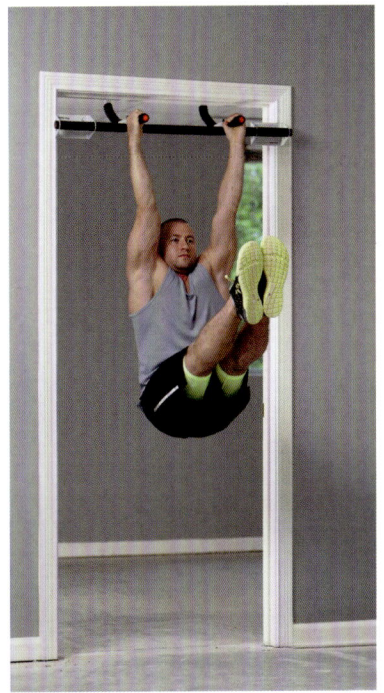

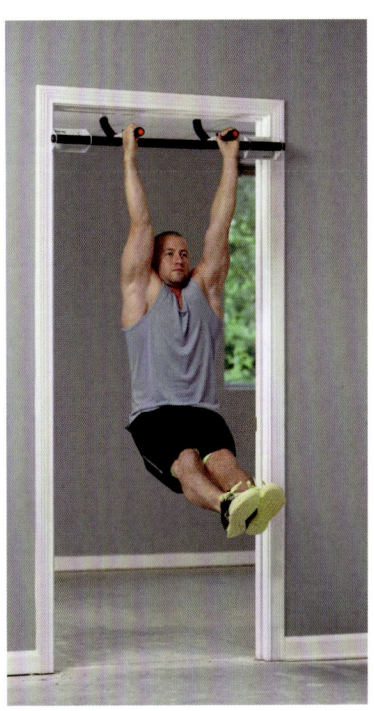

02 Tuck the knees to the chest without causing the body to swing on the bar.

03 Straighten the legs until they're just beyond parallel to the floor, forming an L with the torso. Toes should be pointed, thighs squeezed together, and knees locked.

04 Keep the legs straight and lower them slowly with control until your body forms a straight line, returning to the dead hang position.

DIAGONAL PIKE

Leg raises are a simple yet highly effective way to target your lower abs and hip flexors. The addition of the diagonal movement increases the workload of your obliques.

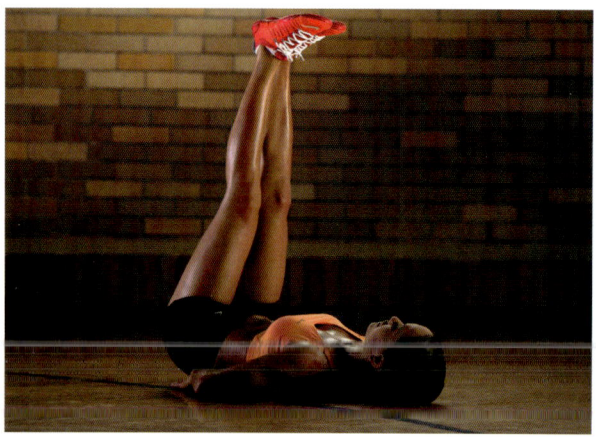

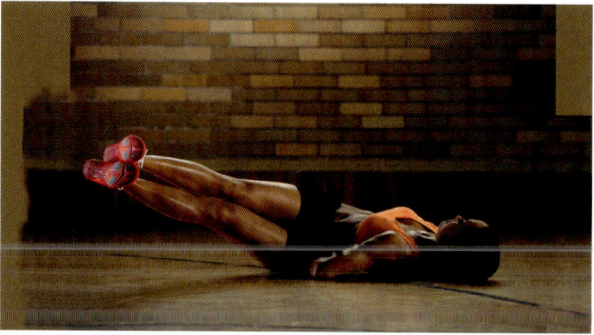

01 Lie on your back with hands under glutes, palms down. Squeeze your legs together and raise, legs straight, until they are perpendicular to the floor.

02 Lower your legs to the left at a 45-degree angle, until feet are just above the floor. Pause before returning to the starting position.

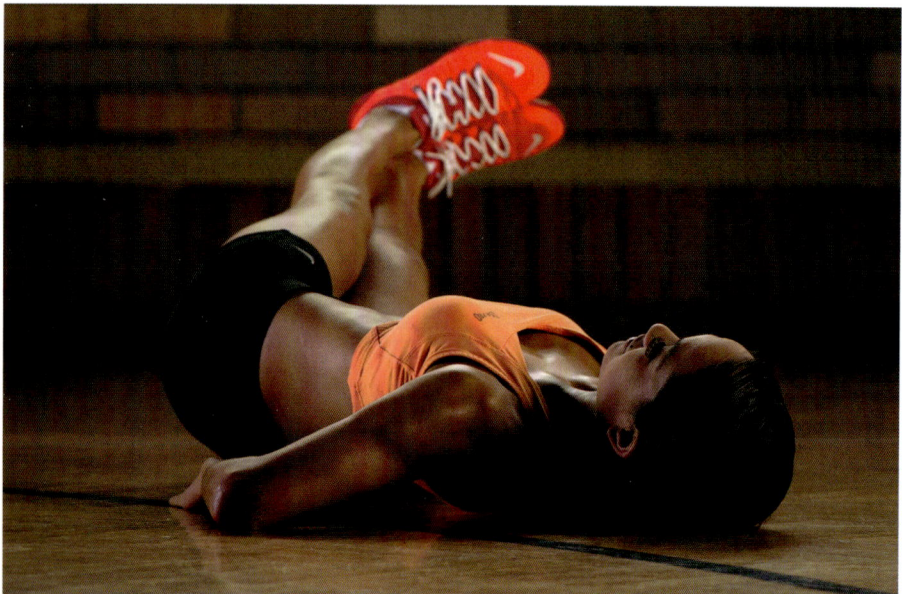

03 Lower your legs to the right at a 45-degree angle, until feet are just above the floor. Pause before returning to the starting position and repeat.

V-UP

The V-up takes its name from the shape your body forms during the exercise. This advanced ab exercise engages the six-pack abdominal muscles, the erector muscles of the spine, and the hip flexors. V-ups require great coordination as well as balance.

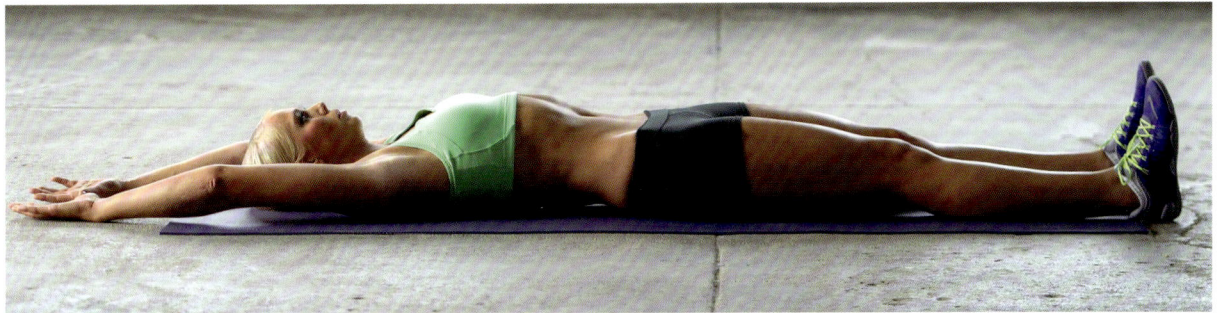

01 Lie on your back with arms and legs straight. Extend your arms above your head. Keep your pelvis flat and a natural arch to your back.

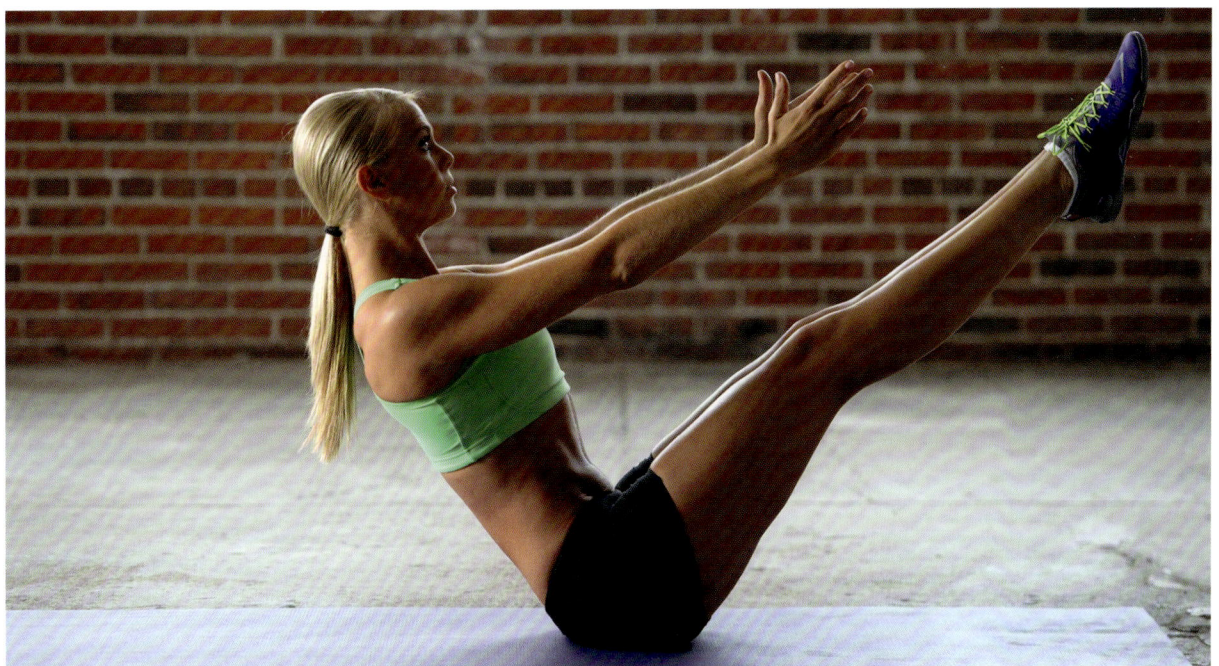

02 In one fluid motion, simultaneously lift your torso and legs. Extend your arms so they are parallel to the legs and keep your head in line with your body. Control the body back to the starting position and repeat.

ROUTINES

LEG PURGATORY

This basic yet torturous leg routine consists of just two exercises. It's the precursor to Leg Hell (page 148) and will target your quads and glutes in an "every minute, on the minute" (EMOM) format.

Complete both exercises in 1 minute. Perform 10 rounds.
Total time: 10 minutes

SQUAT
10x   **p072**

FRONT LUNGE
20x (10x each leg)   **p080**

The goal is to perform 10 squats and 20 total front lunges within 1 minute.

If you finish early, enjoy the well-earned rest. At the start of the next minute, begin again for 10 consecutive minutes.

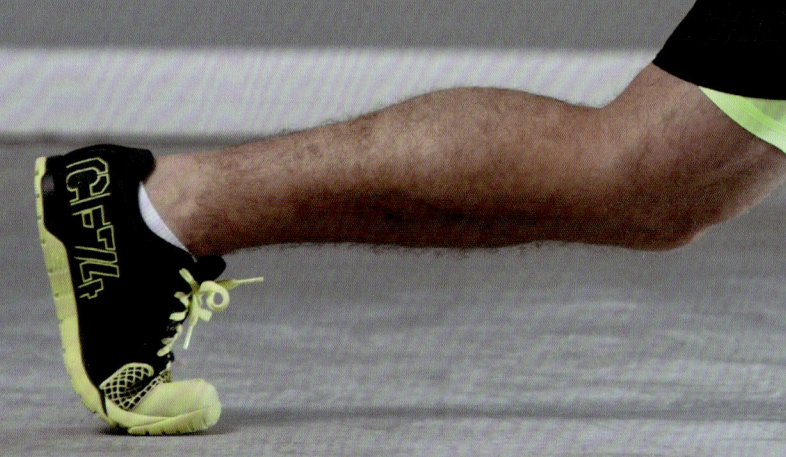

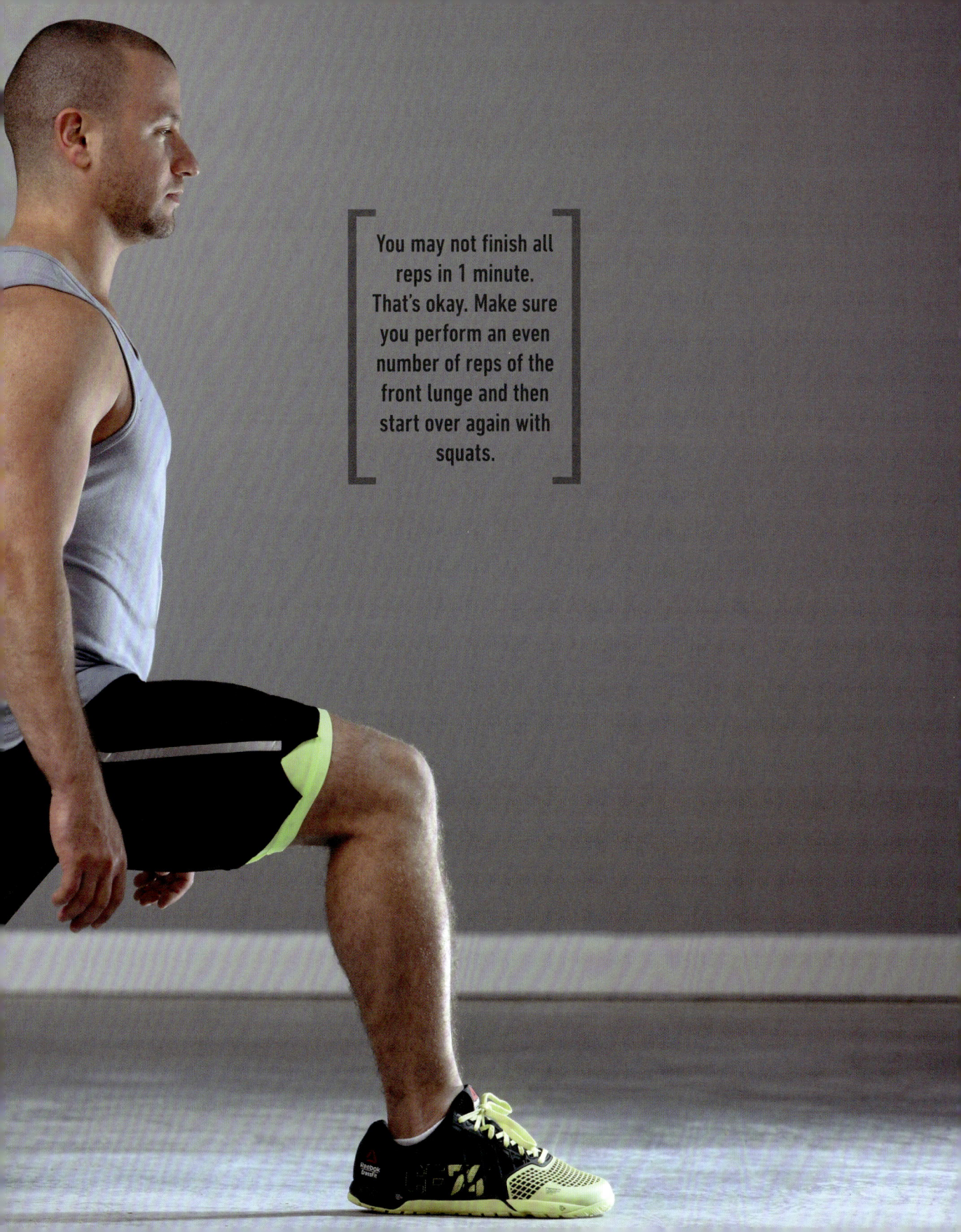

You may not finish all reps in 1 minute. That's okay. Make sure you perform an even number of reps of the front lunge and then start over again with squats.

LEG HELL

This routine adds explosive plyometric movements to push your legs to their limits. It targets the quads, glutes, hamstrings, and calves. At a 4:1 work-to-rest ratio, it will also drive up your heart rate.

Perform 3 rounds with little to no rest between exercises.
Rest for 30 seconds between each round. Total time: 7 minutes

SQUAT
0:30   p072

JUMP LUNGE
0:30   p062

REVERSE LUNGE
0:30   p078

SQUAT JUMP
0:30   p066

🕐 **REST** 0:30
🔁 **REPEAT** for a total of 3 rounds

[It's okay to slow down the exercise to ensure correct form. Always remember: form first, speed second!]

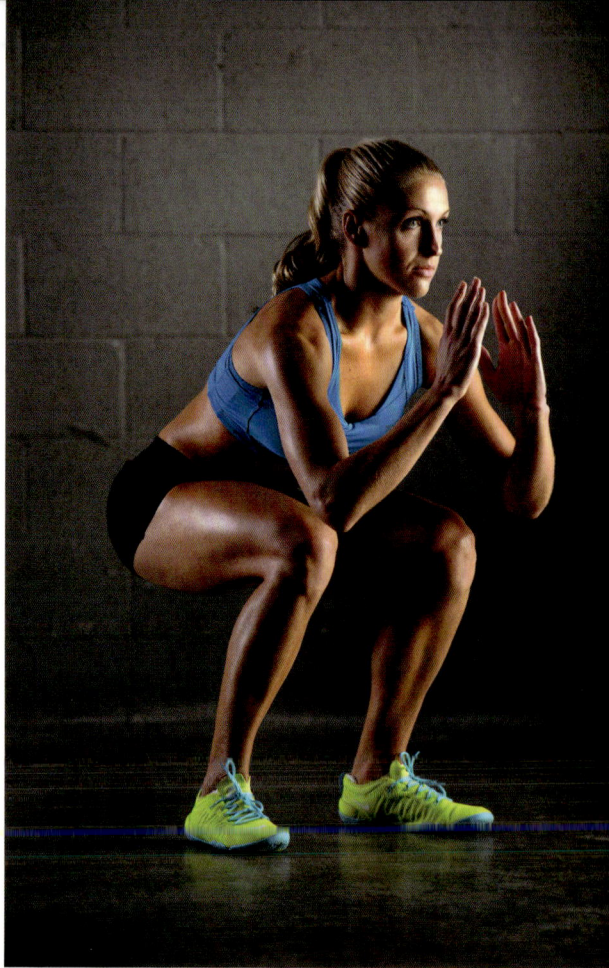

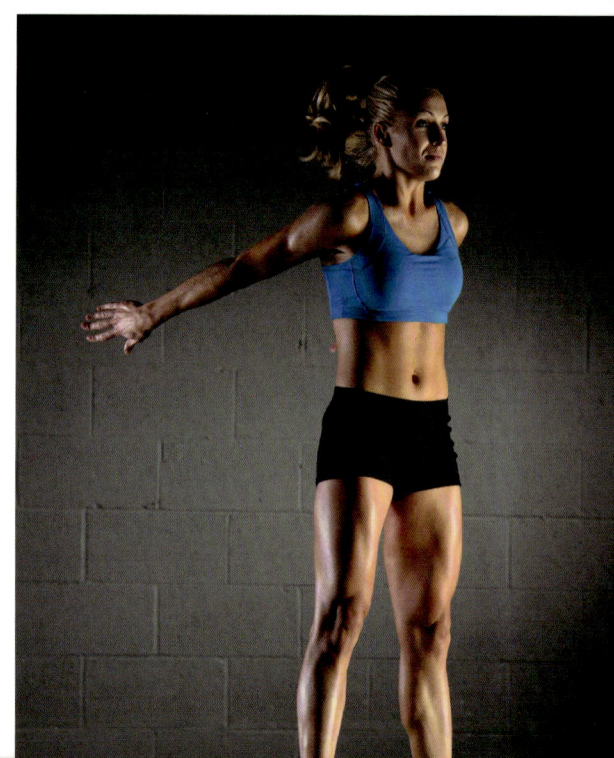

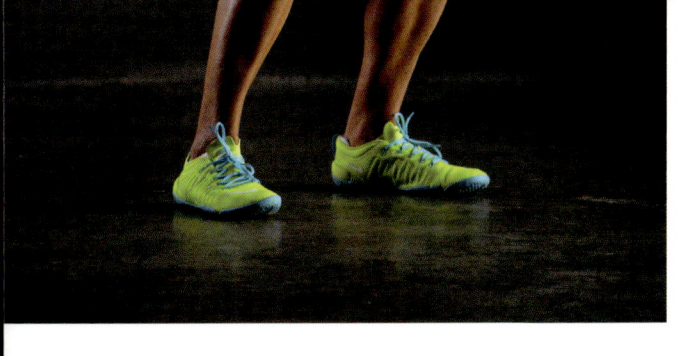

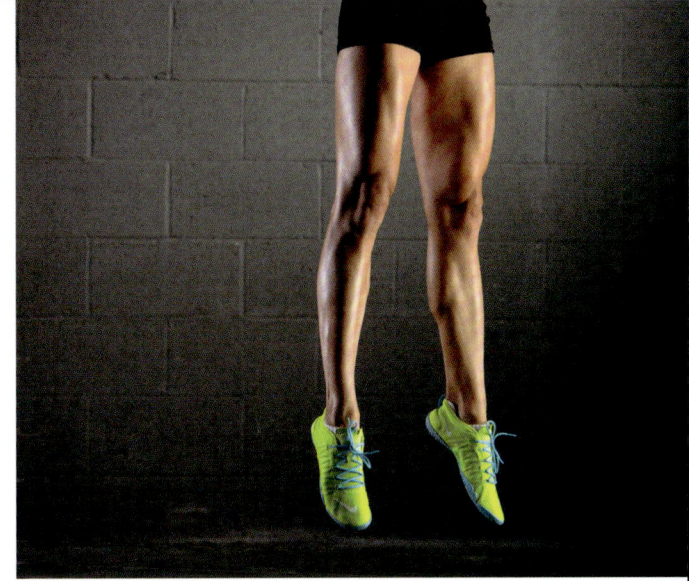

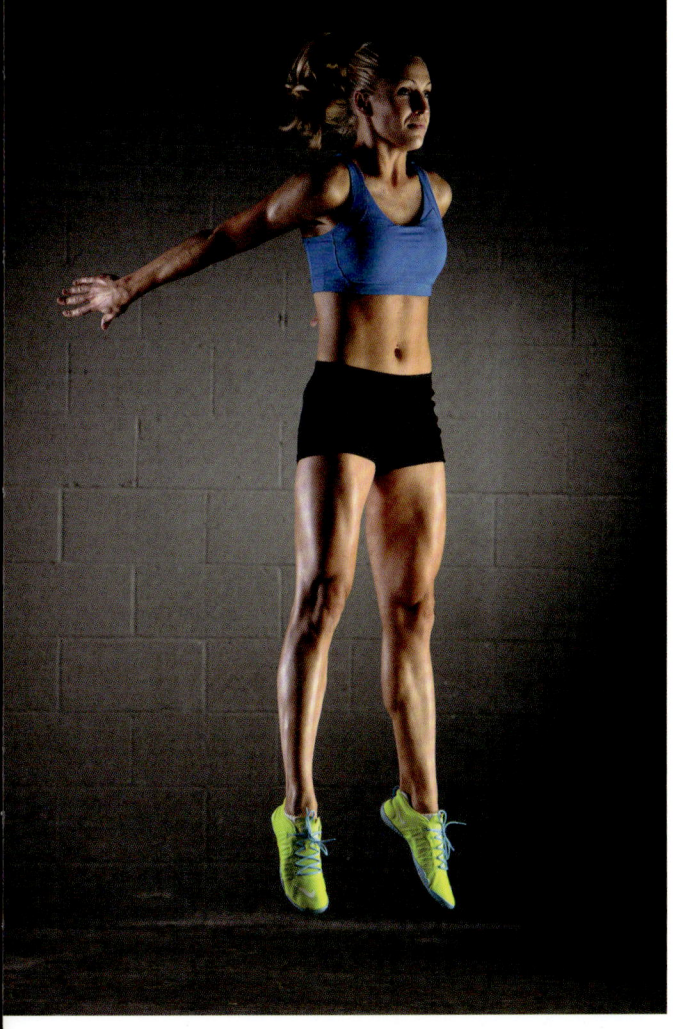

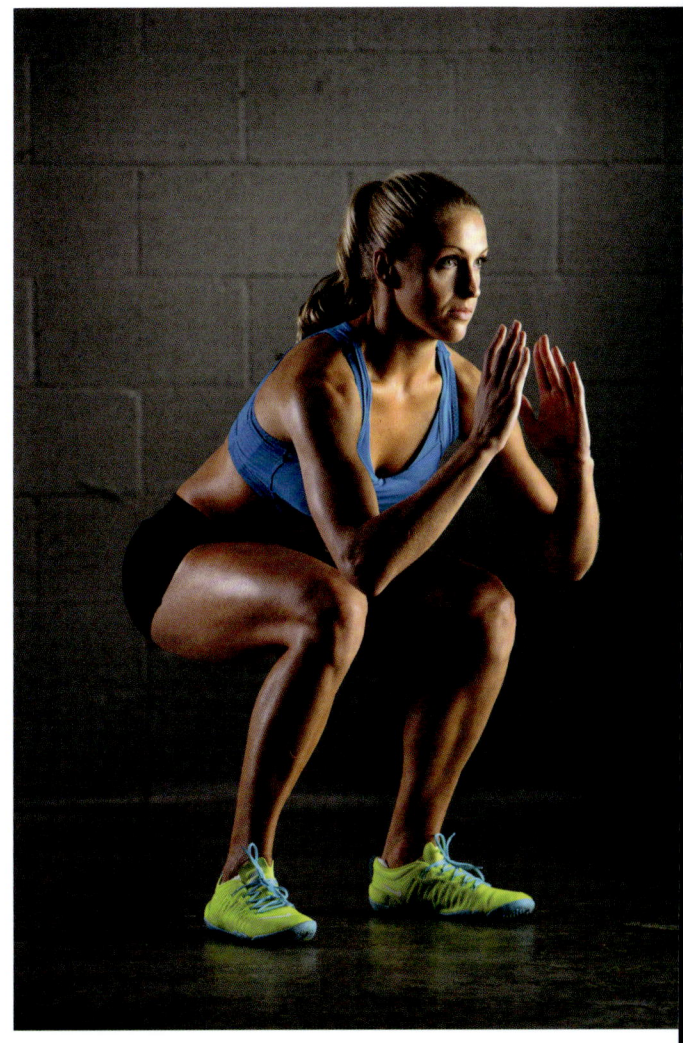

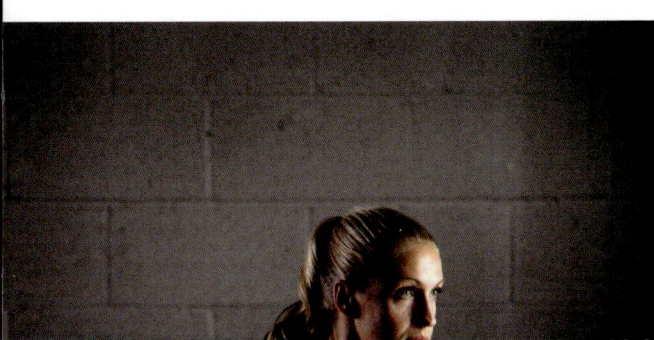

ROUND THE WORLD

This workout is named after the circular motion of the first three exercises and the cyclical circuit-style repetition of the two sets. It will engage the large muscles of the lower body, forging a strong foundation while simultaneously supercharging the metabolism.

[This may be a lower body–focused workout, but keep your core engaged at all times by tightening the abdominals as if readying to take a blow to the body.]

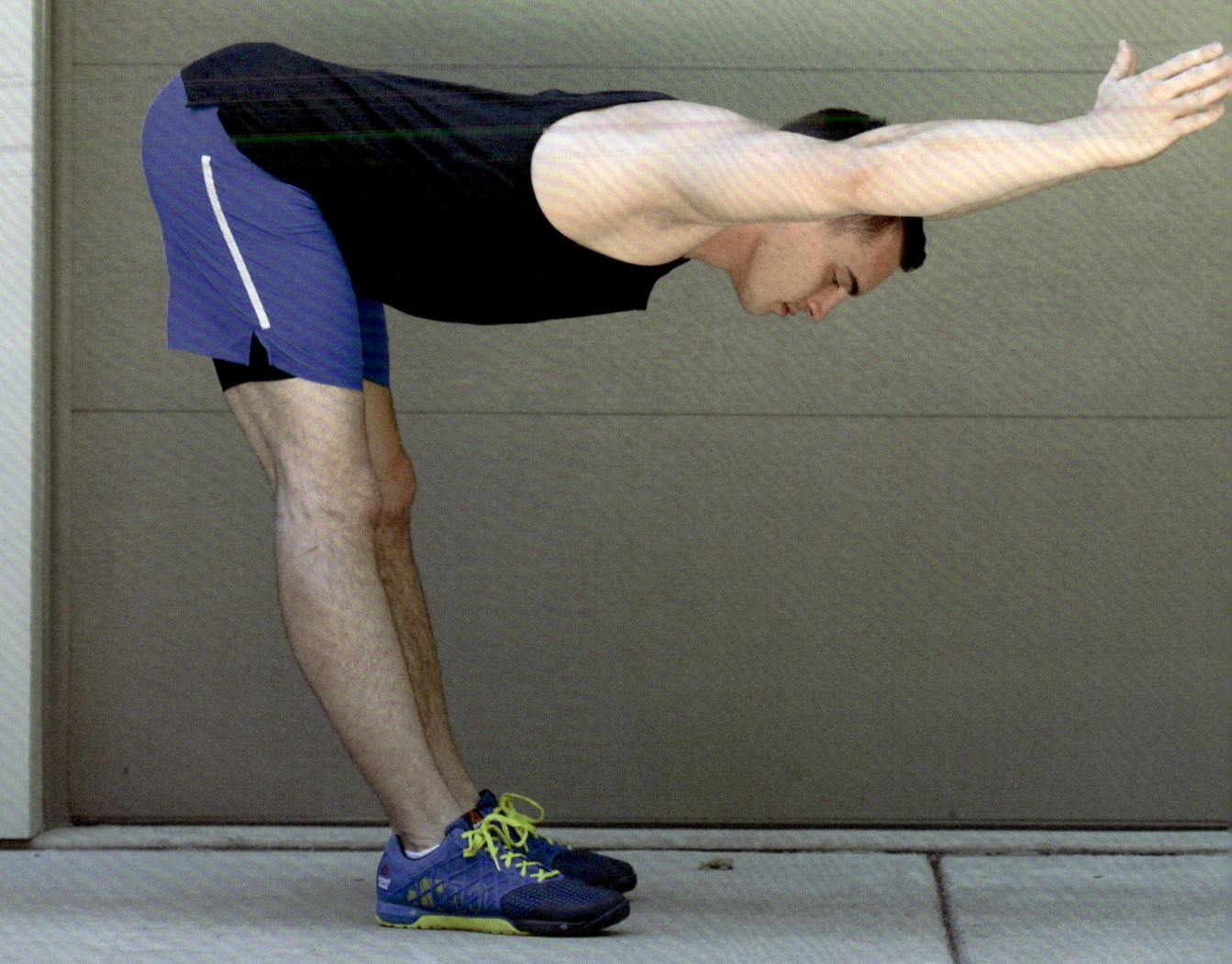

Perform as many reps as you can of all exercises within the prescribed periods of time, and rest for 30 seconds after each set. Repeat sets A–B for a total of 3 rounds. Total time: 13 minutes

 SET A

SQUAT
0:30   p072

ALTERNATING LATERAL LUNGE
0:30   p068

REVERSE LUNGE
0:30   p078

IN-AND-OUTS
0:30   p054

🕐 **REST** 0:30

 SET B

SKATER JUMP
0:30   p055

BRIDGE KICK
0:30 each side   p074

FORWARD HINGE
0:30   p052

🕐 **REST** 0:30

🔁 **REPEAT** sets A–B for a total of 3 rounds

CORE CHAOS

Perform 6 rounds. Rest 30 seconds after each round. Total time: 9 minutes

PIKE
0:30   p134

RUSSIAN TWIST
0:30   p139

SUPER CIRCUIT

With 300 reps, it might take a superhuman effort to get to the end of this routine! The Super Circuit is designed to test your strength, stamina, and willpower.

Perform the exercises in order—15 pull-ups, 15 butterfly peels, 15 push-ups, etc.—then repeat the set for a total of 3 rounds, decreasing by 5 reps per round.

Bonus round: Perform 1 rep as slowly as you possibly can; aim for it to take 10 seconds to perform that rep—5 seconds up and 5 seconds down.

PULL-UP 15x, 10x, 5x, bonus 1x	p114
BUTTERFLY PEEL 15x, 10x, 5x, bonus 1x	p061
PUSH-UP 15x, 10x, 5x, bonus 1x	p096
BURPEE 0:30 all rounds	p086
PIKE 15x, 10x, 5x, bonus 1x	p134
SQUAT 15x, 10x, 5x, bonus 1x	p072
DOWN DOG PUSH-UP 15x, 10x, 5x, bonus 1x	p090
MOUNTAIN CLIMBER 0:30 all rounds	p131
INVERTED BODYWEIGHT ROW 15x, 10x, 5x, bonus 1x	p110
CHIN-UP 15x, 10x, 5x, bonus 1x	p106

🕐 **REST** 2:00

🔁 **REPEAT** for a total of 3 rounds + 1 bonus round (optional)

> When performing the burpees and mountain climbers, aim to do at least the number of reps of the current round within the 30-second time. frame.

COUNTDOWN

When combined in one workout, pull-ups, dips, and squats work almost every muscle in your body, including some of the largest.

Perform the exercises in order—10 squats, 10 pull-ups, 10 push-ups—then repeat the set for a total of 10 rounds, decreasing by 1 rep per round. No rest between rounds.

SQUAT
10x, 9x, 8x, 7x, 6x, 5x, 4x, 3x, 2x, 1x   **p072**

PULL-UP
10x, 9x, 8x, 7x, 6x, 5x, 4x, 3x, 2x, 1x   **p114**

PUSH-UP
10x, 9x, 8x, 7x, 6x, 5x, 4x, 3x, 2x, 1x   **p096**

↻ **REPEAT** for a total of 10 rounds

It's okay to modify this routine based on your current strength and confidence. Push-ups can be performed on your knees, and pull-ups can be substituted for dead hangs for the same number of seconds as the rep count, e.g. 10x reps = 10 seconds.

CORE CHAOS

Perform 3 rounds. Rest 1 minute. Repeat for 3 more rounds. Total time: 7 minutes.

PIKE
0:20   **p134**

MOUNTAIN CLIMBER
0:20   **p131**

REVERSE PLANK BRIDGE
0:20   **p136**

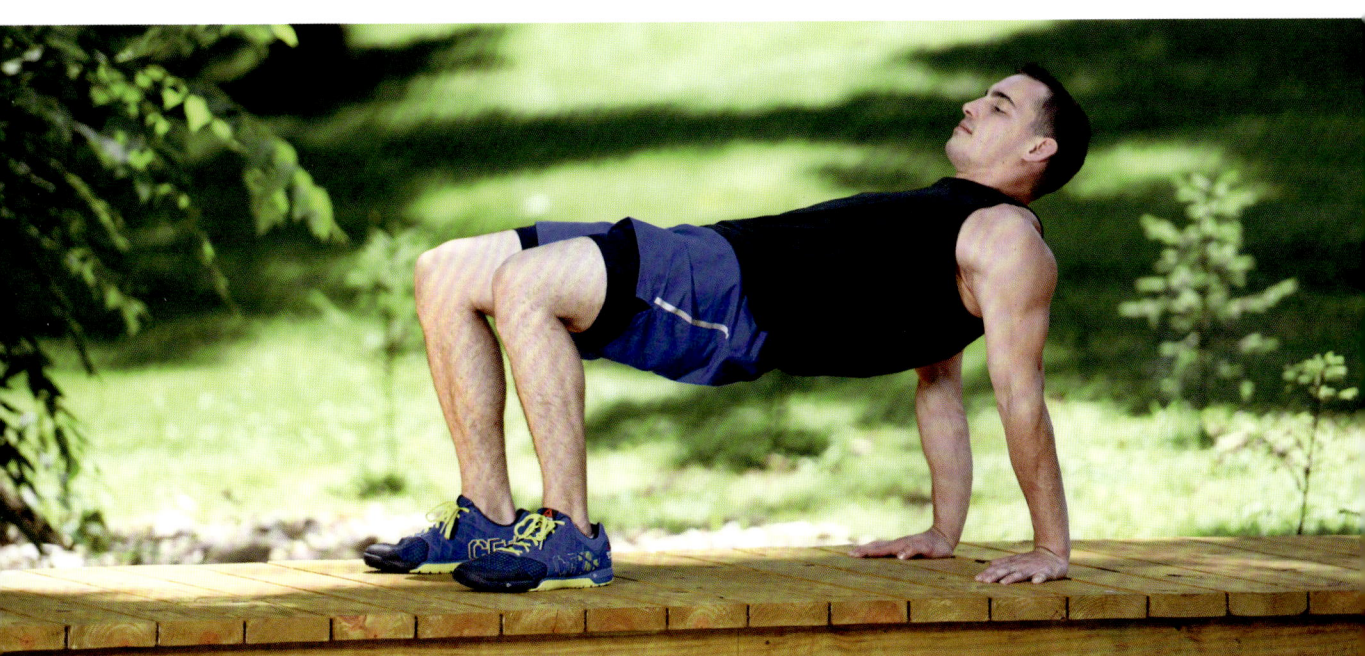

PUSH VS PULL

Concentric versus eccentric muscle contractions; chest versus back; the anterior muscles of the body versus those on the posterior side—Push vs Pull is the body's very own battle of the heavyweight champions. This workout utilizes the pyramid format of decreasing reps per round, which you'll do twice. Can you make it go the distance?

> Attempt to perform the final rep of each exercise as slowly as possible, e.g. 5 seconds to lower, 5 seconds to raise.

Perform the exercises in order—5 push-ups, 5 pull-ups, 5 military push-ups, etc.—then repeat the set, decreasing by 1 rep per round.

PUSH-UP
5x, 4x, 3x, 2x, 1x   p096

PULL-UP
5x, 4x, 3x, 2x, 1x   p114

MILITARY PUSH-UP
5x, 4x, 3x, 2x, 1x   p102

INVERTED BODYWEIGHT ROW
5x, 4x, 3x, 2x, 1x   p110

DOWN DOG PUSH-UP
5x, 4x, 3x, 2x, 1x   p090

CHIN-UP
5x, 4x, 3x, 2x, 1x   p106

↻ **REPEAT** for 5 rounds in pyramid format
🕐 **REST** 2:00

CORE CHAOS
Perform 6 rounds. Rest 30 seconds after each round. Total time: 9 minutes

PIKE
0:30   p134

HOLLOW BODY ROCKER
0:30   p122

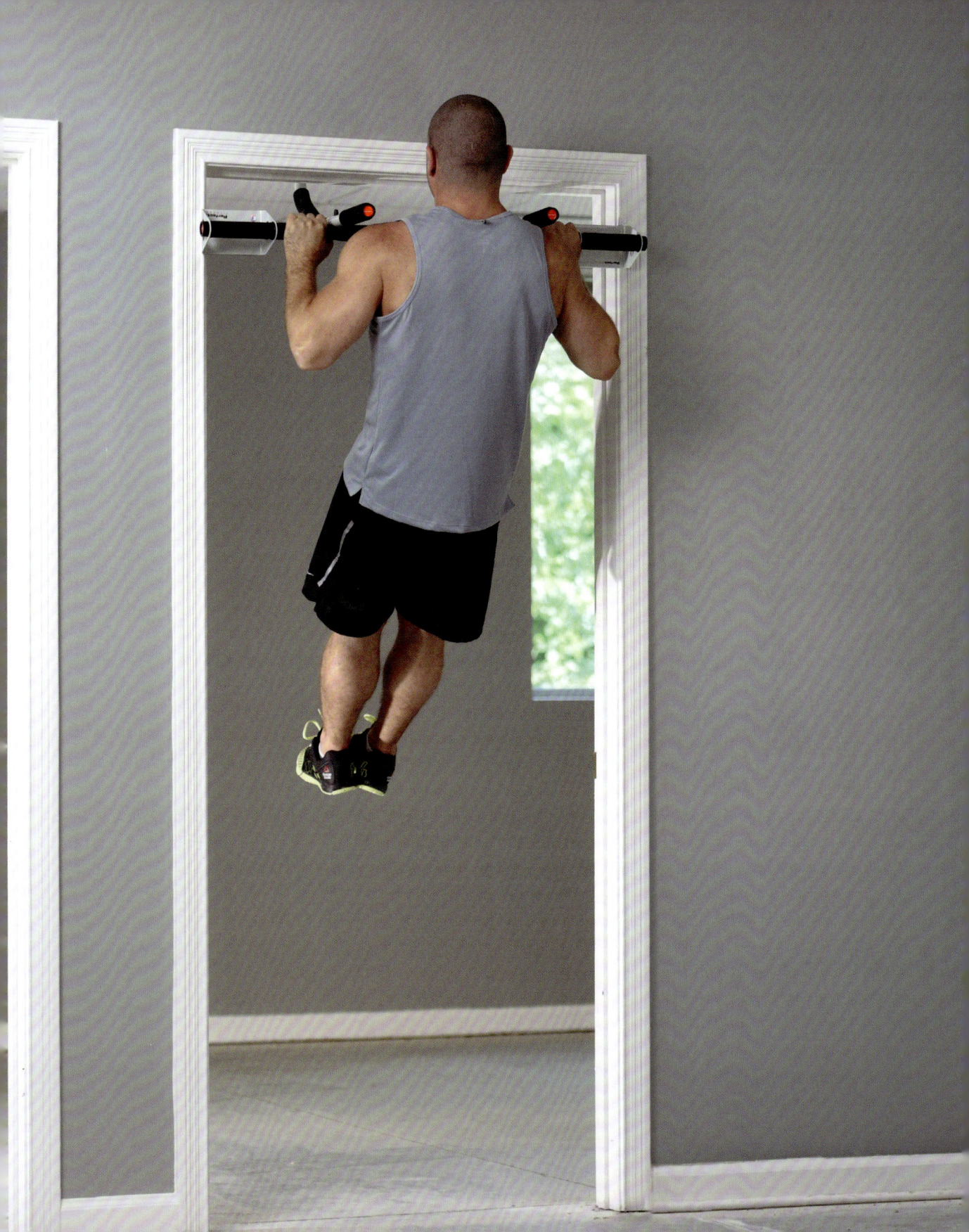

DYNAMIC DUOS

A couplet is a pairing of two functional movements. The two should complement each other in the sense that one is a pull movement and the other a push movement. The benefit of couplets is that by offsetting a push movement with a pull movement, you give yourself time to "rest" as you're actively working, which decreases your downtime and makes the workout more effective.

> If you begin to fatigue on the chin-ups, jump up to the bar, using momentum to help lift you, and slowly control your descent over a count of four. This eccentric contraction helps build strength.

Perform the exercises as couplets (such as 10 dips followed immediately by 10 chin-ups). Don't rest between reps; move immediately to 8 reps of each exercise. Complete all 5 rounds of the couplet set before resting 1 minute and moving on to the next set.

SET A

TRICEPS DIP
10x, 8x, 6x, 4x, 2x   p089

CHIN-UP
10x, 8x, 6x, 4x, 2x   p106

🕐 **REST** 1:00

SET B

SQUAT
10x, 8x, 6x, 4x, 2x   p072

SKATER JUMP
10x, 8x, 6x, 4x, 2x   p055

🕐 **REST** 1:00

SET C

SPHINX
10x, 8x, 6x, 4x, 2x   p108

INVERTED BODYWEIGHT ROW
10x, 8x, 6x, 4x, 2x   p110

🕐 **REST** 1:00

CORE CHAOS

Perform 3 rounds. Rest 1 minute after each round. Total time: 5 minutes

PIKE
0:20   p134

MOUNTAIN CLIMBER
0:20   p131

REVERSE PLANK BRIDGE
0:20   p136

HI-LO

Triplets, as the name suggests, combine three functional exercises—often complementary push and pull exercises. For this routine, we add a third dynamic, high-intensity exercise to each triplet as a metabolic booster, and also to improve endurance and athletic performance.

> If you're having a hard time recovering between sets, increase the rest period to 2 minutes.

Perform 5 rounds of each set in order, decreasing reps by 2 each round. Rest 1 minute between sets.

SET A

| PUSH-UP | p096 |
| 10x, 8x, 6x, 4x, 2x | |

| HANGING SCAPULA RETRACTION | p093 |
| 10x, 8x, 6x, 4x, 2x | |

| MOUNTAIN CLIMBER | p131 |
| 0:45 | |

🕐 **REST** 1:00

SET B

| SQUAT | p072 |
| 10x, 8x, 6x, 4x, 2x | |

| SKATER JUMP | p055 |
| 10x, 8x, 6x, 4x, 2x | |

| X-JACK | p073 |
| 0:45 | |

🕐 **REST** 1:00

SET C

| TRICEPS DIP | p089 |
| 10x, 8x, 6x, 4x, 2x | |

| INVERTED BODYWEIGHT ROW | p110 |
| 10x, 8x, 6x, 4x, 2x | |

| PUSH-UP JACK | p098 |
| 0:45 | |

🕐 **REST** 1:00

SET D

| REVERSE LUNGE | p078 |
| 10x, 8x, 6x, 4x, 2x | |

| CHIN-UP | p106 |
| 10x, 8x, 6x, 4x, 2x | |

| BURPEE | p086 |
| 0:45 | |

🕐 **REST** 1:00

BURN

Based on intervals of 20 seconds of all-out exercise followed by 10 seconds of rest, Tabata training workouts incinerate body fat. Performing as many reps as you possibly can in 20 seconds will make your heart rate skyrocket. The high-energy output allows you to tap the post-workout benefits of Tabata and high-intensity interval training, which allows you to burn calories for up to 48 hours after the workout.

[
Always remember: form first, speed second. Push for maximum reps but not at the cost of your form, as this may lead to injury.
]

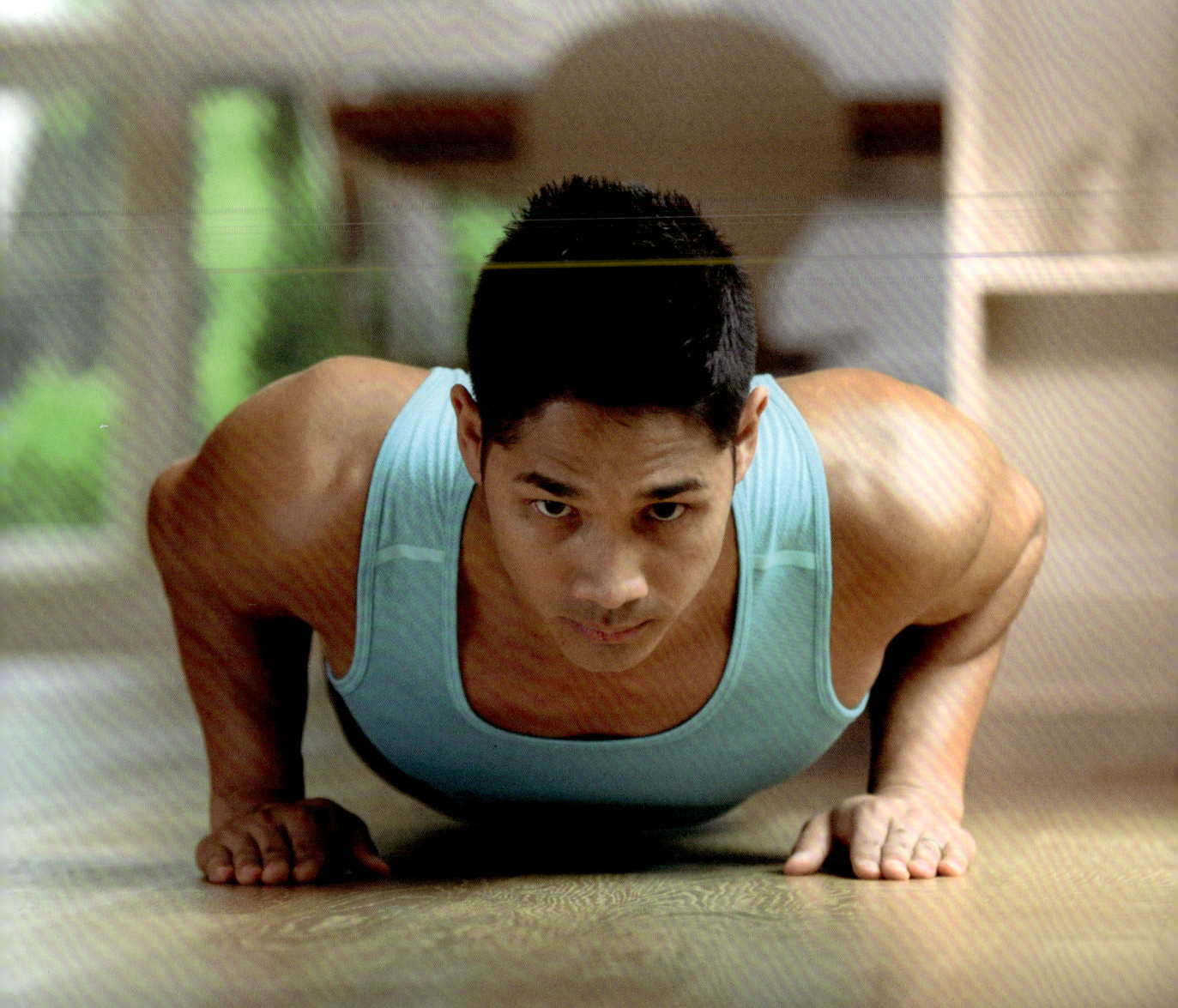

Perform 3 rounds of each set. Rest 1 minute between each set. Total time: 27 minutes

SET A

PUSH-UP JACK
work 0:20, rest 0:10   p098

SQUAT JUMP
work 0:20, rest 0:10   p066

↻ **REPEAT** for 3 rounds
◷ **REST** 1:00 before set B

SET B

CHIN-UP
work 0:20, rest 0:10   p106

PUSH-UP
work 0:20, rest 0:10   p096

↻ **REPEAT** for 3 rounds
◷ **REST** 1:00 before set C

SET C

BURPEE
work 0:20, rest 0:10   p086

1-2 PUSH
work 0:20, rest 0:10   p112

↻ **REPEAT** for 3 rounds
◷ **REST** 1:00 before set D

SET D

PULL-UP
work 0:20, rest 0:10   p114

MILITARY PUSH-UP
work 0:20, rest 0:10   p102

↻ **REPEAT** for 3 rounds
◷ **REST** 1:00 before set E

SET E

REVERSE LUNGE
work 0:20, rest 0:10   p078

MOUNTAIN CLIMBER
work 0:20, rest 0:10   p131

↻ **REPEAT** for 3 rounds
◷ **REST** 1:00 before set F

SET F

SKATER JUMP
work 0:20, rest 0:10   p055

DOWN DOG PUSH-UP
work 0:20, rest 0:10   p090

↻ **REPEAT** for 3 rounds
◷ **REST** 1:00 before set G

SET G

BALL PRESS
work 0:20, rest 0:10   p105

INVERTED BODYWEIGHT ROW
work 0:20, rest 0:10   p110

↻ **REPEAT** for 3 rounds
◷ **REST** 1:00

PUSH-PULL PAIRS

Pushing exercises help improve upper-body strength and muscle definition. Pulling exercises can help improve posture and reduce the risk of injury. Both utilize some of the largest muscle groups in the body, which means big gains in strength and an extended metabolic impact after the workout is complete.

If 10 reps is too many on any exercise, make things easier to allow you to continue. For example, for push-ups, drop to your knees and finish the remaining reps.

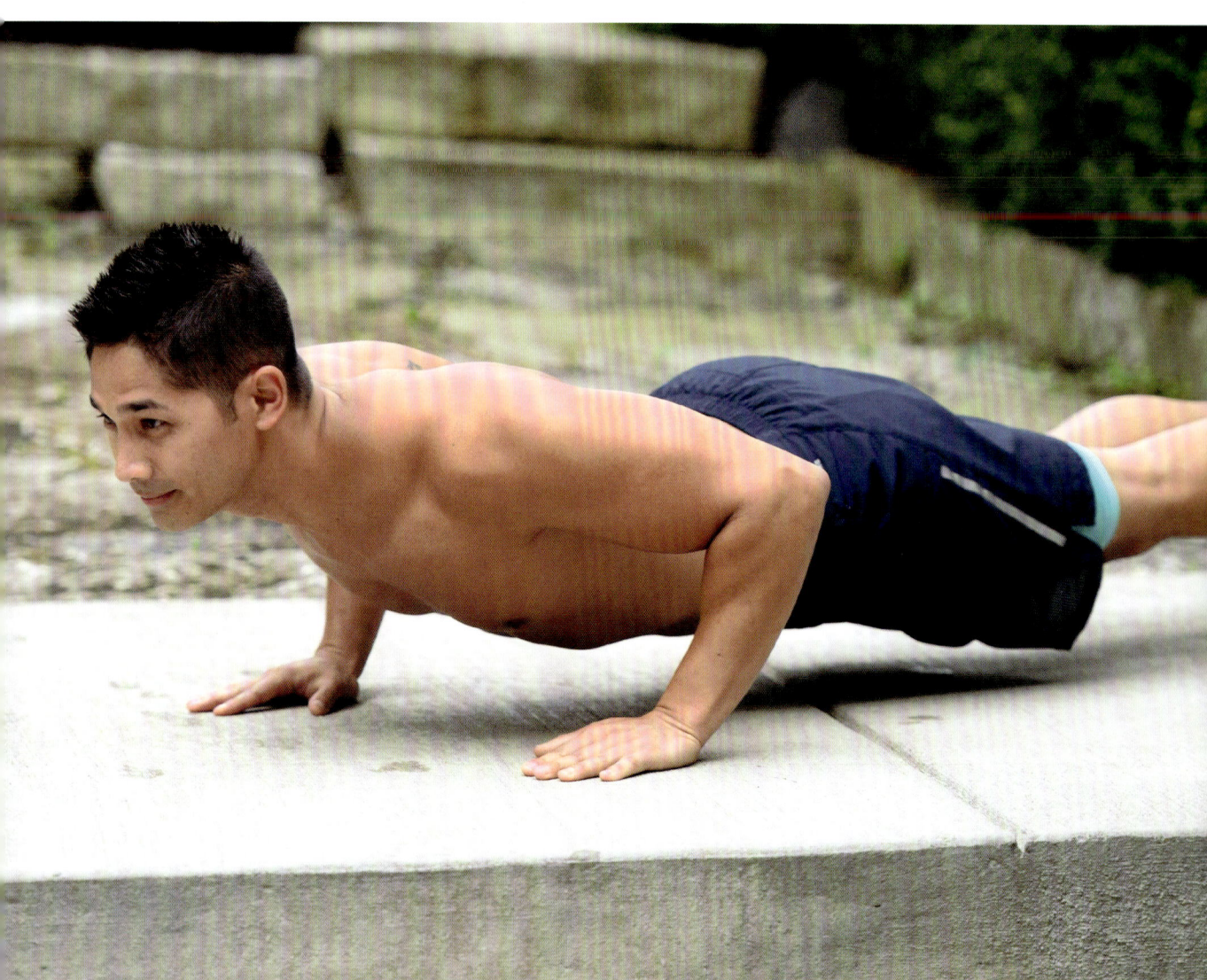

Perform 5 rounds of each set, decreasing reps by 2 each round. Rest 30 seconds after each round.

 SET A

PUSH-UP JACK
10x, 8x, 6x, 4x, 2x   p098

PULL-UP
10x, 8x, 6x, 4x, 2x   p114

🕐 **REST** 0:30 after each round of the set
🔁 **REPEAT** for 5 rounds in pyramid format

 SET B

DOWN DOG PUSH-UP
10x, 8x, 6x, 4x, 2x   p090

INVERTED BODYWEIGHT ROW
10x, 8x, 6x, 4x, 2x   p110

🕐 **REST** 0:30 after each round of the set
🔁 **REPEAT** for 5 rounds in pyramid format

 SET C

SPHINX
10x, 8x, 6x, 4x, 2x   p108

KNEE TUCK EXTENSION
10x, 8x, 6x, 4x, 2x   p140

🕐 **REST** 0:30 after each round of the set
🔁 **REPEAT** for 5 rounds in pyramid format

RIP IT

Perform 2 rounds. Rest 1 minute. Repeat for 2 more rounds. Total time: 9 minutes

HANGING REVERSE CURL
work 0:20, rest 0:10   p132

BURPEE
work 0:20, rest 0:10   p086

1-2 PUSH
work 0:20, rest 0:10   p112

HANGING LEG RAISE
work 0:20, rest 0:10   p119

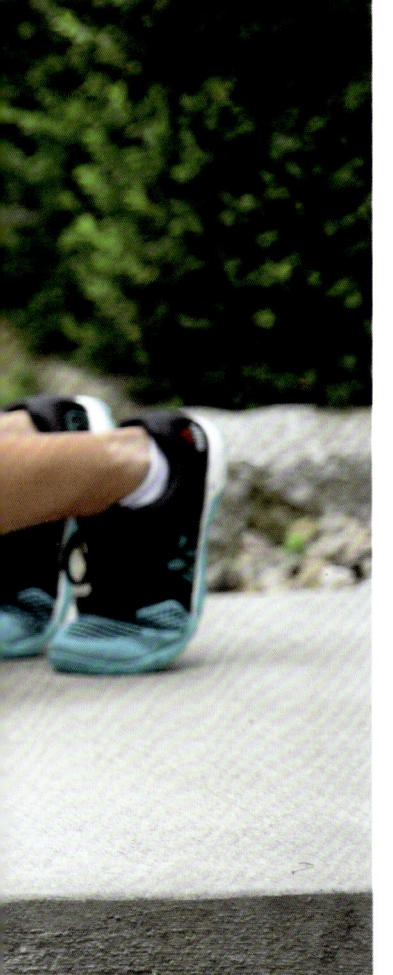

CRAZY 8s

There are any number of rep schemes you can follow when working out, but one of the absolute best I have ever used to gain strength and power is affectionately known as "Crazy 8s" in my gym. It consists of 8 sets of an exercise, performing just 5 reps followed by a 30-second to 1-minute rest. This low-rep but high-volume style of training will build your strength and help you gain muscle.

Avoid working to failure in the latter sets or on very challenging exercises such as pull-ups. If 3 or 4 reps is your max with good form, stop at that point and rest.

For each exercise, perform 8 sets of 5 reps, resting for 30 seconds to 1 minute between sets. Perform all 8 sets before moving to the next.

SQUAT JUMP
8 sets × 5 reps (a.k.a. 8 × 5)　　p066

DOWN DOG PUSH-UP
8 × 5　　p090

SQUAT PEDAL
8 × 5　　p056

SINGLE-LEG BURPEE
8 × 5 (4 sets per leg,
alternate each set)　　p084

PULL-UP
8 × 5　　p114

INVERTED BODYWEIGHT ROW
8 × 5　　p110

V-UP
8 × 5　　p143

BACK BRIDGE
8 × 5 (Hold to a count of
3 at the top of each rep.)　　p124

FANTASTIC FOUR

The four exercises in this routine provide a head-to-toe workout! If pressed for time, there are few exercises that can provide as much bang for your buck as the "fantastic four." This routine is an AMRAP, meaning the goal is to complete "as many rounds as possible" in 20 minutes.

Perform each exercise 10 times with little to no rest between exercises. Repeat for as many rounds as possible in 20 minutes.

PUSH-UP
10x   p096

PULL-UP
10x   p114

SQUAT
10x   p072

INVERTED BODYWEIGHT ROW
10x   p110

↻ **REPEAT** AMRAP

[
AMRAPs can often create a sense of urgency that will cause people to sacrifice form for speed. Remember the golden rule: form first, speed second.
]

RIP IT
Perform 4 rounds, resting 1 minute after each round. Total time: 11 minutes

HANGING REVERSE CURL
work 0:20, rest 0:10   p132

BURPEE
work 0:20, rest 0:10   p086

1–2 PUSH
work 0:20, rest 0:10   p112

HANGING LEG RAISE
work 0:20, rest 0:10   p119

ALL-IN

Are you all-in? This workout is going to test your mental resolve as much as your physical prowess. Each exercise has a lower number of reps, allowing you to accomplish each with good form. The speed at which you perform the exercises and the rest after each is up to you. Can you go three rounds with no rest?

> Don't perform half reps–all-in or modify! If you know you can't complete 10 archer pull-ups, perform as many complete reps as possible and then either assist with a chair or perform any easier pull such as standard pull-ups or inverted rows.

SHRIMP SQUAT 10x (5x each leg)		p118
DEEP SQUAT 20x		p102
FRONT LUNGE 20x (10x each leg)		p104
SINGLE-LEG BURPEE 20x (10x each leg)		p134
PIKE PUSH-UP TO PUSH-UP 10x		p140
ARCHER PULL-UP 10x		p108
DIP 10x		p073
CHIN-UP 10x		p050
HOLLOW BODY HOLD 0:30		p113

🕐 **REST** 1:00

🔁 **REPEAT** the set for a total of 3 rounds

RIP IT
Perform 2 rounds. Rest 1 minute, then repeat for 2 more rounds. Total time: 9 minutes

HANGING REVERSE CURL work 0:20, rest 0:10		p132
BURPEE work 0:20, rest 0:10		p086
1-2 PUSH work 0:20, rest 0:10		p112
HANGING LEG RAISE work 0:20, rest 0:10		p119

FIRE

It's time to light a fire under you! This workout is a metabolic powerhouse, utilizing high-intensity intervals and multi-muscle compound exercises to torch body fat and build lean muscle. Your aim during each 20 seconds of work is to reach 80–90 percent of your maximum heart rate.

> At 80–90 percent of maximum heart rate you should feel slightly uncomfortable, unable to hold a conversation, out of breath, and in need of each 10-second rest.

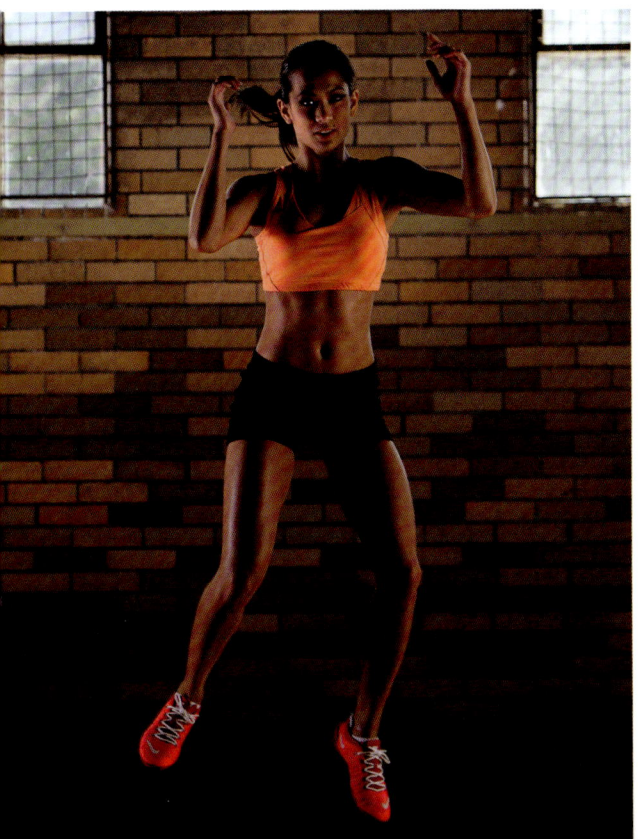

Perform 3 rounds of each set, followed by 1 minute of rest before moving to the next set.
Total time: 20 minutes

 SET A

1–2 PUSH
work 0:20, rest 0:10   p112

SINGLE-LEG BURPEE (RIGHT)
work 0:20, rest 0:10   p084

DEAD HANG
work 0:20, rest 0:10   p092

SINGLE-LEG BURPEE (LEFT)
work 0:20, rest 0:10   p084

🔁 **REPEAT** the set for a total of 3 rounds
🕐 **REST** 1:00 before set B

 SET B

PUSH-UP
work 0:20, rest 0:10   p096

SKI JUMP
work 0:20, rest 0:10   p079

SQUAT PEDAL
work 0:20, rest 0:10   p056

SPRINTER SIT-UP
work 0:20, rest 0:10   p128

🔁 **REPEAT** the set for a total of 3 rounds
🕐 **REST** 1:00 before set C

 SET C

PUSH-UP JACK
work 0:20, rest 0:10   p098

IN-AND-OUT ABS
work 0:20, rest 0:10   p054

SPHINX
work 0:20, rest 0:10   p108

TUCK JUMP BURPEE
work 0:20, rest 0:10   p094

🔁 **REPEAT** the set for a total of 3 rounds

THE BODYWEIGHT 500

This grueling total-body workout will demand 500 total reps of exercises from all levels. It will push you both mentally and physically. In exchange, you'll get increased endurance and improved athletic performance, and you'll shred fat. You have what it takes, but it will take all you've got!

[
Don't substitute any exercises or reduce the reps. Instead, when necessary, use a less difficult modification for each exercise to make the workout easier.
]

Perform all exercises in order and try to minimize rest time between exercises.

SQUAT
50x   p072

PUSH-UP
50x   p096

SQUAT JUMP
25x   p066

SKATER JUMP
25x   p055

PIKE
50x   p134

ALTERNATING LATERAL LUNGE
50x   p060

PULL-UP
25x   p114

REVERSE LUNGE
50x (25x each leg)   p078

MILITARY PUSH-UP
50x   p102

INVERTED BODYWEIGHT ROW
50x   p110

JUMP LUNGE
50x   p062

BURPEE
25x   p086

ABDOMINATION

Even though your core is engaged and working during all the compound exercises found in this book, a dedicated abs routine to target and isolate the core is always fun! Perform the exercises in order for the best results.

[
If the hanging reverse curls and hanging leg raises are too challenging—or if you lack the required pull-up bar—replace both with 20 hollow body rockers (page 122).
]

⟳ **REPEAT** the set for a total of 3 rounds

🕐 **REST** 2 minutes after each round

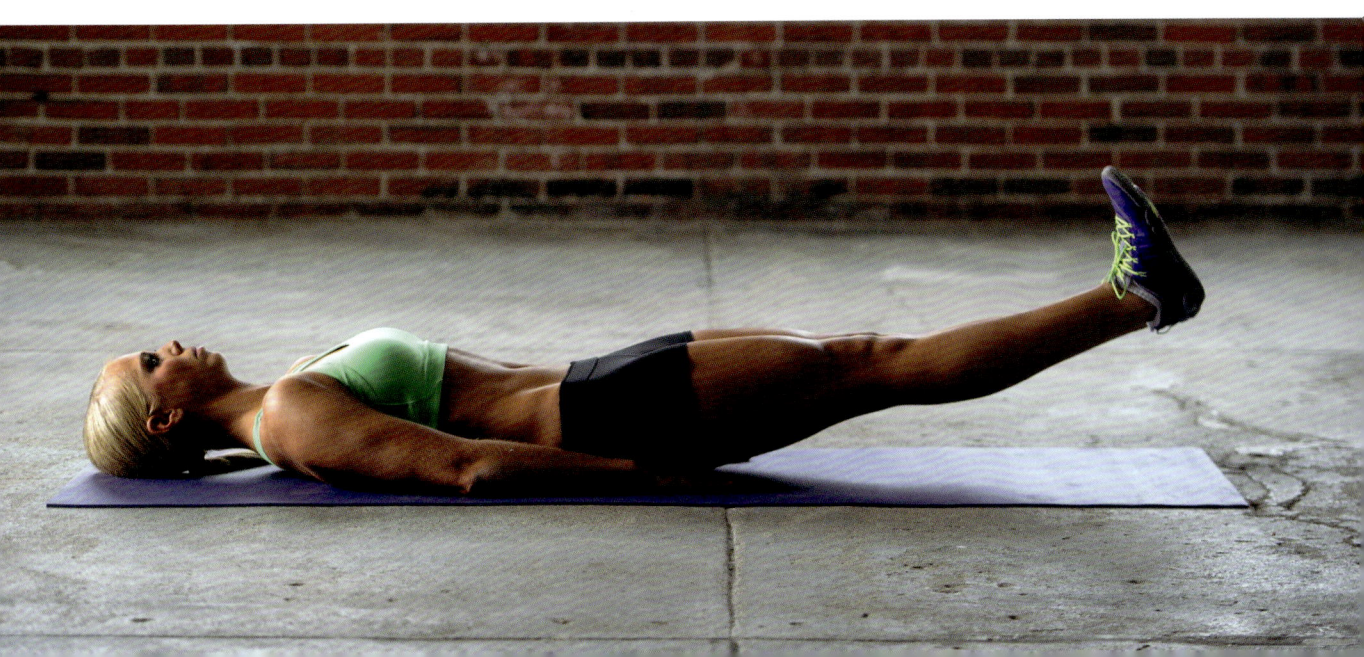

REDLINE

To "redline" means to push until you hit your limits. This fusion of high-intensity interval training and bodyweight resistance exercises will take you to your redline.

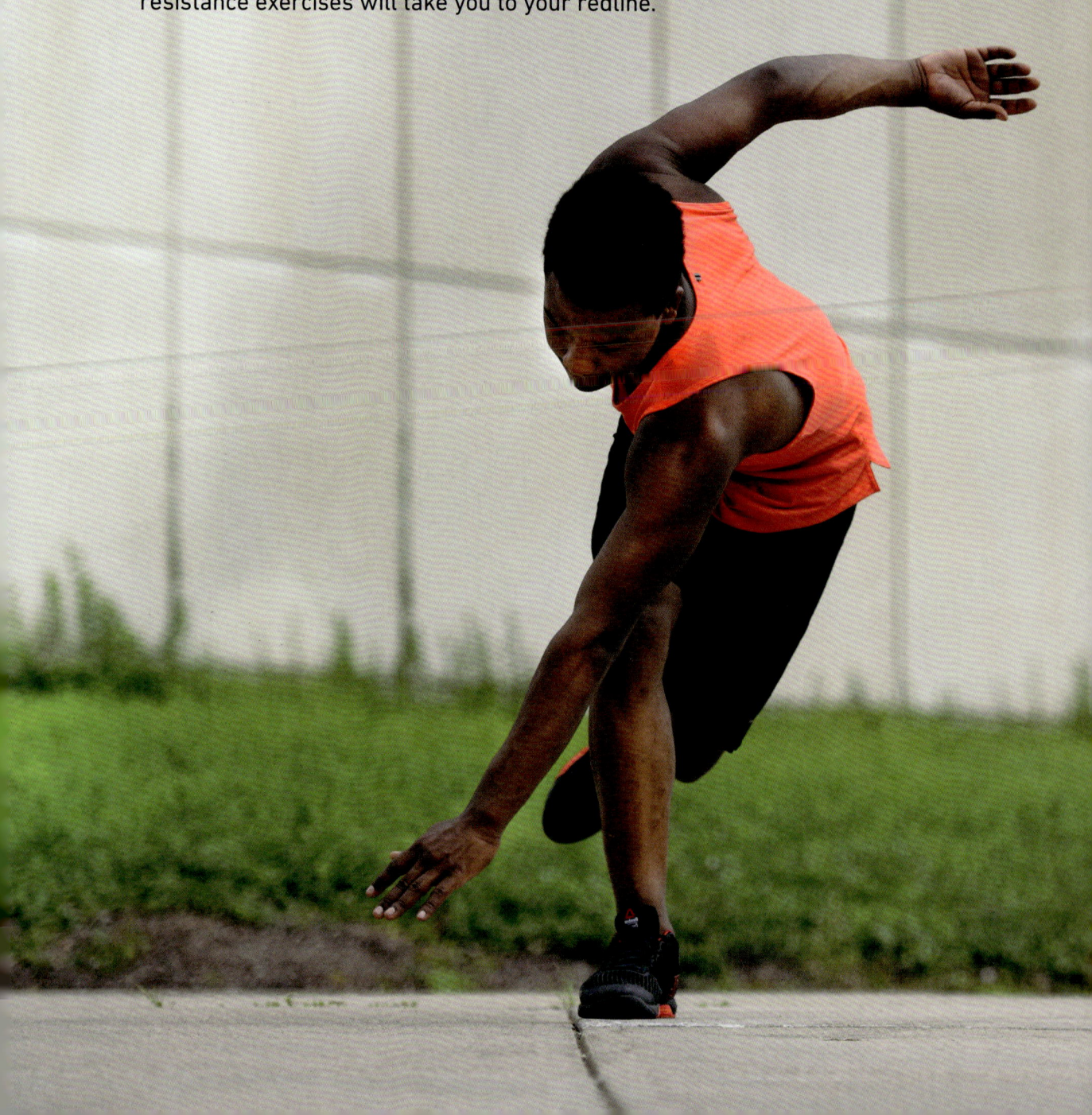

Perform 5 rounds of each set. Rest for 30 seconds after each round. Total time: 25 minutes

 SET A

| **X-JACK** | |
| 0:30 | p073 |

| **TUCK JUMP BURPEE** | |
| 0:30 | p094 |

| **MOUNTAIN CLIMBER** | |
| 0:30 | p131 |

| **BURPEE** | |
| 0:30 | p086 |

🕐 **REST** 0:30 before set B

 SET B

| **PUSH-UP JACK** | |
| 0:30 | p098 |

| **SKI JUMP** | |
| 0:30 | p079 |

| **1-2 PUSH** | |
| 0:30 | p112 |

| **INVERTED BODYWEIGHT ROW** | |
| 0:30 | p110 |

🕐 **REST** 0:30

🔁 **REPEAT** sets A–B for a total of 5 rounds

[
If you struggle to recover between sets, extend the rest period to 1 minute.
]

THE CYCLE

Multi-muscle exercises that constantly change your elevation will drive your heart rate up and challenge your cardiovascular fitness. This routine has a "stair step" format, with the number of rounds increasing for each set.

> If the explosive tuck jump in set A is too challenging, replace it with the standard burpee.

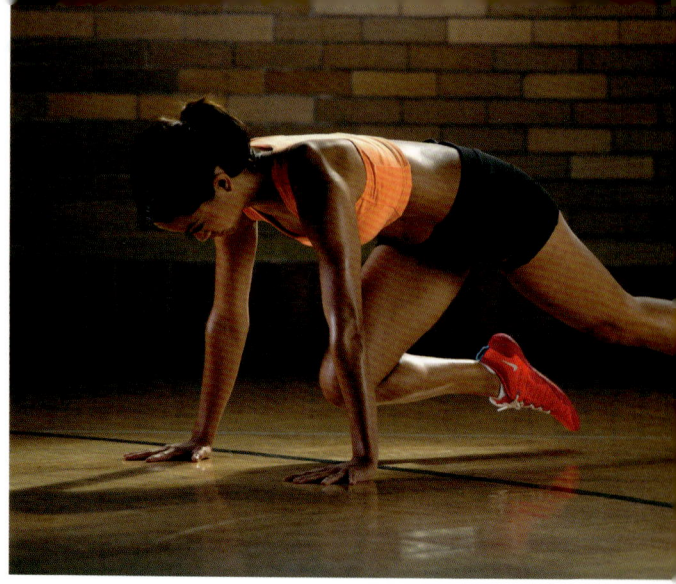

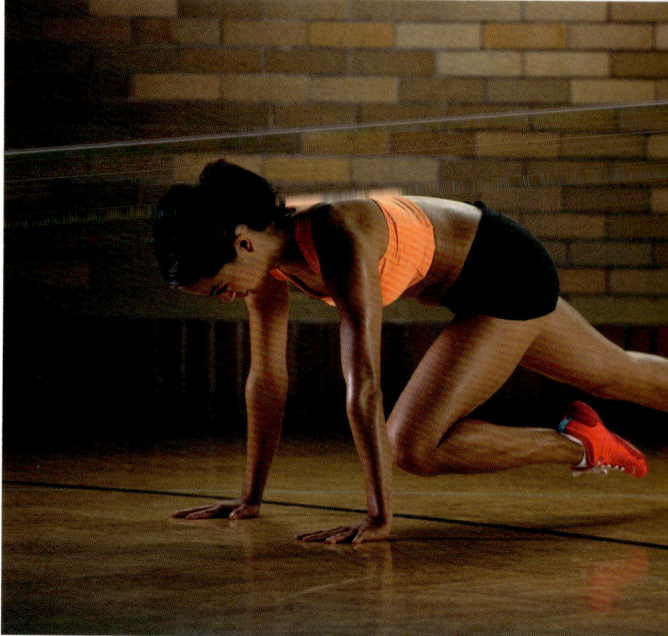

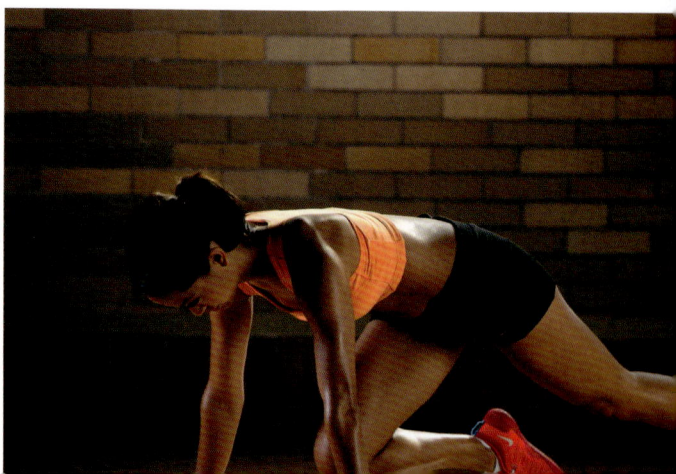

Perform 1 round for set A, 2 rounds for set B, and 3 rounds for set C. Rest for 10 seconds after each exercise.
Total time: 12 minutes

SET A

HIGH KNEES
work 0:30, rest 0:10   p118

1-2 PUSH
work 0:30, rest 0:10   p112

TUCK JUMP BURPEE
work 0:30, rest 0:10   p094

SET B

X-JACKS
work 0:30, rest 0:10   p073

CROSS PUSH
work 0:30, rest 0:10   p100

SQUAT PEDAL
work 0:30, rest 0:10   p056

↻ **REPEAT** set B for a total of 2 rounds

SET C

MOUNTAIN CLIMBER
work 0:30, rest 0:10   p131

TRICEPS DIP
work 0:30, rest 0:10   p089

BURPEE
work 0:30, rest 0:10   p086

↻ **REPEAT** set C for a total of 3 rounds

TOTAL-BODY BLAST

Fusing exercises of varying levels of difficulty, Total-Body Blast evolves with each set to take you from the base motion in set A to the dynamic version in set C.

[
If 3 rounds of this workout is too challenging for you, perform only 2 rounds, or adjust the reps on rounds 2 and 3 so you're working at 80% of your max effort.
]

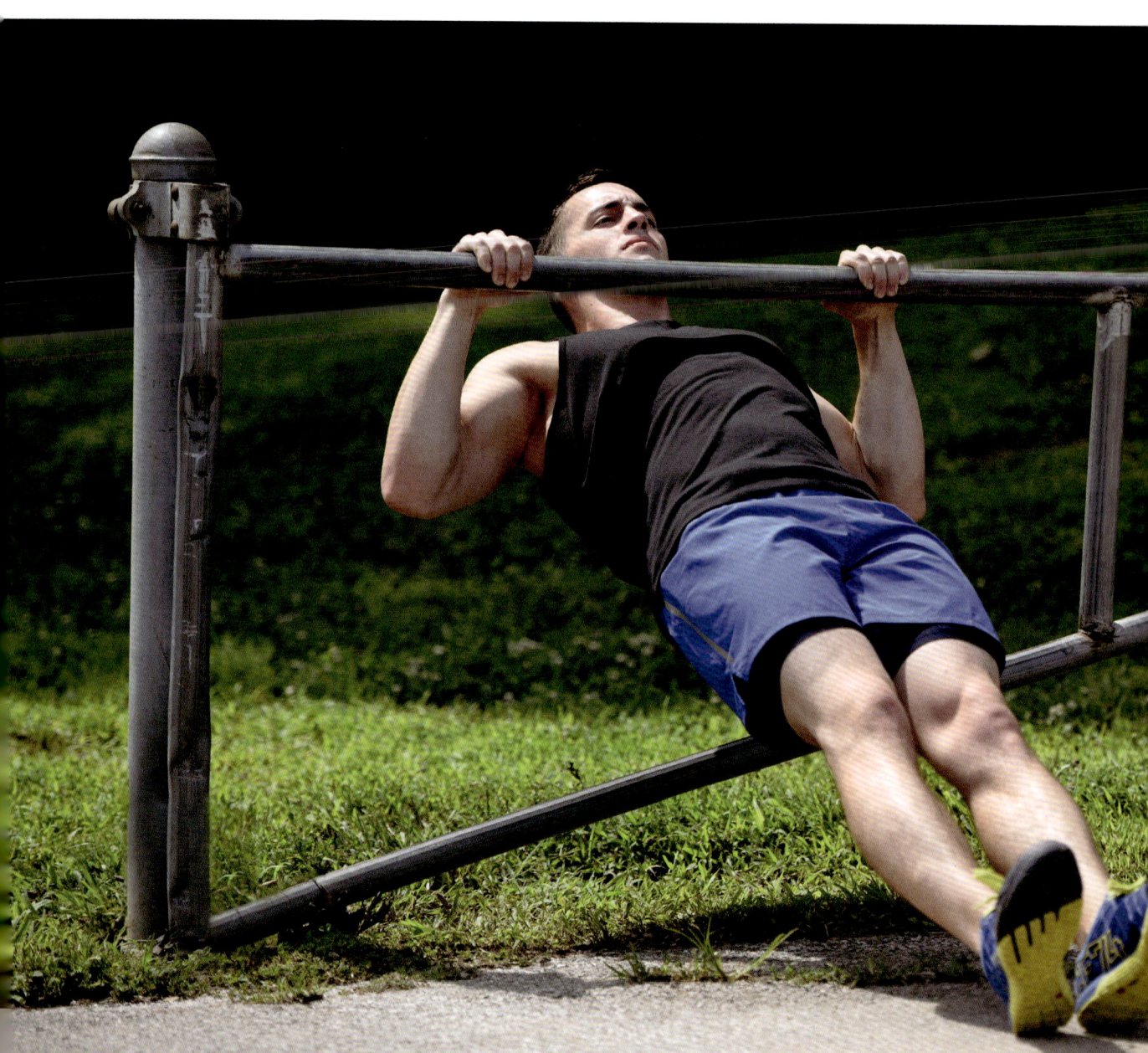

Perform sets A–C in order with little to no rest between exercises. Rest for 1 minute between sets. Repeat 3 times.

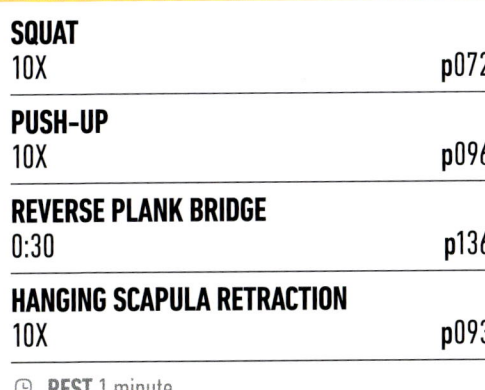

 SET A

SQUAT
10X   p072

PUSH-UP
10X   p096

REVERSE PLANK BRIDGE
0:30   p136

HANGING SCAPULA RETRACTION
10X   p093

🕐 **REST** 1 minute

 SET B

SQUAT JUMP
10X   p066

SPIDERMAN
10X   p109

BACK BRIDGE
0:30   p124

CHIN-UP
10X   p106

🕐 **REST** 1 minute

 SET C

SQUAT PEDAL
10X   p056

PUSH-UP JACK
10X   p098

BRIDGE KICK
10X (alternate legs)   p074

ARCHER PULL-UP
10X   p104

🕐 **REST** 1 minute
🔁 **REPEAT** Sets A–C 3 times

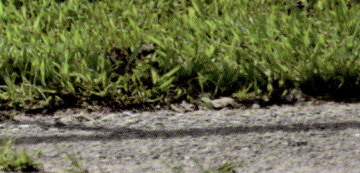

TRI-PHASE

A phase is a distinct period or stage in a process of change, or a part of something's development. Each triplet in this workout features exercises geared to sculpt lean muscle, build strength, burn fat, and evolve your body.

> [If the pull-up is too challenging, replace it with hanging scapula retraction (page 93).]

Perform 3 rounds of each set. Rest for 2 minutes between rounds and 1 minute between sets.

 SET A

BULGARIAN SPLIT SQUAT	
20x (10x each leg)	p076
DOWN DOG PUSH-UP	
10x	p090
1-2 PUSH	
20x	p112

↻ **REPEAT** for a total of 3 rounds
◷ **REST** 1:00 before set B

 SET B

T-STAND	
20x (10x each leg)	p067
CROSS PUSH	
20x	p100
SKI JUMP	
20x	p079

↻ **REPEAT** for a total of 3 rounds
◷ **REST** 1:00 before set C

 SET C

SQUAT	
20x	p072
PULL-UP	
20x	p114
SPIDERMAN	
0:45	p109

↻ **REPEAT** for a total of 3 rounds
◷ **REST** 1:00 before set D

 SET D

BUTTERFLY PEEL	
20x	p061
INVERTED BODYWEIGHT ROW	
20x	p110
MOUNTAIN CLIMBER	
20x	p131

↻ **REPEAT** for a total of 3 rounds
◷ **REST** 1:00

CORE CHAOS
Perform 4 rounds. Rest 30 seconds after each round.

V-UP		**HANGING REVERSE CURL**	
10x	p143	10x	p132
HOLLOW BODY ROCKER		**MOGUL JUMP**	
0:30	p122	0:30	p130

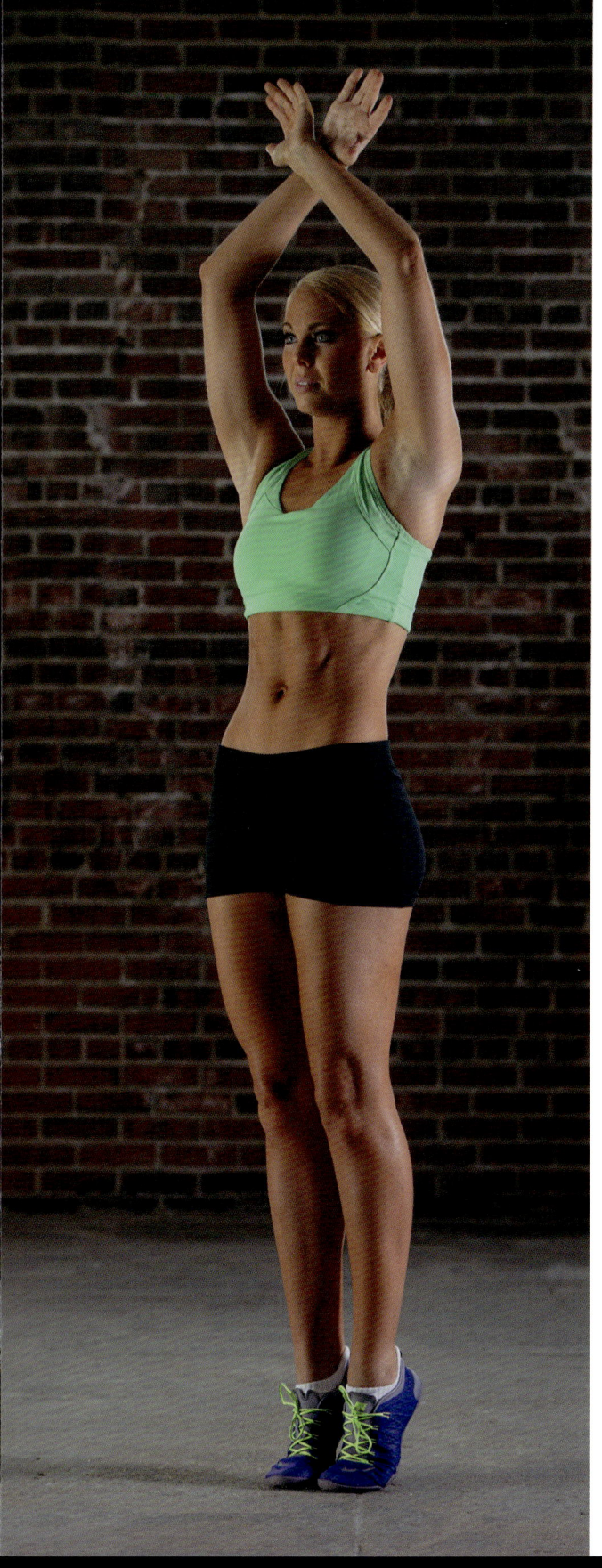

JACKED UP

We all know the infamous jumping jack. It's a wonderful cardio exercise that features heavily in high-intensity interval training workouts. This routine features three evolutions of that exercise to challenge your lower body, upper body, and core.

Perform 5 rounds. Don't rest between each exercise. Rest for 1 minute after each round.

X-JACK
20x   p073

PUSH-UP JACK
20x   p098

SHOULDER PRESS JACK
1:00   p088

↻ **REPEAT** for a total of 5 rounds
⏲ **REST** 1:00 after each round

CORE CHAOS
Perform 6 rounds. Rest 30 seconds after each round. Total time: 9 minutes

PIKE
0:30   p134

HOLLOW BODY ROCKER
0:30   p122

TOTAL-BODY BURN

This routine features three exercises per set: one lower-body, one upper-body, and one core exercise. The reps decrease each round, allowing you to focus on form and range of motion. The goal is for each round to take the same amount of time despite the decreasing reps. Slow down and let it BURN!

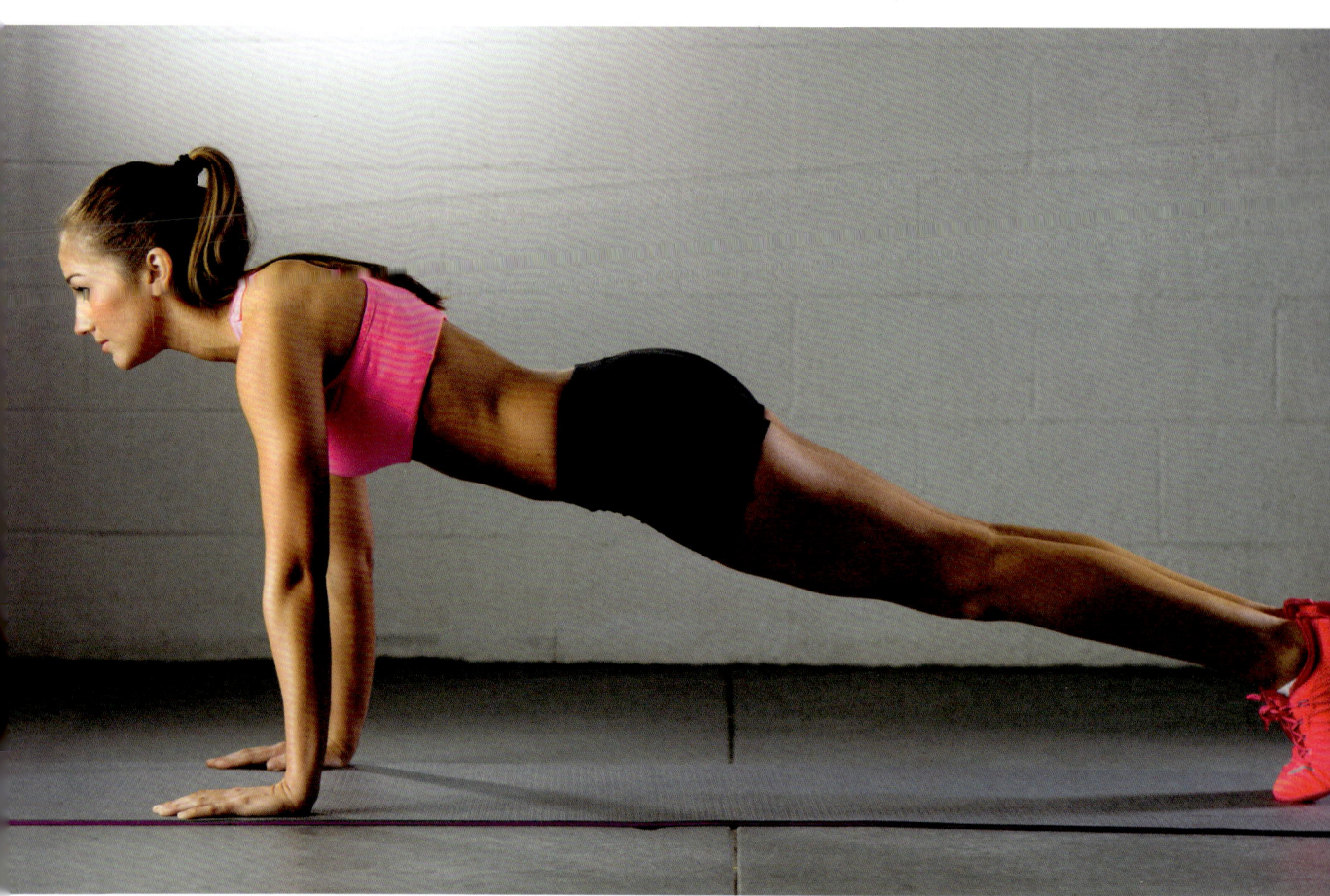

Perform each set in order, starting with 20 reps per exercise, then 12, and finally 10. Rest for 2 minutes after each set.

 SET A

SQUAT
20x, 12x, 10x   p072

PUSH-UP
20x, 12x, 10x   p096

V-UP
20x, 12x, 10x   p143

🕐 **REST** 2 minutes

 SET B

REVERSE LUNGE
20x, 12x, 10x   p078

TRICEPS DIP
20x, 12x, 10x   p089

SPRINTER SIT-UP
20x, 12x, 10x   p128

🕐 **REST** 2 minutes

 SET C

ALTERNATING LATERAL LUNGE
20x, 12x, 10x   p068

PULL-UP
20x, 12x, 10x   p114

RUSSIAN TWIST
20x, 12x, 10x   p139

🕐 **REST** 2 minutes

 SET D

FORWARD HINGE
20x, 12x, 10x   p052

CHIN-UP
20x, 12x, 10x   p106

SQUAT TO L-SIT
20x, 12x, 10x   p120

🕐 **REST** 2 minutes

SET E

T-STAND
20x, 12x, 10x   p067

MILITARY PUSH-UP
20x, 12x, 10x   p102

HANGING REVERSE CURL
20x, 12x, 10x   p132

🕐 **REST** 2 minutes

Try to minimize rest between the descending reps of each exercise. This will challenge endurance and stoke the body's fat-burning furnace—but not at the expense of your form: form first, speed second!

CORE KILLER

Each exercise in this series will challenge the muscles of the core (six-pack abs, obliques, transverse abs, back, and hips) to work together to stabilize the spine and resist the forces generated by moving your body through space. Unlike doing endless crunches that focus only on the six-pack abs (rectus abdominis), these exercises together create a set that will attack your entire core.

> Focus on keeping the triangle of your pelvis flat on the floor whenever you're lying on your back. If the curve in your spine becomes exaggerated, you can injure your lower back.

Perform 6 rounds. Don't rest between exercises.
Rest for 30 seconds after each round.
Total time: 18 minutes

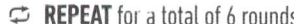

V-UP
0:30   p143

SPRINTER SIT-UP
0:30   p128

FLUTTER UP
0:30   p126

PLANK
0:30   p123

DIAGONAL PIKE
0:30   p142

↻ **REPEAT** for a total of 6 rounds

⏱ **REST** 0:30 after each round

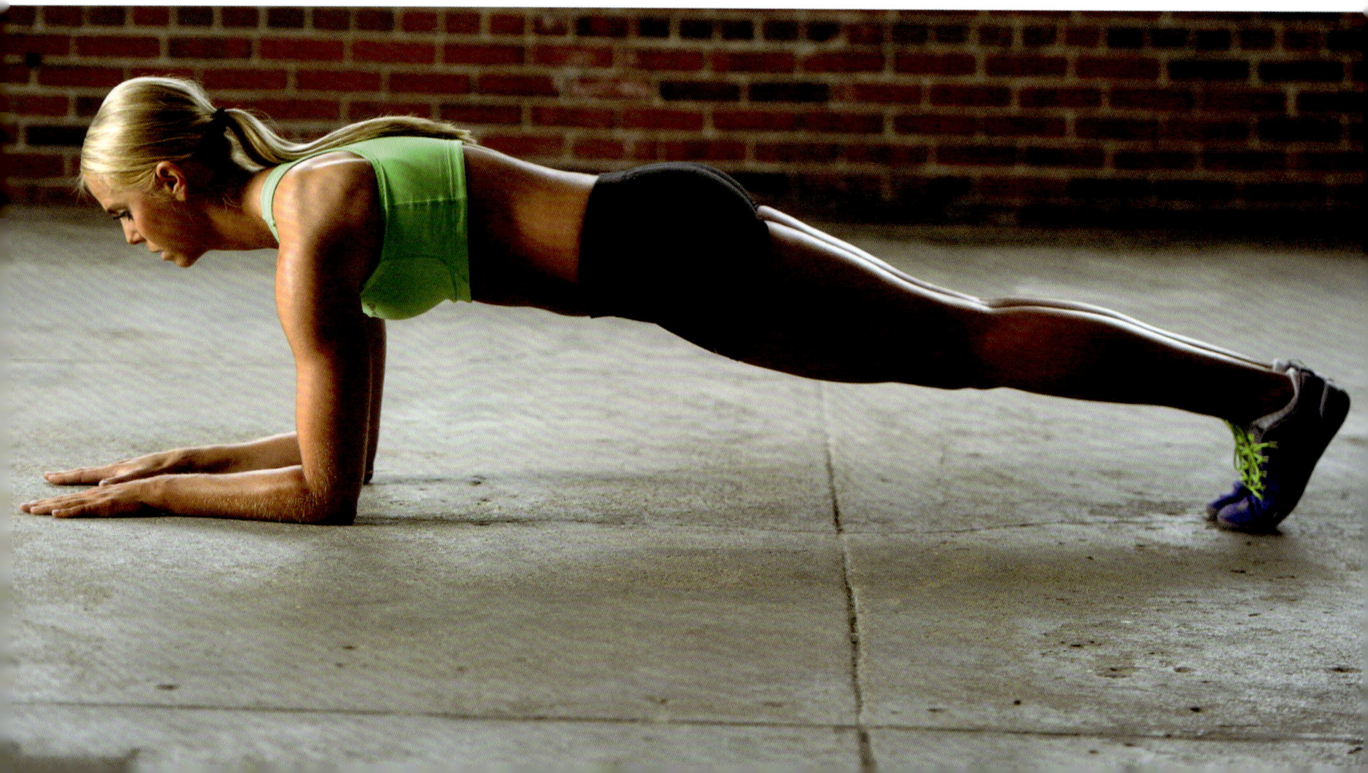

HARD-CORE

The core muscles work as stabilizers for the entire body and help the body function more effectively. Core muscles, like the rectus abdominis, internal obliques, transverse abdominis, and erector spinae, work together to supply strength and coordinated movement.

[
For an advanced challenge, replace the pike and the Russian twist with the hanging reverse curl (page 132) and the knee tuck extension (page 140), respectively.
]

Perform 5 rounds. Don't rest between exercises. Rest for 30 seconds after each round.
Total time: 13 minutes

V-UP
0:30   p143

PLANK ROTATION
0:30   p127

PIKE
0:30   p134

RUSSIAN TWIST
0:30   p139

↻ **REPEAT** for a total of 5 rounds
🕑 **REST** 0:30 after each round

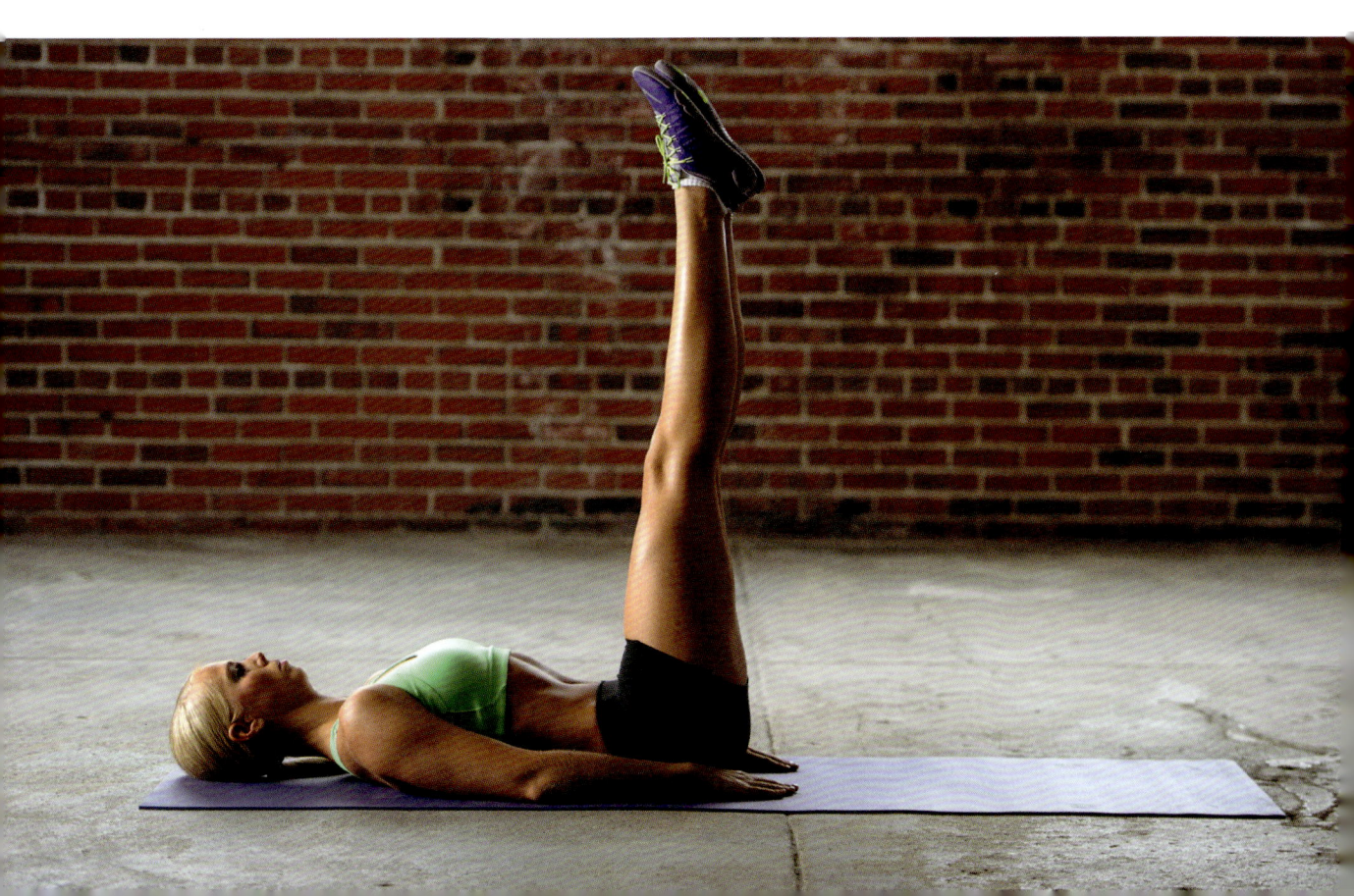

TERRIBLE TRIO

This routine boasts 3 exercises × 3 sets × 3 rounds. Each set blends high-output, high-intensity interval training with multi-muscle compound exercises to build strength and stamina.

Perform each set 3 times before moving to the next set. Don't rest between exercises. Rest for 30 seconds after each set. Total time: 18 minutes

 SET A

BURPEE
0:30   p086

JUMP LUNGE
0:30   p062

PUSH-UP JACK
0:30   p098

↻ **REPEAT** the set for a total of 3 rounds
🕐 **REST** 0:30 before set B

 SET B

TUCK JUMP BURPEE
0:30   p094

1-2 PUSH
0:30   p112

SQUAT JUMP
0:30   p066

↻ **REPEAT** the set for a total of 3 rounds
🕐 **REST** 0:30 before set C

 SET C

SPHINX
0:30   p108

UP DOWN
0:30   p064

MOUNTAIN CLIMBER
0:30   p131

↻ **REPEAT** the set for a total of 3 rounds

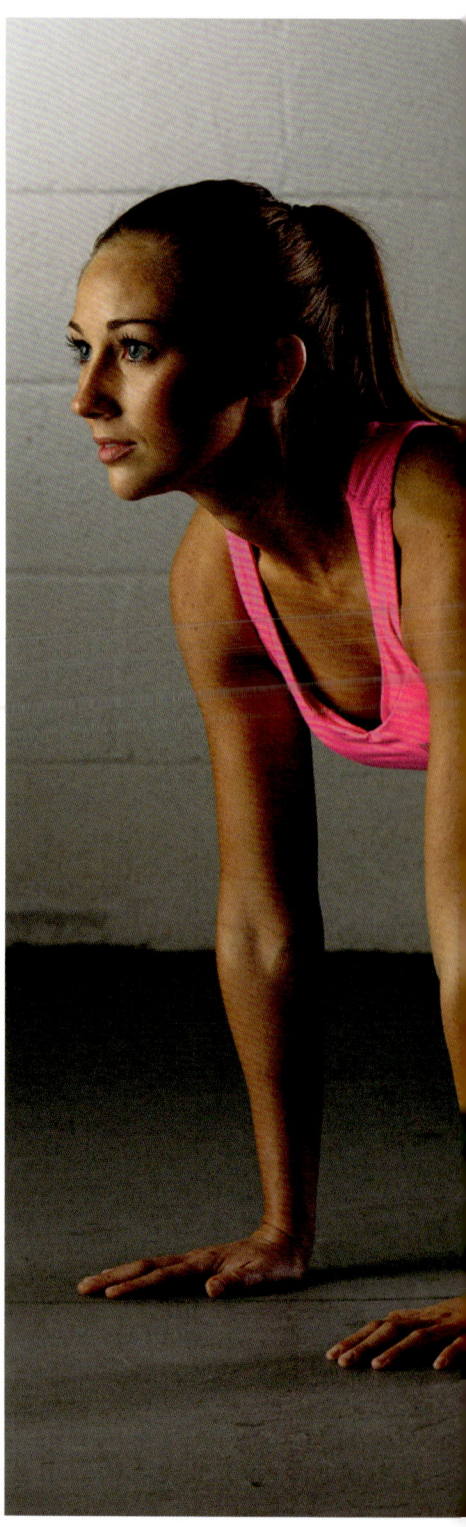

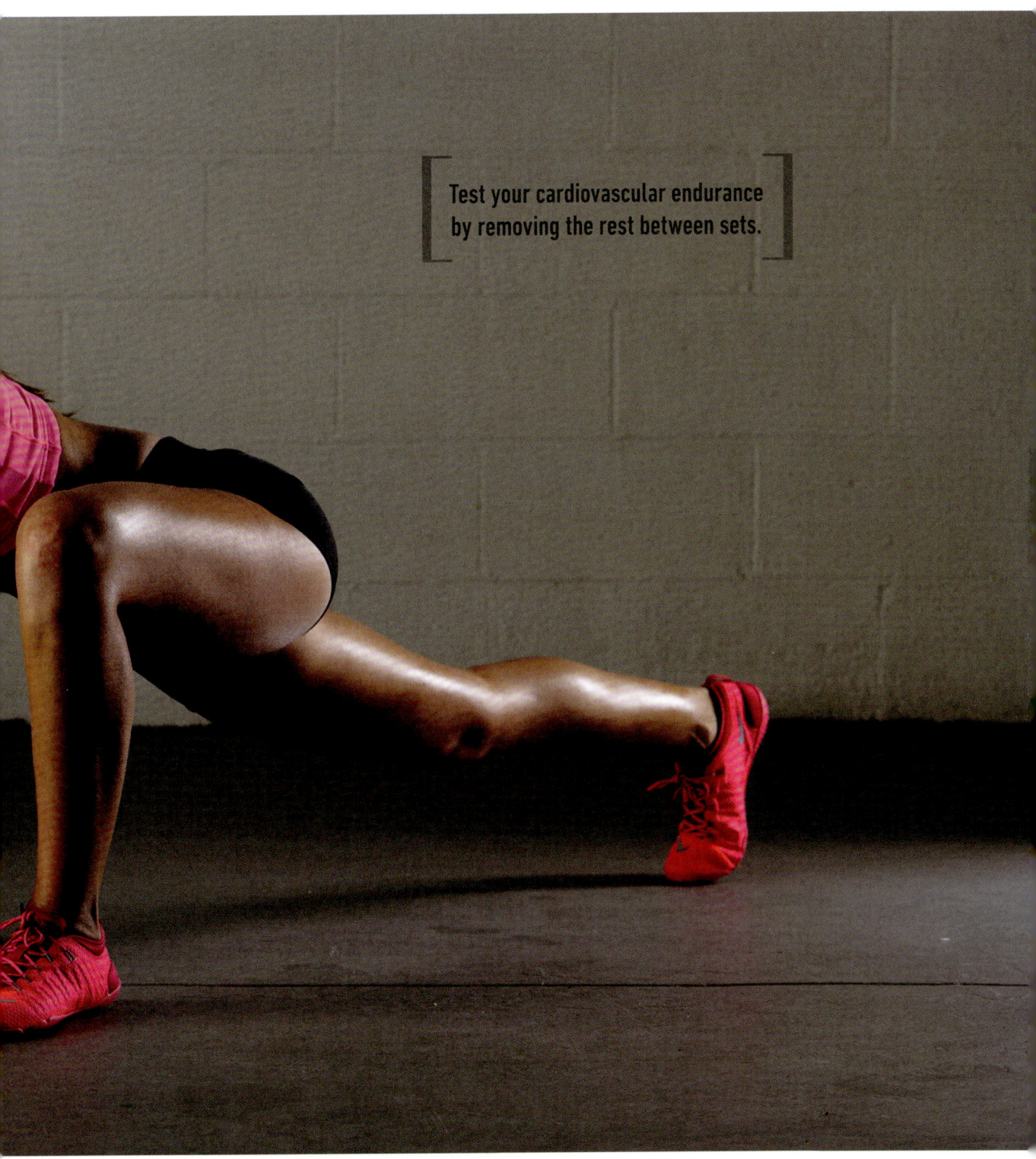

Test your cardiovascular endurance by removing the rest between sets.

METABOLIC MAYHEM

Metabolism is the process by which your body converts what you eat and drink into energy. This high-intensity interval training workout is all about boosting your metabolism to burn more calories. Multiple fast-paced compound exercises performed back-to-back will ignite your body's fat-burning furnace.

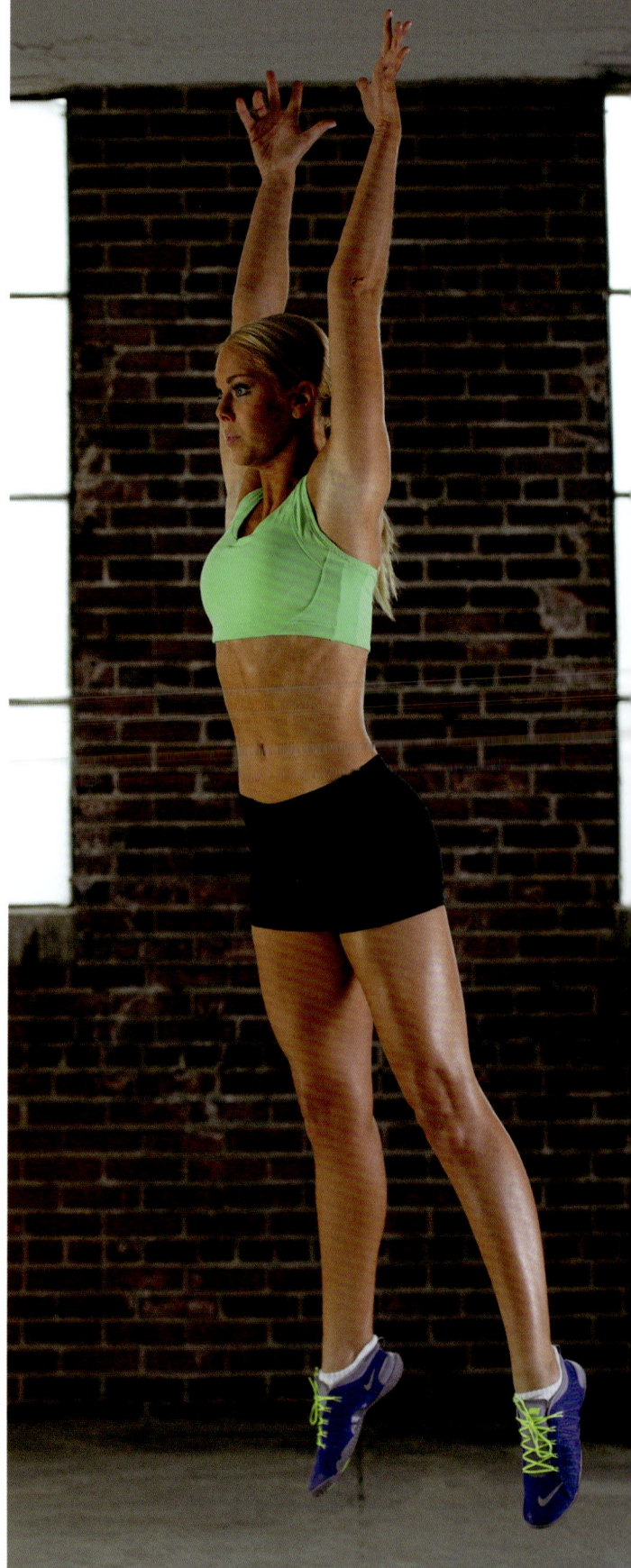

Perform Level 1 for 1 round, Level 2 for 2 rounds, and Level 3 for 3 rounds. Rest for 1 minute after each round.

	LEVEL 1	LEVEL 2	LEVEL 3	
SQUAT JUMP	work 0:30, rest 0:30	work 0:30, rest 0:15	work 0:30, rest 0:10	p066
MOUNTAIN CLIMBER	work 0:30, rest 0:30	work 0:30, rest 0:15	work 0:30, rest 0:10	p131
SQUAT PEDAL	work 0:30, rest 0:30	work 0:30, rest 0:15	work 0:30, rest 0:10	p056
MILITARY PUSH-UP	work 0:30, rest 0:30	work 0:30, rest 0:15	work 0:30, rest 0:10	p102
IN AND OUTS	work 0:30, rest 0:30	work 0:30, rest 0:15	work 0:30, rest 0:10	p054
BURPEE	work 0:30, rest 0:30	work 0:30, rest 0:15	work 0:30, rest 0:10	p086
PUSH-UP JACK	work 0:30, rest 0:30	work 0:30, rest 0:15	work 0:30, rest 0:10	p098
	⏱ **REST** 1:00	⏱ **REST** 1:00	⏱ **REST** 1:00	
TOTAL TIME	**8:00**	**12:00**	**16:00**	

HORSEPOWER

Horsepower refers to the power an engine produces. You're going to need your engine firing on all cylinders to complete this bodyweight circuit, followed by an explosive HIIT finisher that will give you a Tabata-inspired 2:1 work-to-rest ratio.

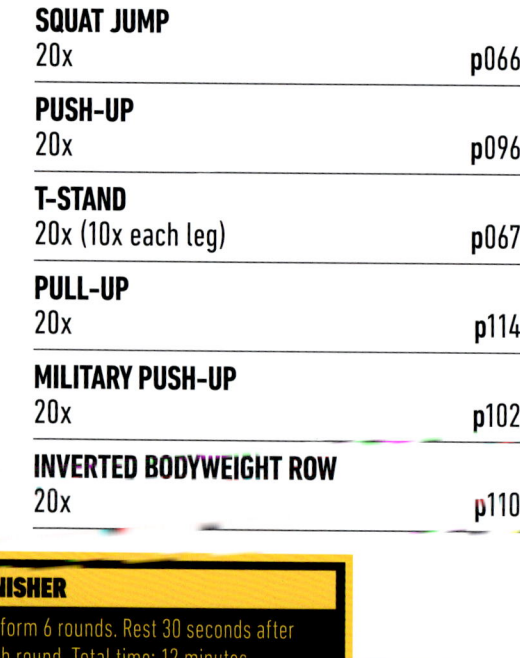

SQUAT JUMP
20x   p066

PUSH-UP
20x   p096

T-STAND
20x (10x each leg)   p067

PULL-UP
20x   p114

MILITARY PUSH-UP
20x   p102

INVERTED BODYWEIGHT ROW
20x   p110

FINISHER
Perform 6 rounds. Rest 30 seconds after each round. Total time: 12 minutes

SINGLE-LEG BURPEE (LEFT LEG)
work 0:20, rest 0:10   p084

X-JACK
work 0:20, rest 0:10   p073

SINGLE-LEG BURPEE (RIGHT LEG)
work 0:20, rest 0:10   p084

MULTI-

This workout features a tri-set format and includes multiplanar motions (movement on multiple axes) to add complication and challenge. A fixed number of reps in each set challenges endurance, and the reverse-pyramid format requires you to perform the greatest number of reps first, so you can continue to complete reps with correct form even as you fatigue.

Perform sets A–C in order with little to no rest between exercises. Rest for 1 minute between sets. Repeat 5 times.

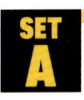 **SET A**

BULGARIAN SPLIT SQUAT
20x (10x each leg) — p076

SPIDERMAN
5x, 4x, 3x, 2x, 1x — p109

PULL-UP
5x, 4x, 3x, 2x, 1x — p114

🕐 **REST** 1:00
🔁 **REPEAT** 5 times

 SET B

ALTERNATING CROSSOVER LUNGE
20x (10x each leg) — p058

SPHINX
5x, 4x, 3x, 2x, 1x — p108

CHIN-UP
5x, 4x, 3x, 2x, 1x — p106

🕐 **REST** 1:00
🔁 **REPEAT** 5 times

 SET C

PIGEON PEEL
10x — p060

BUTTERFLY PEEL
10x — p061

DOWN DOG PUSH-UP
5x, 4x, 3x, 2x, 1x — p090

INVERTED BODYWEIGHT ROW
5x, 4x, 3x, 2x, 1x — p110

🕐 **REST** 1:00
🔁 **REPEAT** set 5 times

> The pigeon peel and butterfly peel are considered one exercise for the purposes of the tri-set format. Changing the foot position and the internal vs. external rotation of the legs activates and challenges different muscle groups.

FINISHER

Perform 3 rounds. Don't rest between each exercise or after each round.

1-2 PUSH
10x — p112

SQUAT JUMP
20x — p066

BURPEE
30x — p086

MOUNTAIN CLIMBER
40x — p131

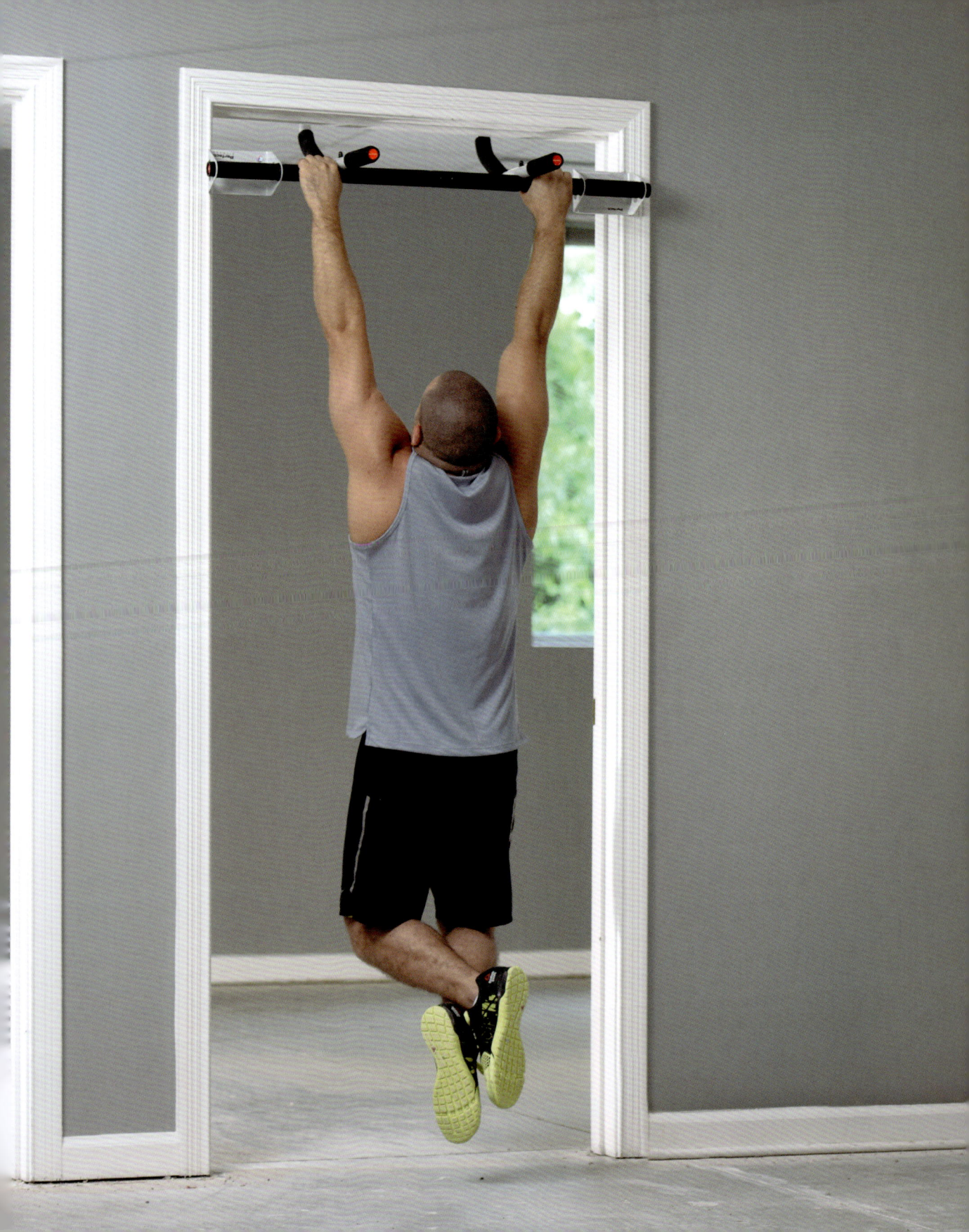

HANG TIME

Hanging for 30 seconds might sound simple, but when performed with correct form, dead hangs and scapular retraction decompress the spine, engage multiple muscles, and build grip strength. These foundational exercises if performed regularly will improve posture and set you up to be able to undertake more advanced exercises such as hanging leg raises and knee tuck extensions.

Perform 3 rounds. Rest 2 minutes after each round.
Total time: 18 minutes

DEAD HANG
work: 0:30, rest 0:30   p092

PIKE
work: 0:30, rest 0:30   p134

HANGING SCAPULA RETRACTION
work: 0:30, rest 0:30   p093

DIAGONAL PIKE
work: 0:30   p142

↻ **REPEAT** for a total of 3 rounds

⏲ **REST** 2:00 after each round

4 IN 4

Short on time or in need of a metabolic boost? These 4-minute "finishers" are made to spike your heart rate and kick your metabolism into high gear. Perform each set as a standalone workout if pressed for time or combine them for a brutal 16-minute circuit.

Perform 2 rounds of sets A and B and then perform 1 round of sets C and D. Don't rest between sets or exercises. Total time: 16 minutes (4 minutes per set)

SET A

X-JACK 0:30		p073
SQUAT 0:30		p072
PUSH-UP 0:30		p096
SPRINTER SIT-UP 0:30		p128

⟳ **REPEAT** the set for a total of 2 rounds

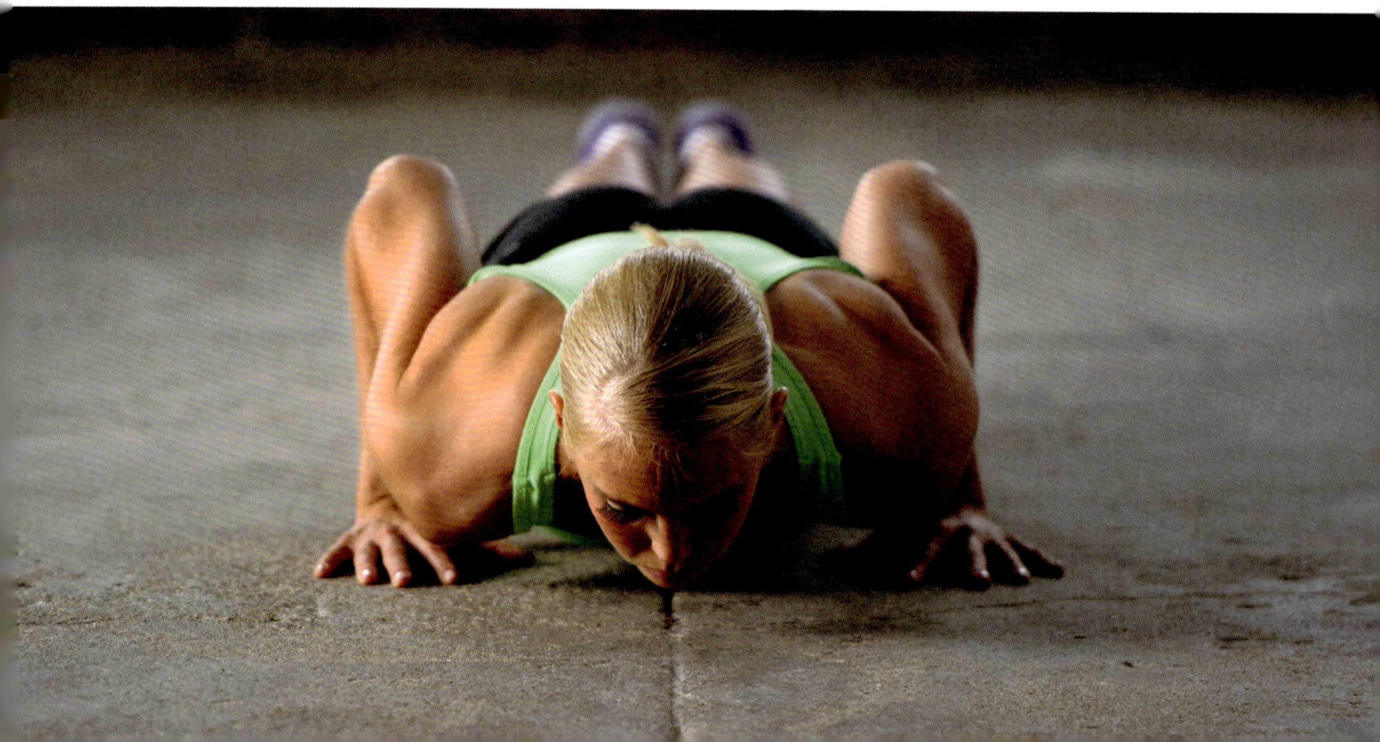

SET B

HIGH KNEES 0:30	p118
BURPEE 0:30	p086
SQUAT JUMP 0:30	p066
1-2 PUSH 0:30	p112

↻ **REPEAT** the set for a total of 2 rounds

 SET C

JUMP LUNGE 0:30	p062
SPIDERMAN 0:30	p109
PIGEON PEEL 0:30	p060
1-2 PUSH 0:30	p112
V-UP 0:30	p143
SPHINX 0:30	p108
SQUAT LIFT 0:30	p070
ARCHER PULL-UP 0:30	p104

 SET D

SINGLE-LEG BURPEE (LEFT LEG) 0:30	p084
CROSS PUSH 0:30	p100
SINGLE-LEG BURPEE (RIGHT LEG) 0:30	p084
BULGARIAN SPLIT SQUAT (LEFT LEG) 0:30	p076
MOUNTAIN CLIMBER 0:30	p131
BULGARIAN SPLIT SQUAT (RIGHT LEG) 0:30	p076
DOWN DOG PUSH-UP 0:30	p090
FLUTTER UP 0:30	p126

PROGRAMS

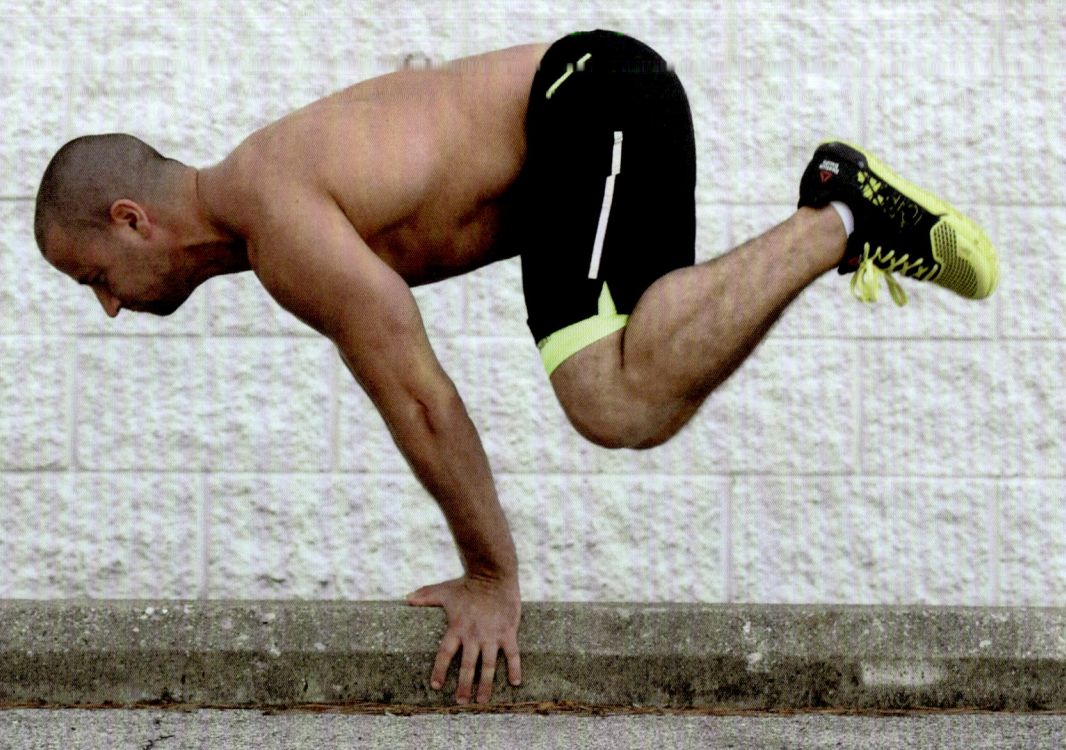

LEVEL 1
PROGRAM

Programs are structured so weeks 1 and 3 are the same, as are weeks 2 and 4. Each week has 6 work days and 1 day off. Ideally, you'd structure it Monday to Saturday and rest Sunday, but if your schedule prevents this or you need a midweek rest at first because of muscle soreness, schedule your rest day accordingly. Avoid switching the workouts within the program, as this might adversely affect your rest time for a specific muscle group.

WEEK 1

WEEK 2

WEEK 3

WEEK 4

DAY 01	DAY 02	DAY 03	DAY 04	DAY 05	DAY 06
• The Cycle **P170**	• Hang Time **P186**	• Leg Purgatory **P146**	• Tri-Phase **P174**	• Hi-Lo **P157**	• Jacked Up **P175**

DAY 08	DAY 09	DAY 10	DAY 11	DAY 12	DAY 13
• Dynamic Duos **P156**	• Abdomination **P167**	• Leg Hell **P148**	• Push vs Pull **P154**	• Burn **P158**	• Super Circuit **P152**

DAY 15	DAY 16	DAY 17	DAY 18	DAY 19	DAY 20
• The Cycle **P170**	• Hang Time **P186**	• Leg Purgatory **P146**	• Tri-Phase **P174**	• Hi-Lo **P157**	• Jacked Up **P175**

DAY 22	DAY 23	DAY 24	DAY 25	DAY 26	DAY 27
• Dynamic Duos **P156**	• Abdomination **P167**	• Leg Hell **P148**	• Push vs Pull **P154**	• Burn **P158**	• Super Circuit **P152**

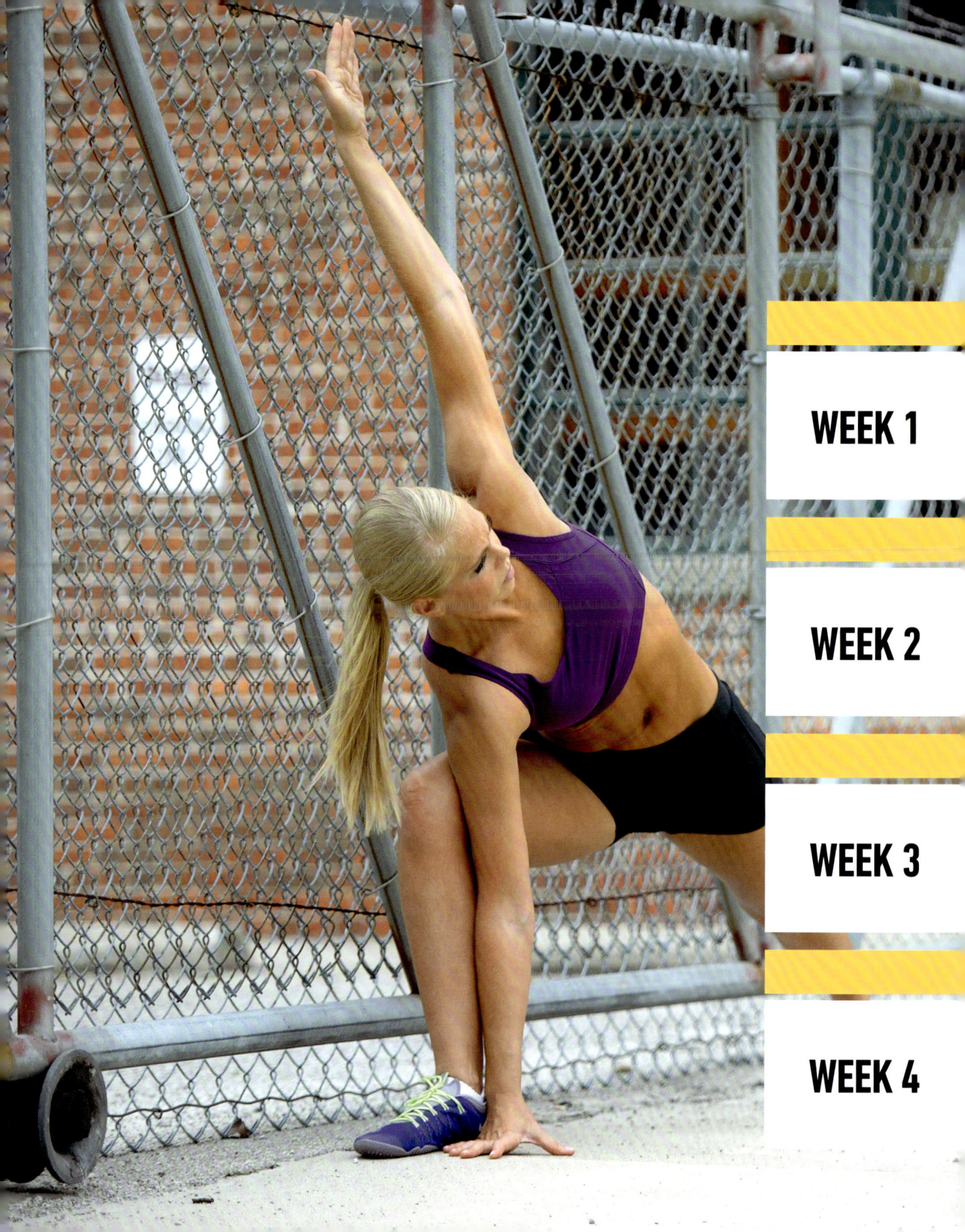

WEEK 1

WEEK 2

WEEK 3

WEEK 4

LEVEL 2
PROGRAM

Level 2 follows the same schedule as Level 1, but it incorporates more explosive, plyometric exercises that might increase fatigue and muscle soreness. If an exercise is too challenging, you can substitute it for a Level 1 equivalent. If frequent substitutions are necessary, consider repeating Level 2 to master the exercises and gain strength before graduating to Level 3. There is nothing wrong with taking more time to gain strength and coordination and to prevent injury.

DAY 01	DAY 02	DAY 03	DAY 04	DAY 05	DAY 06
• Horsepower P184	• Crazy 8s P162	• Leg Hell P148	• Push–Pull Pairs P160	• Total-Body Burn P176	• 4 in 4 P188

DAY 08	DAY 09	DAY 10	DAY 11	DAY 12	DAY 13
• Fire P165	• All-In P164	• Fantastic Four P163	• Hard-Core P179	• Terrible Trio P180	• The Bodyweight 500 P166

DAY 15	DAY 16	DAY 17	DAY 18	DAY 19	DAY 20
• Horsepower P184	• Crazy 8s P162	• Leg Hell P148	• Push–Pull Pairs P160	• Total-Body Burn P176	• 4 in 4 P188

DAY 22	DAY 23	DAY 24	DAY 25	DAY 26	DAY 27
• Fire P165	• All-In P164	• Fantastic Four P163	• Hard-Core P179	• Terrible Trio P180	• The Bodyweight 500 P166

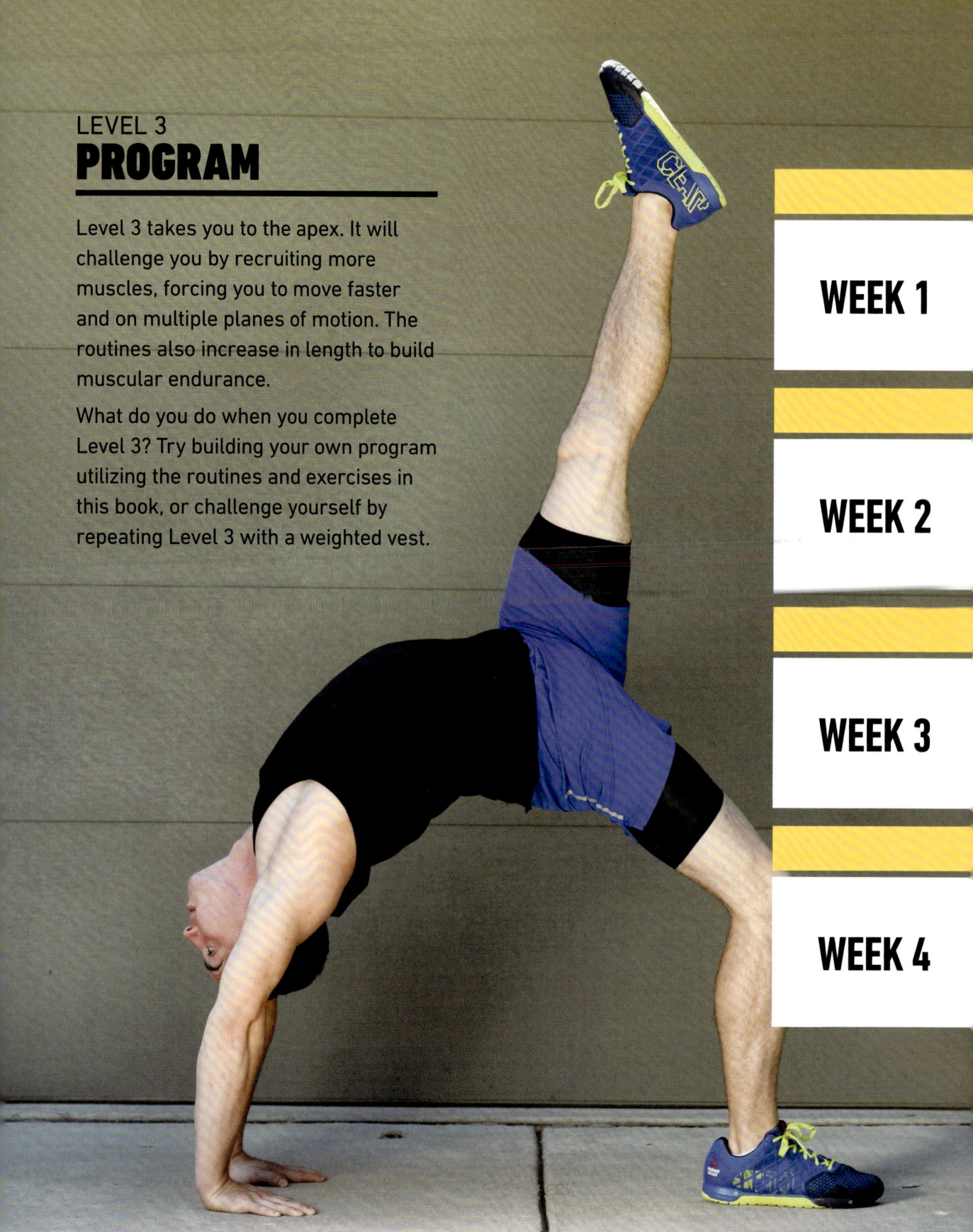

LEVEL 3
PROGRAM

Level 3 takes you to the apex. It will challenge you by recruiting more muscles, forcing you to move faster and on multiple planes of motion. The routines also increase in length to build muscular endurance.

What do you do when you complete Level 3? Try building your own program utilizing the routines and exercises in this book, or challenge yourself by repeating Level 3 with a weighted vest.

WEEK 1

WEEK 2

WEEK 3

WEEK 4

DAY 01	DAY 02	DAY 03	DAY 04	DAY 05	DAY 06
• Total-Body Blast **P172**	• All-In **P164**	• 4 in 4 **P188**	• Countdown **P153**	• Fire **P165**	• The Bodyweight 500 **P166**

DAY 08	DAY 09	DAY 10	DAY 11	DAY 12	DAY 13
• Multi- **P185**	• Metabolic Mayhem **P182**	• Redline **P168**	• The Bodyweight 500 **P166**	• Round the World **P150**	• Total-Body Burn **P176**

DAY 15	DAY 16	DAY 17	DAY 18	DAY 19	DAY 20
• Super Circuit **P152**	• All-In **P164**	• 4 in 4 **P188**	• Countdown **P153**	• Fire **P165**	• The Bodyweight 500 **P166**

DAY 22	DAY 23	DAY 24	DAY 25	DAY 26	DAY 27
• Multi- **P185**	• Metabolic Mayhem **P182**	• Crazy 8s **P162**	• Bodyweight 500 **P166**	• Round the World **P150**	• Total-Body Burn **P176**

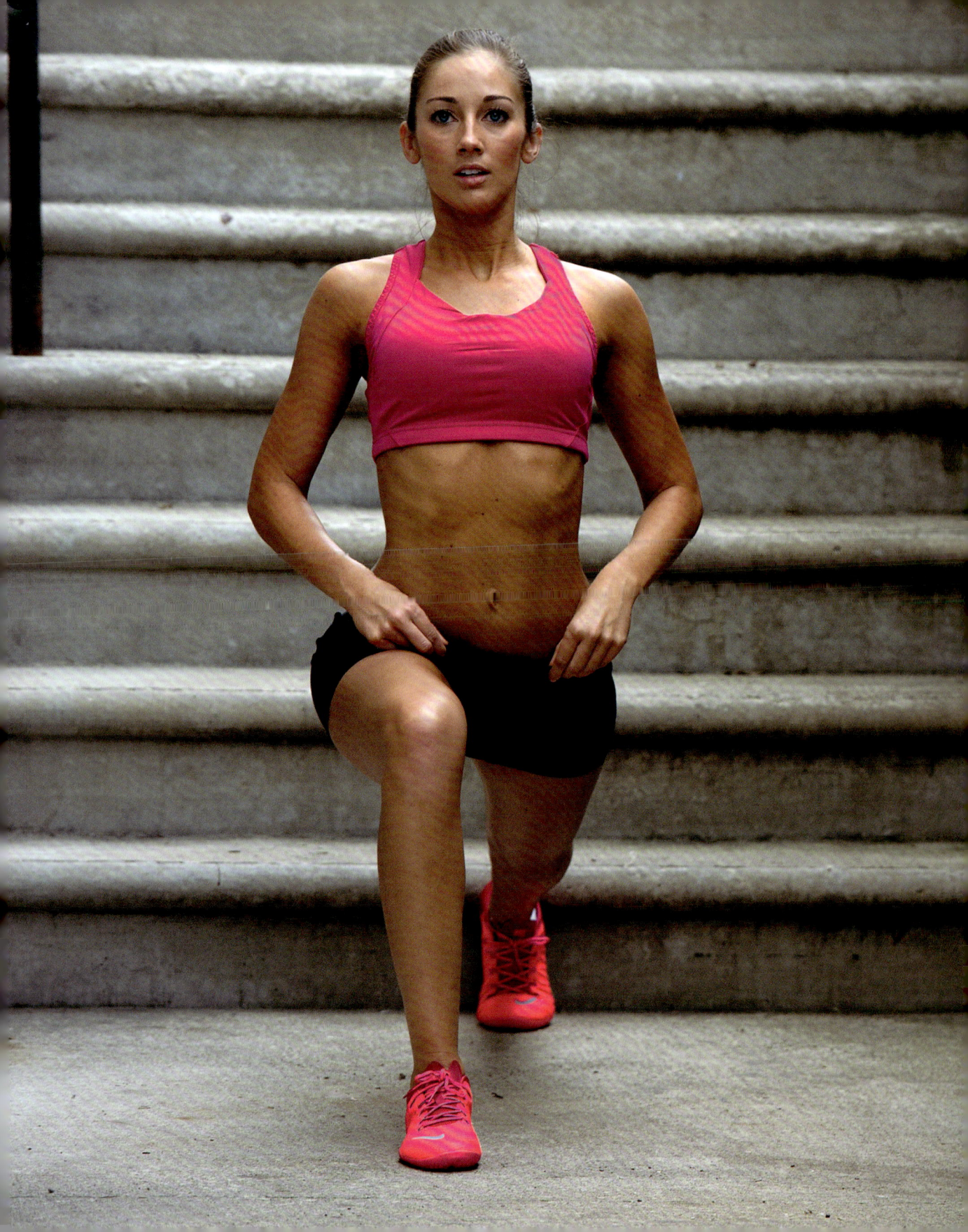

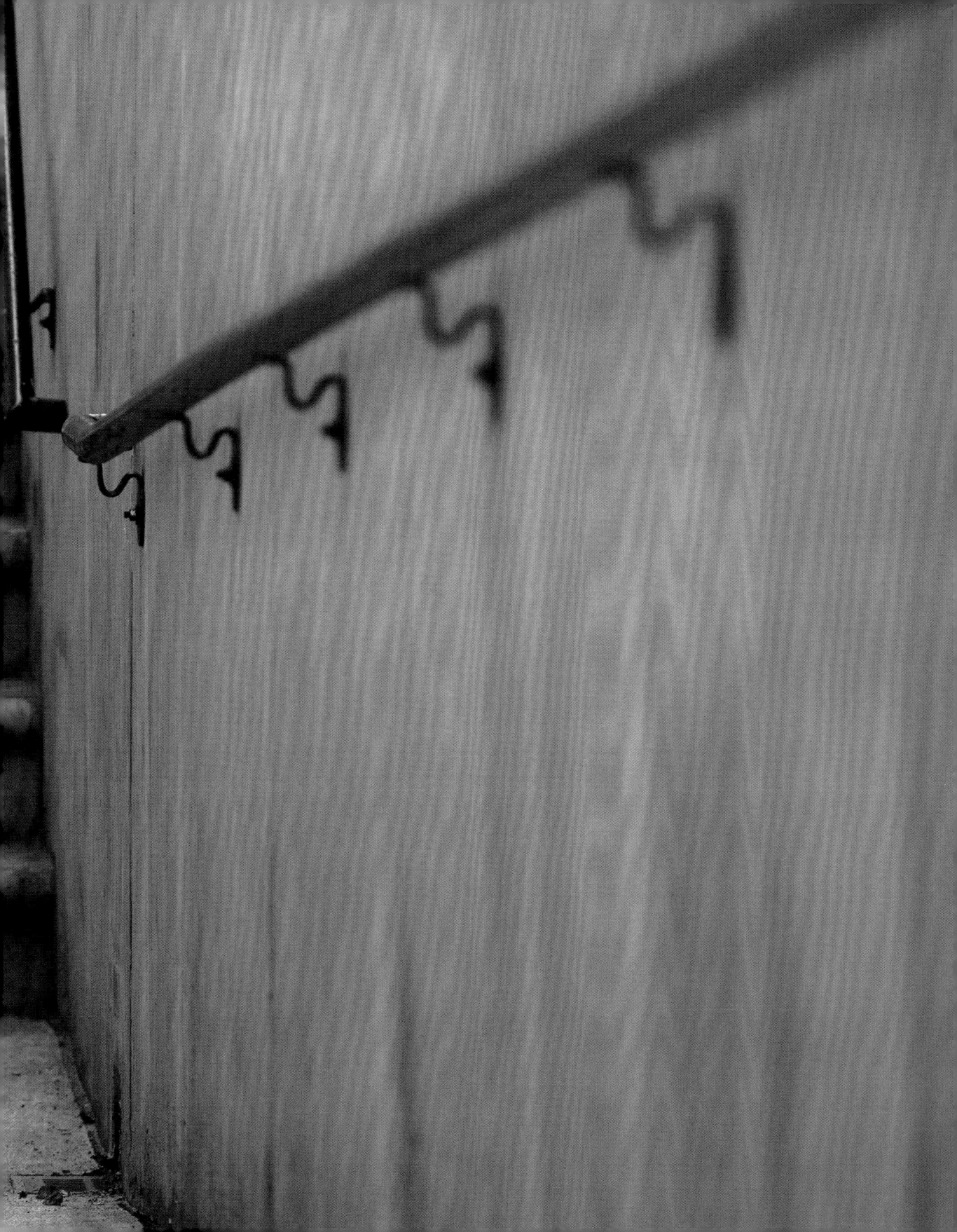

INDEX

ACKNOWLEDGMENTS

A HUGE thank you to everyone at DK for this opportunity. It's still mind-blowing to me that I have been fortunate enough to write a single book, let alone four! I don't know that I have the words to express my gratitude to all the countless people who work behind the scenes to bring the books to life.

A very sincere thank you to my editors: to Chris Stolle, for hunting me down and persuading me to be part of this project, and to Ann Barton, with whom I worked on *HIIT for Women*. It's been a pleasure working with you both—let's do it again!

I have so many friends and family to thank that I could not possibly list them all but it's essential I start with my biggest supporters—Rochelle and Chloe. None of this is possible without your love, support, and faith.

I would also like to thank the wonderful people and companies who have partnered with me, most of all James and Blanca at SOS Rehydrate who have supported my journey since day one.

I lost my mum in 2020, but she showed me what true strength, grit, perseverance, and love look like. There isn't a day I don't miss her. To my dad and sister—love you. We don't say it enough; now it's in print!

ABOUT THE AUTHOR

SEAN BARTRAM instructs and trains athletes on two continents and has been featured by *Shape, Popsugar, The Huffington Post*, Fox, CBS, and Reuters. He is the author of *High Intensity Interval Training for Women, Idiot's Guides: High-Intensity Interval Training*, and *Bodyweight Workouts for Men*. Sean lives in Westfield, Indiana.